D0439240

Stockley's Drug Interactions
Pocket Companion

Stockley's Drug Interactions Pocket Companion 2009

Editor
Karen Baxter, BSc, MSc, MRPharmS

Editorial Staff
Mildred Davis, BA, BSc, PhD, MRPharmS
Samuel Driver, BSc
Rebecca E Garner, BSc
C Rhoda Lee, BPharm, PhD, MRPharmS
Alison Marshall, BPharm, DipClinPharm,
  PGCertClinEd, MRPharmS
Rosalind McLarney, BPharm, MSc, MRPharmS
Jennifer M Sharp, BPharm, DipClinPharm, MRPharmS

Digital Products Team
Julie McGlashan, BPharm, DipInfSc, MRPharmS
Elizabeth King, Dip BTEC PharmSci

Consultant Editorial Advisor
Ivan H Stockley, BPharm, PhD, FRPharmS, CBiol,
  MIBiol

London • Chicago

Pharmaceutical Press

Published by the Pharmaceutical Press
An imprint of RPS Publishing

1 Lambeth High Street, London SE1 7JN, UK
100 South Atkinson Road, Suite 200, Grayslake, IL 60030-7820, USA

© Pharmaceutical Press 2009

(PP) is a trade mark of RPS Publishing

RPS Publishing is the publishing organisation of the Royal
Pharmaceutical Society of Great Britain

First published 2009

Typeset by Data Standards Ltd, Frome, Somerset
Printed in Italy by LEGO S.p.A.

ISBN 978 0 85369 795 4

A catalogue record for this book is available from the British Library

Contents

Preface

What is *Stockley's Drug Interactions Pocket Companion*?

Stockley's Drug Interactions is a reference work that provides concise, accurate, and clinically relevant information to healthcare professionals. Monographs are based on published sources including clinical studies, case reports, and systematic reviews, and are fully referenced. *Stockley's Drug Interactions Pocket Companion* has summarised this comprehensive work to create a small and conveniently sized quick-reference text.

Stockley's Drug Interactions Pocket Companion provides the busy healthcare professional with quick and easy access to clinically relevant, evaluated and evidence-based information about drug interactions. As with the full reference work this publication attempts to answer the following questions:

- Are the drugs or substances in question known to interact or is the interaction only theoretical and speculative?
- If they do interact, how serious is it?
- Has it been described many times or only once?
- Are all patients affected or only a few?
- Is it best to avoid some drug combinations altogether or can the interaction be accommodated in some way?
- What alternative and safer drugs can be used instead?

Coverage

Stockley's Drug Interactions Pocket Companion 2009 contains over 1500 interaction monographs pertaining to specific drugs or drug groups, an increase of about 200 from the previous edition. Each monograph in *Stockley's Drug Interactions* was assessed by practising clinical pharmacists for its suitability for inclusion in the *Pocket Companion*. Broadly speaking interactions involving anaesthesia, the specialist use of multiple antiretrovirals, the specialist use of multiple antineoplastics or intravenous antineoplastics, and non-interactions were omitted. However, exceptions were made, particularly where there has been controversy over whether or not a drug interacts. All herbal interactions were included as this is a growing area about which we get many questions, and so we felt that even sparse data was worthy of comment. All these interactions are discussed under the general heading of Herbal medicines or Dietary supplements.

Monographs

Following the familiar format of the Stockley products, the information in this publication is organised into a brief summary of the evidence for the interaction and a description of how best to manage it. The information is based on the most recent quarterly update of *Stockley's Drug Interactions* at the time of going to press. This data is fully referenced and available at www.medicinescomplete.com. These references have not been included in the *Pocket Companion* to keep size to a minimum. Anyone interested in seeing our sources can consult *MedicinesComplete*, or the full reference work of *Stockley's Drug Interactions*.

Ratings

Each monograph has been assigned a rating symbol to offer guidance to the user on the clinical significance of the interaction. These ratings are the same as those used in Stockley's *Interaction Alerts*. The *Alerts* are rated using three separate categories:

- Action – This describes whether or not any action needs to be taken to accommodate the interaction. This category ranges from 'avoid' to 'no action needed'.
- Severity – This describes the likely effect of an unmanaged interaction on the patient. This category ranges from 'severe' to 'nothing expected'.
- Evidence – This describes the weight of evidence behind the interaction. This category ranges from 'extensive' to 'theoretical'.

These ratings are combined to produce one of four symbols:

❌ For interactions that have a life-threatening outcome, or where concurrent use is contraindicated by the manufacturers.

🅰 For interactions where concurrent use may result in a significant hazard to the patient and so dosage adjustment or close monitoring is needed.

❓ For interactions where there is some doubt about the outcome of concurrent use, and therefore it may be necessary to give patients some guidance about possible adverse effects, and/or consider some monitoring.

✅ For interactions that are not considered to be of clinical significance, or where no interaction occurs.

We put a lot of thought in to the original design of these symbols, and have deliberately avoided a numerical or colour coding system as we did not want to imply any relationship between the symbols or colours. Instead we chose internationally recognisable symbols, which in testing were intuitively understood by our target audience of healthcare professionals.

Structure

Stockley's Drug Interactions Pocket Companion is structured alphabetically for ease of use, with International Nonproprietary Names (INNs) to identify drug names. Cross references to US Approved Names (USANs) are also included where drug names differ significantly. Consequently an interaction between aspirin and beta blockers will appear under A, and an interaction between beta blockers and digoxin will appear under B. We have only used drug groups where they are considered to be widely recognised, hence beta blockers is used, but alpha agonists is not. In contrast to previous editions, *Stockley's Drug Interactions Pocket Companion* has been fully indexed to help those less familiar with drugs and their groupings with searching. The alphabetical format has proven popular, and so this has been maintained.

Acknowledgements

Aside from the editorial staff many other people have contributed to this publication and the Editor gratefully acknowledges the assistance and guidance they have provided. In particular, we would like to express our gratitude to Michael Evans for his continued support in producing the final data and developing the content for release as a PDA version, and to John Wilson and Tamsin Cousins who have handled the various aspects of the production of this book. Thanks are also due to Ivan Stockley, Sean Sweetman, Paul Weller and Charles Fry for their support with this project.

Individual users of this product continue to take the time to provide us with feedback on the contents and structure of the data, and for that we are grateful. These comments are always useful to us in developing the products to better meet the needs of end-users.

Contact details

We are always very pleased to receive feedback from those using our products. Anyone wishing to comment can contact us at the following e-mail address: stockley@rpsgb.org

Abbreviations

ACE	angiotensin-converting enzyme
ALT	alanine aminotransferase
AST	aspartate aminotransferase
AUC	area under the time–concentration curve
BPH	benign prostatic hyperplasia
bpm	beats per minute
CNS	central nervous system
CSF	cerebrospinal fluid
CSM	Committee on Safety of Medicines (now the Commission on Human Medicines)
DMARD	disease modifying antirheumatic drug
e.g.	*exempli gratia* (for example)
ECG	electrocardiogram
HIV	human immunodeficiency virus
HRT	hormone replacement therapy
i.e.	*id est* (that is)
INR	international normalised ratio
IUD	intrauterine device
LFT	liver function test
MAO	monoamine oxidase
MAO-A	monoamine oxidase, type A
MAO-B	monoamine oxidase, type B
MAOI	monoamine oxidase inhibitor
mg	milligrams
MHRA	Medicines and Healthcare products Regulatory Agency
mL	millilitres
mmHg	millimetres of mercury
mol	mole
NNRTI	non-nucleoside reverse transcriptase inhibitor
NRTI	nucleoside reverse transcriptase inhibitor
NSAID	non-steroidal anti-inflammatory drug
PCP	*Pneumocystis carinii* (now *Pneumocystis jirovecii*) pneumonia
pH	the negative logarithm of the hydrogen ion concentration
PPI	proton pump inhibitor
RNA	ribonucleic acid
SSRI	selective serotonin reuptake inhibitor
TSH	thyroid stimulating hormone
UK	United Kingdom
US	United States of America
WHO	World Health Organization

About the Editor

Karen Baxter studied pharmacy at De Montfort University, Leicester, graduating in 1995 and then completing her pre-registration year in Yeovil, Somerset. She then moved to Derby where she was a resident pharmacist for 3 years, during which time she completed her Clinical Diploma and MSc. She then worked in a variety of clinical roles, before taking on an education and training role, during which time she undertook a joint appointment with the University of Derby, working on their postgraduate pharmacy programme. Karen started at the Pharmaceutical Press in 2001 as the Assistant Editor of *Stockley's Drug Interactions*, working under the guidance of Dr Ivan Stockley and the Martindale team. She became the Editor of *Stockley's Drug Interactions* in 2005.

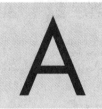

ACE inhibitors

Most ACE inhibitor interactions are pharmacodynamic, that is, interactions that result in an alteration in drug effects rather than drug disposition, so in most cases interactions of individual drugs will be applicable to the group as a whole.

ACE inhibitors + Allopurinol

Three cases of Stevens-Johnson syndrome (one fatal) and two cases of hypersensitivity have been attributed to the use of captopril with allopurinol. Anaphylaxis and myocardial infarction occurred in one man taking enalapril with allopurinol. The combination of ACE inhibitors and allopurinol may increase the risk of leucopenia and serious infection.

Patients taking both drugs should be very closely monitored for any signs of hypersensitivity (e.g. skin reactions) or low white cell count (sore throat, fever etc.), especially if they have renal impairment.

ACE inhibitors + Alpha blockers

Severe first-dose hypotension, and synergistic hypotensive effects that occurred in a patient taking enalapril with bunazosin have been replicated in healthy subjects. The first-dose effect seen with other alpha blockers (particularly alfuzosin, prazosin and terazosin) is also likely to be potentiated by ACE inhibitors. In one small study tamsulosin did not have any clinically relevant effects on blood pressure that was already well controlled by enalapril.

Acute hypotension (dizziness, fainting) sometimes occurs unpredictably with the first dose of some alpha blockers (particularly alfuzosin, prazosin and terazosin), and this can be exaggerated by beta blockers and calcium-channel blockers. ACE inhibitors would be expected to have a similar effect. Minimise the risk by starting with a low dose of alpha blocker, preferably given at bedtime, and escalate the dose slowly over a couple of weeks. It is recommended that the dose of ACE inhibitor is reduced during initiation. Patients should be warned to lie down if symptoms such as dizziness, fatigue or sweating develop, and to remain lying down until symptoms abate.

A

ACE inhibitors + **Antacids**

Fosinopril ⚠

Mylanta (probably containing aluminium/magnesium hydroxide) reduces the bioavailability of fosinopril by about one-third.

> The manufacturers suggest separating its dosing from that of antacids by at least 2 hours.

Other ACE inhibitors ✅

Antacids are said to reduce the bioavailability of a number of ACE inhibitors but this seems unlikely to be clinically important (except perhaps in the case of fosinopril, see above).

> Several manufacturers of ACE inhibitors warn that antacids may reduce their bioavailability, but there seems to be no evidence of a clinically significant interaction in practice.

ACE inhibitors + **Antidiabetics** ❓

The concurrent use of ACE inhibitors and antidiabetics normally appears to be uneventful. However, hypoglycaemia, marked in some instances, has occurred in a small number of diabetics taking insulin or sulphonylureas with captopril, enalapril, lisinopril or perindopril. This has been attributed, but not proven, to be due to an interaction.

> This interaction remains the subject of considerable study and debate. It would be prudent to warn all patients taking insulin or oral antidiabetics who are just starting any ACE inhibitors that excessive hypoglycaemia has been seen very occasionally and unpredictably. It may be prudent to temporarily increase the frequency of blood glucose monitoring. The problem has been resolved in some patients by reducing the sulphonylurea dosage.

ACE inhibitors + **Aspirin** ❓

The antihypertensive efficacy of captopril and enalapril may be reduced by high-dose aspirin in about 50% of patients. Low-dose aspirin (less than or equal to 100 mg daily) appears to have little effect. It is unclear whether aspirin attenuates the benefits of ACE inhibitors in coronary artery disease and heart failure. The likelihood of an interaction may depend on disease state (more likely with non-ischaemic disease).

> For hypertension, no action needed if low-dose aspirin is used. Suspect an interaction with high-dose aspirin if the ACE inhibitor seems less effective, or blood pressure control is erratic. Consider an alternative analgesic, but note that NSAIDs interact in the same way as high-dose aspirin. For heart failure it is generally advised that concurrent use is best avoided, unless a specific indication (e.g. coronary heart disease, stroke) exists.

ACE inhibitors + **Azathioprine** ⚠

Anaemia has been seen in kidney transplant patients given azathioprine with enalapril or captopril. Leucopenia occasionally occurs when captopril is given with azathioprine. Azathioprine is rapidly and extensively metabolised to mercaptopurine. Mercaptopurine is therefore expected to share the interactions of azathioprine.

> The manufacturer of captopril recommends that it should be used with extreme caution in patients taking immunosuppressants, especially if there is renal impairment. They advise that differential white blood cell counts should be performed before therapy, then every 2 weeks in the first 3 months of captopril use, and periodically thereafter. Any effect seems likely to be a group interaction, and it would therefore seem prudent to consider monitoring with any ACE inhibitor.

ACE inhibitors + Ciclosporin (Cyclosporine) ⚠

Acute renal failure has developed in kidney transplant patients taking ciclosporin with enalapril. Oliguria was seen in another patient taking ciclosporin with captopril. There is a possible risk of hyperkalaemia when ACE inhibitors are given with ciclosporin as both drugs may raise potassium levels.

> The incidence of renal failure appears to be low, nevertheless care and good monitoring are needed if ACE inhibitors and ciclosporin are used concurrently. Monitor potassium levels more closely in the initial weeks of concurrent use.

ACE inhibitors + Clonidine ❓

ACE inhibitors may potentiate the antihypertensive effects of clonidine, and this can be clinically useful. However, limited evidence suggests that the effects of captopril may be delayed when patients are switched from clonidine. Note that sudden withdrawal of clonidine may cause rebound hypertension.

> The general importance of this interaction is unknown, but be aware that it may occur.

ACE inhibitors + Co-trimoxazole ❓

Two reports describe serious hyperkalaemia, apparently caused by the concurrent use of trimethoprim and enalapril or quinapril, in association with renal impairment.

> Trimethoprim or ACE inhibitors alone can cause hyperkalaemia, particularly with other factors such as renal impairment. Monitor potassium levels if this combination is used in those with renal impairment. Note that co-trimoxazole is a combination preparation containing trimethoprim, and may therefore interact similarly. It has been suggested that patients with AIDS taking an ACE inhibitor for associated nephropathy should probably discontinue this treatment during treatment with high-dose co-trimoxazole.

ACE inhibitors + Digoxin ✅

No significant interaction has been seen between digoxin and most ACE inhibitors. Some studies have found that serum digoxin levels rise by about 20% or more if captopril is used, but others have found no significant changes. It has been suggested

ACE inhibitors

A

that any interaction is likely to occur only in those patients who have pre-existing renal impairment.

> No action usually needed. In patients with renal impairment given digoxin and captopril it may be prudent to be alert for increased digoxin effects (e.g. bradycardia).

ACE inhibitors + Diuretics

Loop diuretics and Thiazides ❓

The use of ACE inhibitors with loop or thiazide diuretics is normally safe and effective, but 'first-dose hypotension' (dizziness, fainting) can occur, particularly if the dose of diuretic is high (greater than furosemide 80 mg daily or equivalent) and often in association with predisposing conditions (heart failure, renovascular hypertension, haemodialysis, high levels of renin and angiotensin, low-sodium diet, dehydration, diarrhoea or vomiting, etc.). In addition, renal impairment, and even acute renal failure, have been reported, and diuretic-induced hypokalaemia may occur when ACE inhibitors are used with potassium-depleting diuretics.

> First-dose hypotension is well established. For those with risk factors consider temporarily stopping the diuretic or reducing its dosage a few days before the ACE inhibitor is added, but if this is not clinically appropriate give the first dose of the ACE inhibitor under close supervision. ACE inhibitors should be started with a very low dose, even in patients at low risk (e.g. those with uncomplicated essential hypertension taking low-dose thiazides). All patients should be given a simple warning about what can happen and what to do if hypotension occurs. The immediate problem (dizziness etc.) can usually be solved by the patient lying down. Any marked hypotension is normally transient, but if not it may be necessary to temporarily reduce the diuretic dosage. Severe reactions (e.g. renal impairment or hypokalaemia) are rare, and routine monitoring during the initiation of the ACE inhibitor should suffice. However, if increases in urea and creatinine occur, a dosage reduction and/or discontinuation of the diuretic and/or ACE inhibitor may be required.

Potassium-sparing diuretics ⚠️

The use of ACE inhibitors with potassium-sparing diuretics, such as amiloride, eplerenone, spironolactone and triamterene can result in hyperkalaemia, particularly in the presence of other risk factors (e.g. advanced age, diabetes, doses of spironolactone greater than 25 mg daily, and particularly renal impairment).

> The concurrent use of ACE inhibitors and amiloride or triamterene is normally not advised, but if both drugs are appropriate potassium levels should be closely monitored. The presence of a loop or thiazide diuretic may not necessarily prevent hyperkalaemia. The combination of an ACE inhibitor and spironolactone or eplerenone is beneficial in some indications, but close monitoring of serum potassium and renal function is needed, especially with any changes in treatment or in the patient's clinical condition. It has been suggested that spironolactone should not be given with ACE inhibitors in those with a glomerular filtration rate of less than 30 mL/minute.

ACE inhibitors + Epoetin [?]

Epoetin may cause hypertension and thereby reduce the effects of ACE inhibitors, and an additive hyperkalaemic effect is theoretically possible. ACE inhibitors appear to reduce the efficacy of epoetin, but any interaction may take many months to develop.

As the epoetin dosage is governed by response, no immediate intervention is necessary. Blood pressure should be routinely monitored in those taking epoetin, but increased monitoring of potassium levels may be warranted.

ACE inhibitors + Food ✓

Food reduces the absorption of imidapril and moexipril, and reduces the conversion of perindopril to its active metabolite, perindoprilat.

It is recommended that imidapril and perindopril should be given before food. The US manufacturers suggest taking moexipril one hour before food, although the interaction is of doubtful clinical significance. Food has little or no clinically important effect on the absorption of captopril, cilazapril, enalapril, fosinopril, lisinopril, moexipril, quinapril, ramipril, spirapril, and trandolapril.

ACE inhibitors + Gold ✓

Peripheral vasodilatation (facial flushing, nausea, dizziness, and occasionally, hypotension) has occurred in some patients treated with gold whilst taking ACE inhibitors.

The general importance of this interaction is unclear, but it is worth bearing in mind in case of an unexpected response to treatment.

ACE inhibitors + Heparin ⚠

An extensive review of the literature found that heparin (both unfractionated and low-molecular-weight heparins) and heparinoids inhibit the secretion of aldosterone, which can cause hyperkalaemia. This may be additive with the hyperkalaemic effects of ACE inhibitors.

The CSM in the UK suggests that potassium should be measured in all patients with risk factors (e.g. renal impairment, diabetes mellitus, pre-existing acidosis and those taking potassium-sparing drugs) before starting heparin, and monitored regularly thereafter (every 4 days has been suggested) particularly in patients receiving heparin for more than 7 days.

ACE inhibitors + Herbal medicines or Dietary supplements [?]

A patient taking lisinopril developed marked hypotension and became faint after taking garlic capsules.

The general importance of this interaction is unknown (probably minor), but bear it in mind in case of an unexpected response to treatment.

ACE inhibitors + Lithium ⚠

ACE inhibitors can raise lithium levels, and in some individuals 2- to 4-fold increases have occurred. Cases of lithium toxicity have been reported in patients given captopril, enalapril or lisinopril (and possibly perindopril). One analysis found an increased relative risk of 7.6 for lithium toxicity requiring hospitalisation, in elderly patients, newly started on an ACE inhibitor. Risk factors for this interaction seem to be poor renal function, heart failure, volume depletion, and increased age.

Even though the interaction appears rare, patients should have their lithium levels monitored to avoid a potentially severe adverse interaction. The development of the interaction may be delayed, and so it has been advised that lithium levels should be monitored weekly for several weeks. Patients taking lithium should be aware of the symptoms of lithium toxicity (e.g. increased nausea, weakness, fine tremor, drowsiness, lethargy) and told to immediately report them should they occur. This should be reinforced when they are given ACE inhibitors.

ACE inhibitors + Low-molecular-weight heparins ⚠

An extensive review of the literature found that heparin (both unfractionated and low-molecular-weight heparins) and heparinoids inhibit the secretion of aldosterone, which can cause hyperkalaemia. This may be additive with the hyperkalaemic effects of ACE inhibitors.

The CSM in the UK suggests that potassium should be measured in all patients with risk factors (e.g. renal impairment, diabetes mellitus, pre-existing acidosis and those taking potassium-sparing drugs) before starting a low-molecular-weight heparin, and monitored regularly thereafter (every 4 days has been suggested) particularly in patients receiving a low-molecular-weight heparin for more than 7 days.

ACE inhibitors + NSAIDs ❓

There is evidence that most NSAIDs (including the coxibs) can increase blood pressure in patients taking antihypertensives, including ACE inhibitors, although some studies have not found the increase to be clinically relevant. Indometacin appears to have the most significant effect. The combination of an NSAID and an ACE inhibitor may increase the risk of renal impairment, and rarely, hyperkalaemia has been associated with the combination.

Only some patients are affected. Consider increasing the frequency of blood pressure monitoring if an NSAID is started. Monitor renal function and electrolytes periodically.

ACE inhibitors + Potassium ⚠

ACE inhibitors can raise potassium levels. Hyperkalaemia is therefore a possibility if potassium supplements or potassium-containing salt substitutes are given, particularly in those patients where other risk factors are present, such as decreased renal function.

Monitor potassium levels, adjusting supplementation as necessary.

ACE inhibitors + **Probenecid** ✅

Probenecid decreases the renal clearance of captopril and raises enalapril serum levels.

These changes do not appear to result in a significant clinical effect.

ACE inhibitors + **Procainamide** ⚠️

The combination of captopril (or other ACE inhibitors) and procainamide possibly increases the risk of leucopenia, especially in patients with renal impairment. No pharmacokinetic interaction occurs between captopril and procainamide.

It is recommended that white cell counts are monitored before concurrent use, every 2 weeks during the first 3 months of combined treatment, and then periodically thereafter.

ACE inhibitors + **Rifampicin (Rifampin)** ❓

An isolated report describes a rise in blood pressure in one hypertensive patient, which was attributed to an interaction between enalapril and rifampicin. Rifampicin may reduce the plasma levels of the active metabolites of imidapril and spirapril.

The general importance of these interactions is unknown (expected to be minor), but bear them in mind in case of unexpected elevations in blood pressure.

ACE inhibitors + **Sirolimus** ❓

Oedema of the tongue, face, lips, neck and chest has been reported in patients taking sirolimus with enalapril or ramipril who had previously taken these ACE inhibitors without any adverse effects.

Caution should be used when either starting an ACE inhibitor in a patient already taking sirolimus or when starting sirolimus in a patient taking an ACE inhibitor. Higher doses of both drugs may pose a greater risk.

ACE inhibitors + **Tacrolimus** ⚠️

Tacrolimus may cause nephrotoxicity and hyperkalaemia, which may be additive with the effects of the ACE inhibitors.

Renal function and potassium levels should be monitored.

ACE inhibitors + **Tetracyclines** ⚠️

The absorption of oral tetracycline (and therefore probably most tetracyclines) is moderately reduced by the magnesium carbonate excipient in some quinapril formulations (e.g. *Accupro*).

The manufacturers of both drugs recommend avoiding concurrent use. One possible way to accommodate this interaction (as with the interaction between tetracyclines and antacids) is to separate the dosages as much as possible (2 to 3 hours should be sufficient).

A

ACE inhibitors + **Trimethoprim** ❓

Two reports describe serious hyperkalaemia, apparently caused by the concurrent use of trimethoprim and enalapril or quinapril, in association with renal impairment.

> Trimethoprim or ACE inhibitors alone can cause hyperkalaemia, particularly with other factors such as renal impairment. Monitor potassium levels if this combination is used in those with renal impairment.

Acetazolamide

Note that although hypokalaemia may occur with acetazolamide it is said to be transient and rarely clinically significant.

Acetazolamide + **Aspirin** ⚠

Metabolic acidosis can occur in those taking high-dose salicylates if they are given carbonic anhydrase inhibitors (e.g. acetazolamide).

> Carbonic anhydrase inhibitors should probably be avoided in those taking high-dose salicylates. If they are used, the patient should be well monitored for any evidence of toxicity (confusion, lethargy, hyperventilation, tinnitus). In this context NSAIDs or paracetamol (acetaminophen) may be safer alternatives. It is not known whether eye drops interact similarly; there appear to be no reports of an interaction.

Acetazolamide + **Carbamazepine** ⚠

In a very small number of patients rises in serum carbamazepine levels resulting in toxicity have occurred when acetazolamide was also given.

> The general importance of this interaction is unknown, but it may be prudent to monitor for indicators of carbamazepine toxicity (nausea, vomiting, ataxia, drowsiness) and take levels if necessary.

Acetazolamide + **Ciclosporin (Cyclosporine)** ⚠

There is some limited evidence that acetazolamide can cause a marked and rapid rise in ciclosporin serum levels (up to 6-fold in 72 hours), possibly accompanied by renal toxicity.

> Ciclosporin levels and/or effects (e.g. on renal function) should be monitored as a matter of routine, but it may be prudent to increase monitoring if acetazolamide is started or stopped. Adjust the dose of ciclosporin as necessary.

Acetazolamide + Lithium ⚠

There is some evidence to suggest that the excretion of lithium can be increased by acetazolamide, but lithium *toxicity* has been seen in one patient given the combination.

> The general importance of this interaction is unclear. Bear it in mind in case of an unexpected response to treatment.

Acetazolamide + Mexiletine ✕

Large changes in urinary pH caused by the concurrent use of alkalinising drugs such as acetazolamide can, in some patients, have a marked effect on the plasma levels of mexiletine.

> The effect does not appear to be predictable. The manufacturer of mexiletine recommends that concurrent use should be avoided.

Acetazolamide + Opioids ❓

Theoretically, urinary alkalinisers such as acetazolamide may increase the effects of methadone.

> The clinical significance of this interaction is unclear, but bear it in mind in case of an unexpected response to methadone.

Acetazolamide + Phenobarbital ⚠

Severe osteomalacia and rickets have been seen in a few patients taking phenobarbital or primidone with acetazolamide. A marked reduction in serum primidone levels with a loss in seizure control has also been described in a very small number of patients.

> The general importance of this interaction is unknown, but bear it in mind in case of an unexpected response to treatment.

Acetazolamide + Phenytoin ⚠

Severe osteomalacia and rickets have been seen in a few patients taking phenytoin with acetazolamide. Rises in phenytoin levels have also been described in a very small number of patients. Fosphenytoin, a prodrug of phenytoin, may interact similarly.

> The clinical importance of this interaction is unknown, but bear it in mind in case of an unexpected response to treatment. Indicators of phenytoin toxicity include blurred vision, nystagmus, ataxia or drowsiness.

Acetazolamide + Quinidine ⚠

Large rises in urinary pH due to the concurrent use of acetazolamide could cause the retention of quinidine, which could lead to quinidine toxicity. Also note that hypokalaemia, which may rarely be caused by acetazolamide, can increase the toxicity of QT-prolonging drugs such as quinidine.

> Monitor the effects if acetazolamide is started or stopped and adjust the quinidine

dosage as necessary. Also consider monitoring potassium to ensure it is within the accepted range.

Aciclovir

Valaciclovir is a prodrug of aciclovir and therefore has the potential to interact similarly.

Aciclovir + Ciclosporin (Cyclosporine) ⚠

Aciclovir does not normally seem to affect ciclosporin levels nor worsen renal function, but a very small number of cases of nephrotoxicity and increased ciclosporin levels have been seen following concurrent use. Valaciclovir, a prodrug of aciclovir, is expected to interact similarly.

> The handful of cases where problems have arisen clearly indicate that renal function should be well monitored if both drugs are given. The manufacturers of valaciclovir recommend that renal function is closely monitored if high doses (more than 4 g daily) are given with ciclosporin.

Aciclovir + H₂-receptor antagonists ✔

Single-dose studies have found that cimetidine increases the AUC of valaciclovir but this is thought unlikely to be clinically important.

> No action is generally needed. However, the manufacturers of valaciclovir recommend considering an alternative H₂-receptor antagonist if high-dose valaciclovir is used. A similar interaction seems possible with aciclovir.

Aciclovir + Mycophenolate ❓

No clinically significant pharmacokinetic interaction appears to occur between aciclovir and mycophenolate. However, the manufacturers say that in renal impairment there may be competition for tubular secretion and increased concentrations of both drugs may occur. This is also possible with valaciclovir. A case report describes neutropenia in a patient taking valaciclovir with mycophenolate.

> No action is needed, but increased monitoring may be prudent in patients with reduced renal function. Neutropenia is a rare adverse effect of valaciclovir alone. Nevertheless, bear the possibility of an interaction in mind should neutropenia occur if mycophenolate is also given.

Aciclovir + **Probenecid** ✅

Probenecid reduces the renal excretion of aciclovir and valaciclovir and therefore increases their plasma levels.

> Dose alterations are unlikely to be needed due to the wide therapeutic range of aciclovir and valaciclovir, although the manufacturer recommends that that alternatives to probenecid could be considered if high-dose valaciclovir is given.

Aciclovir + **Theophylline** ⚠

Preliminary evidence suggests that aciclovir can reduce the clearance of theophylline (and therefore possibly aminophylline) by about 30%. Evidence for valaciclovir appears to be lacking although it would be expected to interact similarly.

> Evidence appears to be limited. Be alert for an increase in the adverse effects of theophylline (nausea, headache, tremor) if aciclovir or valaciclovir is added, and consider monitoring theophylline levels.

Acitretin

Acitretin + **Alcohol** ❓

There is evidence that the consumption of alcohol may increase the serum levels of etretinate in patients taking acitretin.

> The clinical significance of this interaction is unknown, but it is suggested that it may have some bearing on the length of the period after acitretin treatment during which women are advised not to conceive.

Acitretin + **Contraceptives** ❓

There seems to be no evidence that the reliability of the combined oral contraceptives is affected by acitretin, and they are the contraceptive method of choice with teratogenic drugs. Progestogen-only oral contraceptives are not generally considered reliable enough for use with teratogenic drugs.

> Contraceptives should be started one month before acitretin and continued for 2 years after stopping acitretin. In the USA, it is standard practice to recommend that a second form of contraception, such as a barrier method, should also be used. This is because, even though hormonal methods of contraception are highly effective, they do, on rare occasions, fail.

A

Acitretin + **Food** ❓

The absorption of acitretin is approximately doubled by food.

Acitretin should be taken with food or milk to maximise absorption.

Acitretin + **Tetracyclines** ❌

The development of pseudotumour cerebri' (benign intracranial hypertension) has been associated with the concurrent use of acitretin and tetracyclines.

The manufacturer of acitretin contraindicates its use with tetracyclines.

Acitretin + **Vitamin A** ⚠

A condition similar to vitamin A (retinol) overdose may occur if acitretin and vitamin A are given concurrently.

The manufacturer of acitretin says that high doses of vitamin A (more than 4000 to 5000 units daily, the recommended daily allowance) should be avoided.

Adenosine

Adenosine + **Dipyridamole** ❌

Dipyridamole markedly reduces the bolus dose of adenosine necessary to convert supraventricular tachycardia to sinus rhythm (by about 4-fold). Profound bradycardia occurred in a patient taking dipyridamole when an adenosine infusion was given for myocardial stress testing.

The manufacturers advise the avoidance of adenosine in patients taking dipyridamole. If adenosine must be used for supraventricular tachycardia in a patient taking dipyridamole, use an initial bolus dose of 0.5 to 1 mg. If adenosine is considered necessary for myocardial imaging in a patient taking dipyridamole, the dipyridamole should be stopped 24 hours before imaging, or the dose of adenosine should be greatly reduced. This may be insufficient for extended-release dipyridamole preparations, and in this case it has been suggested that the dipyridamole will need to be stopped several days before the test.

Adenosine + **Theophylline** ❌

Theophylline can inhibit the effects of adenosine infusions used in conjunction with radionuclide myocardial imaging. Theophylline may antagonise the effect of adenosine when used to treat supraventricular arrhythmias.

Theophylline, aminophylline and other xanthines should be avoided for 24 hours before using an adenosine infusion for radionuclide myocardial imaging. Adenosine bolus injections for the termination of paroxysmal supraventricular tachycardia may still be effective in patients taking xanthines. The usual dose schedule should be followed. However, note that adenosine has induced bronchospasm and it has been suggested that adenosine should be avoided in patients with asthma, and used cautiously in those with obstructive pulmonary disease. Xanthines, such as intravenous aminophylline, may be used to terminate any persistent adverse effects of adenosine infusions given for myocardial imaging.

Albendazole

Albendazole + **Carbamazepine** ⚠

Carbamazepine approximately halves the levels of albendazole.

For systemic infections it may be necessary to increase the albendazole dosage. Monitor the outcome of concurrent use. This interaction is of no importance in the treatment of intestinal worm infections.

Albendazole + **Contraceptives** ✖

The manufacturer of albendazole recommends that women should use non-hormonal methods of contraception during and for one month after stopping albendazole. This is because there is a theoretical risk of an interaction (albendazole is a liver enzyme inducer) and because albendazole is potentially teratogenic.

Counsel patients on additional/alternative contraception.

Albendazole + **Food** ❓

Giving albendazole with a meal (especially fatty meals) markedly increases its absorption.

Albendazole absorption is poor, and if it is being used for systemic infections, it is advisable to take it with a meal.

Albendazole + **Phenobarbital** ⚠

Phenobarbital approximately halves the levels of albendazole.

For systemic infections it may be necessary to increase the albendazole dosage. Monitor the outcome of concurrent use. This interaction is of no importance in the treatment of intestinal worm infections.

Albendazole + **Phenytoin** ⚠

Phenytoin approximately halves the levels of albendazole. Fosphenytoin, a prodrug of phenytoin, may interact similarly.

For systemic infections it may be necessary to increase the albendazole dosage.

Monitor the outcome of concurrent use. This interaction is of no importance in the treatment of intestinal worm infections.

Alcohol

Probably the most common drug interaction of all occurs if alcohol is drunk by those taking other drugs that have CNS depressant activity, the result being even further CNS depression. Blood alcohol levels well within the legal driving limit may, in the presence of other CNS depressants, be equivalent to blood alcohol levels at or above the legal limit in terms of worsened driving and other skills. A less common interaction that can occur between alcohol and some drugs, chemicals, and fungi is the flushing reaction. This is exploited in the case of disulfiram (*Antabuse*) as an alcohol deterrent. However, it can occur unexpectedly with some other drugs and can be both unpleasant and possibly frightening, but it is not usually dangerous. See also antihypertensives, page 77, for general comments about hypertension and alcohol consumption.

Alcohol + Alpha blockers ?

Alpha blockers may enhance the hypotensive effect of alcohol in subjects susceptible to the alcohol flush syndrome. This appears to be rare in whites and blacks, but more common in Orientals. The serum levels of both indoramin and alcohol may be raised by concurrent use, which could lead to increased drowsiness.

The general significance of the hypotensive effects are unclear, but it may be prudent to warn susceptible patients when they start treatment. The degree of impairment caused by drinking alcohol whilst taking indoramin will depend on the individual patient. However, warn all patients of the potential effects, and counsel against driving or undertaking other skilled tasks. See also antihypertensives, page 77, for general comments about hypertension and alcohol consumption.

Alcohol + Amfetamines and related drugs ⚠

Dexamfetamine, and related drugs such as ecstasy, may reduce the deleterious effects of alcohol on driving skills, although reports are conflicting. Tests with metamfetamine suggest that it increases the feeling of intoxication caused by alcohol. Alcohol may increase the cardiac adverse effects of amfetamines.

The effects of this interaction are not clear, but as some psychomotor impairment occurs warn all patients of the potential effects, and counsel against driving or undertaking other skilled tasks.

Alcohol + Antidiabetics ?

Diabetics receiving insulin, oral antidiabetics, or diet alone need not abstain from alcohol, but they should drink only in moderation and accompanied by food. Alcohol makes the signs of hypoglycaemia less clear, and delayed hypoglycaemia can occur. The CNS depressant effects of alcohol in association with hypoglycaemia can make driving or the operation of dangerous machinery much more hazardous. Metformin does not carry the same risk of lactic acidosis seen with phenformin and it is suggested by the British Diabetic Association that one or two drinks a day are unlikely to be harmful to those taking metformin. A flushing reaction is common in patients taking chlorpropamide who drink alcohol, but is rare with other sulphonylureas.

Diabetics are advised not to exceed 2 drinks (for women) or 3 drinks (for men) daily and limit the intake of drinks with high-carbohydrate content (e.g. sweet sherries, liqueurs). Diabetics should not drink on an empty stomach and they should know that the warning signs of hypoglycaemia may possibly be obscured by the effects of the alcohol and that the hypoglycaemic effects of alcohol may occur several hours after drinking. The chlorpropamide-alcohol interaction (flushing reaction) is very well documented, but of minimal importance. It is a nuisance and possibly socially embarrassing but normally requires no treatment. Patients should be warned.

Alcohol + Antihistamines ❓

Some antihistamines cause drowsiness, which can be increased by alcohol. The detrimental effects of alcohol on driving skills are considerably increased by the use of the older more sedative antihistamines (e.g. diphenhydramine, hydroxyzine) and appear to be minimal or absent with the newer non-sedating antihistamines (e.g. cetirizine, loratadine). Note that some of the more sedative antihistamines are common ingredients of cough, cold and influenza remedies.

The degree of impairment will depend on the individual patient. However, warn all patients taking sedating antihistamines of the potential effects, and counsel against driving or undertaking other skilled tasks.

Alcohol + Antipsychotics ❓

The detrimental effects of alcohol on the skills related to driving are greatly increased by chlorpromazine, increased by flupentixol and thioridazine, and possibly increased by olanzapine, prochlorperazine and quetiapine. Any interaction with amisulpride, haloperidol, sulpiride or tiapride seems to be mild. The postural hypotension seen with antipsychotics is likely to be worsened by alcohol. There is evidence that drinking can precipitate extrapyramidal adverse effects in patients taking antipsychotics.

It has been suggested that patients should routinely be advised to abstain from alcohol during antipsychotic treatment in order to avoid potentiating extrapyramidal adverse effects, although note that cases of a problem seem rare. The degree of sedation will depend on the antipsychotic given and the individual patient. However, warn all patients of the potential effects, and counsel against driving or undertaking other skilled tasks. Patients should also be warned about postural hypotension and counselled on how to manage it (i.e. lay down, raise the legs, and on recovering to get up slowly).

Alcohol + Apomorphine ❓

The manufacturers say that interaction studies in subjects given apomorphine (for erectile dysfunction) found that alcohol increased the incidence and extent of hypotension (one of the adverse effects of apomorphine). They also point out that alcohol can diminish sexual performance.

Concurrent use need not be avoided, but warn patients they may feel dizzy if they drink, and to sit or lie down if this occurs.

Alcohol + Aspirin ✅

The combined effect of aspirin and alcohol on the stomach wall is established. Aspirin 3 g daily for a period of 3 to 5 days induces an average blood loss of about 5 mL. Some increased loss undoubtedly occurs with alcohol, but it seems to be quite small and unlikely to be of much importance in most healthy individuals using moderate doses of aspirin. In one study it was found that alcohol was a mild damaging agent or a mild potentiating agent for other gastrointestinal damaging drugs. It should be remembered that chronic and/or gross overuse of aspirin and alcohol may result in gastric ulceration. Other salicylates would be expected to have similar effects to aspirin.

This interaction is only likely to be of significance where high doses of aspirin or other oral salicylates are given to heavy drinkers.

Alcohol + Azoles ❓

A few cases of disulfiram-like reactions (nausea, vomiting, facial flushing) have been seen in patients who drank alcohol while taking ketoconazole.

The incidence of this reaction appears to be very low and its importance is probably small. Reactions of this kind are usually more unpleasant than serious. Nevertheless, the manufacturer of ketoconazole advises avoiding alcohol.

Alcohol + Benzodiazepines ⚠

Benzodiazepine and related hypno-sedatives increase the CNS depressant effects of alcohol to some extent. Alcohol modestly affects the pharmacokinetics of some benzodiazepines, and may increase aggression or amnesia, and/or reduce their anxiolytic effects.

The deterioration in the skills related to driving (as a result of the increased CNS depression that may occur) will depend on the particular drug in question, its dosage and the amounts of alcohol taken. The risk is heightened because the patient may be unaware of being affected. Some benzodiazepines used at night for sedation are still present in appreciable amounts the next day and therefore may continue to interact. Anyone taking any of these drugs should be warned that their usual response to alcohol may be greater than expected, and their ability to drive a car, or carry out any other tasks requiring alertness, may be impaired.

Alcohol + Beta blockers ✅

The effects of atenolol and metoprolol do not appear to be changed by alcohol. Some preliminary evidence suggests that the detrimental effects of alcohol and atenolol (with chlortalidone) or propranolol are additive on the performance of some psychomotor tests, and there is some evidence that alcohol modestly reduces the haemodynamic effects of propranolol. The blood pressure lowering effects of sotalol appear to be increased by alcohol.

The clinical significance of these minor effects is undetermined, but they seem unlikely to be of great importance. See also antihypertensives, page 77, for general comments about antihypertensives and alcohol consumption.

Alcohol + Bupropion ❓

Adverse neuropsychiatric events or reduced alcohol tolerance has been reported in patients taking bupropion. The risk of seizures with bupropion may be increased with both the excessive use and abrupt withdrawal of alcohol.

The manufacturers recommend that the consumption of alcohol should be minimised or avoided. Bupropion is contraindicated during abrupt withdrawal from alcohol.

Alcohol + Buspirone ⚠️

The use of buspirone with alcohol may cause drowsiness and weakness, although it does not appear to impair the performance of a number of psychomotor tests.

The UK manufacturer suggests avoiding concurrent use, and cautions patients of the potential hazards of driving or handling other potentially dangerous machinery until they are certain that buspirone does not adversely affect them. The evidence would appear to support this suggestion.

Alcohol + Calcium-channel blockers

See also antihypertensives, page 77, for general comments about antihypertensives and alcohol consumption.

Felodipine or Nifedipine ✅

Alcohol may increase the AUC of felodipine by 77% and nifedipine by 54%. This resulted in an increase in heart rate in patients taking felodipine but no effects were noted in patients taking nifedipine.

Information about these interactions is limited. Their clinical significance is uncertain, but probably small.

Verapamil ⚠️

Blood alcohol levels were raised by 17%, and remained elevated for five times longer than normal, in patients taking verapamil.

Information about this interaction is limited and unconfirmed. An alcohol concentration rise of almost 17% is quite small, but it could be enough to raise legal blood levels to illegal levels if driving. Moreover, the intoxicant effects of alcohol may persist for a much longer period of time. Warn patients of these potential effects.

A

Alcohol + Carbamazepine ✅

Moderate social drinking does not appear to affect the serum levels of carbamazepine. Heavy drinking may possibly increase the metabolism of carbamazepine, and this may be further increased in alcoholics who abstain from drinking alcohol.

No action needed for moderate social drinking. However, note that the sedative effects of antiepileptics may be additive with those of alcohol. The risk of seizures may be increased in heavy drinkers on tapering or stopping alcohol.

Alcohol + Cephalosporins ❓

Disulfiram-like reactions have been seen in patients taking cefamandole, cefmenoxime, cefoperazone, cefotetan, latamoxef (moxalactam) and possibly cefonicid after drinking alcohol or following an injection of alcohol. This is not a general reaction of the cephalosporins, but is confined to those with particular chemical structures. Due to their structure ceforanide, cefotiam, and cefpiramide also present a risk. Other cephalosporins are not expected to interact.

The reaction appears normally to be more embarrassing or unpleasant and frightening than serious, with the symptoms subsiding spontaneously after a few hours. Treatment is not usually needed although two elderly patients needed treatment for hypotension. Patients taking the interacting cephalosporins should be advised to avoid alcohol during treatment and for up to 3 days (7 in the presence of renal or hepatic impairment) after treatment is finished.

Alcohol + Ciclosporin (Cyclosporine) ✅

An isolated report describes a marked increase in serum ciclosporin levels in a patient after an episode of binge drinking, but a subsequent study found that moderate single doses of alcohol in other patients had no such effect. Red wine appears to decrease ciclosporin bioavailability.

It seems that alcohol in moderation will not affect ciclosporin levels, although greater care should be taken with red wine. However, note that the study with red wine was in patients taking the old *Sandimmun* preparation orally, which is known to have greater fluctuations in bioavailability than the *Neoral* preparation.

Alcohol + Contraceptives ✅

The detrimental effects of alcohol may be reduced to some extent in women taking hormonal contraceptives, but blood alcohol levels do not seem to be altered. Alcohol does not affect the pharmacokinetics of ethinylestradiol.

No action is needed in those taking contraceptives.

Alcohol + Disulfiram ❌

The ingestion of alcohol while taking disulfiram will result in flushing and fullness of the face and neck, tachycardia, breathlessness, giddiness and hypotension, nausea, and vomiting. A mild flushing reaction of the skin may possibly occur in particularly sensitive individuals if alcohol is applied to the skin or if the vapour is inhaled. Note that some products (e.g. *Norvir oral solution*) are formulated with alcohol and, although the volume of alcohol taken with the dose is likely to be small, may still provoke this reaction.

> This interaction is exploited therapeutically to deter alcoholics from drinking. Patients should also be warned about the exposure to alcohol from some unexpected sources such as foods, cosmetics, medicinal remedies, and solvents.

Alcohol + Duloxetine ❓

No important psychomotor interaction normally appears to occur between duloxetine and alcohol. However, additive effects (e.g. drowsiness) are considered possible.

> The degree of impairment will depend on the individual patient. However, warn all patients of the potential effects, and counsel against driving or undertaking other skilled tasks.

Alcohol + Food ✅

Food (particularly milk) may reduce the absorption of alcohol. Foods rich in serotonin (e.g. bananas, pineapples) taken with alcohol may produce adverse effects such as diarrhoea and headache. A disulfiram-like reaction can occur if alcohol is taken up to 24 hours after eating the smooth ink(y) caps fungus (*Coprinus atramentarius*) or certain other edible fungi.

> Whether the interaction leading to reduced alcohol absorption can be regarded as advantageous or undesirable is a moot point. The intensity of the disulfiram-like reaction depends upon the quantity of fungus and alcohol consumed, and the time interval between them. However, reports of this reaction in the medical literature are few and far between. Treatment does not normally appear to be necessary.

Alcohol + Furazolidone ⚠️

A disulfiram-like reaction may occur in patients taking furazolidone if they drink alcohol. One report suggests that about 1 in 5 patients may be affected.

> Reactions of this kind appear to be more unpleasant and possibly frightening than serious, and normally need no treatment. Nevertheless, patients should be warned about what may happen if they drink.

Alcohol + Griseofulvin ❓

An isolated case report describes a very severe disulfiram-like reaction when a man taking griseofulvin drank a can of beer. Two other patients taking griseofulvin developed flushing and tachycardia after drinking. Several other patients have experienced an increase in the effects of alcohol while taking griseofulvin.

> The documentation is extremely sparse, which would seem to suggest that adverse interactions between alcohol and griseofulvin are uncommon. At the risk of being over-cautious, warn all patients of the potential effects, and counsel against driving or undertaking other skilled tasks.

A

Alcohol + H₂-receptor antagonists ✓

Although some studies have found that blood alcohol levels can be slightly raised and possibly remain elevated for longer than usual in those taking H₂-receptor antagonists, other studies report that no significant interaction occurs. Hypoglycaemia, which can occur following alcohol intake, may be enhanced by H₂-receptor antagonists.

> Extensive reviews of the data have concluded that the interaction is not, in general, clinically significant. There are insufficient grounds to justify any general warning regarding alcohol and H₂-receptor antagonists, but note that many of the conditions for which H₂-receptor antagonists are used may be made worse by alcohol, so restriction of drinking may be needed.

Alcohol + Herbal medicines or Dietary supplements

Cannabis ?

Smoking cannabis (marijuana) may reduce and delay peak alcohol levels. The effects of drinking alcohol and smoking cannabis appear to be at least additive on driving performance, although some limited evidence suggests that regular cannabis use does not potentiate the effects of alcohol.

> The degree of impairment will depend on the individual patient. However, patients should be aware of the potential additive effects, and counselled against driving or undertaking other skilled tasks.

Ginseng ✓

Ginseng increases the clearance of alcohol from the body and lowers blood alcohol levels.

> The clinical significance of this interaction is unclear.

Kava ⚠

There is some evidence that kava may worsen the deleterious effects of alcohol.

> The effects of this interaction are not clear, but as some psychomotor impairment occurs warn all patients of the potential effects, and counsel against driving or undertaking other skilled tasks. The use of kava is restricted in the UK because of reports of idiosyncratic hepatotoxicity.

Liv. 52 ?

Liv.52, an Ayurvedic herbal remedy, appears to reduce the hangover symptoms after drinking. However it also raises the blood alcohol levels of moderate drinkers (by about 30%) for the first few hours after drinking.

> Increases of up to 30% may be enough to raise the blood alcohol from legal to illegal levels when driving. Moderate drinkers should be warned.

Alcohol + HRT ✓

Acute ingestion of alcohol markedly increases the levels of circulating estradiol in women using oral HRT. A smaller increase occurs with transdermal HRT. Estradiol does not affect blood alcohol levels.

It has been suggested that women taking HRT should limit their alcohol intake, but more study is needed to confirm any interaction and its importance.

Alcohol + Hyoscine ✔

Although additive CNS effects are possible, a study found no adverse interaction appears to occur if patients using transdermal hyoscine (*Scopoderm TTS*) drink alcohol.

In general, the manufacturers of several hyoscine preparations suggest that alcohol should be avoided, although note that hyoscine butylbromide and hyoscine methobromide do not readily pass the blood-brain barrier, and would not be expected to cause additive adverse effects with alcohol.

Alcohol + Isoniazid ❓

Isoniazid slightly increases the hazards of driving after drinking alcohol. Isoniazid-induced hepatitis may also possibly be increased, and the effects of isoniazid are possibly reduced, by alcohol.

There appear to be some extra risks for patients taking isoniazid who drink, but the effect does not appear to be large. Patients should nevertheless be warned about the potential adverse effects. The clinical significance of the other effects are unclear, but it may be prudent to limit alcohol intake whilst taking isoniazid.

Alcohol + Leflunomide ✖

The UK manufacturers say that concurrent use of alcohol and leflunomide has the potential to cause additive hepatotoxic effects.

It is recommended that alcohol should be avoided by patients taking leflunomide.

Alcohol + Levamisole ❓

There is some evidence that a disulfiram-like reaction can occur if patients taking levamisole drink alcohol.

The clinical significance of this interaction is not known. The reaction, when it occurs, normally seems to be more unpleasant and possibly frightening than serious, and usually requires no treatment.

Alcohol + Lithium ❓

Some limited evidence suggests that taking lithium carbonate and drinking alcohol may impair the performance of skills related to driving, without affecting blood alcohol levels.

At the risk of being over-cautious, warn all patients of the potential effects, and counsel against driving or undertaking other skilled tasks.

A

Alcohol + Macrolides ❓

Alcohol can cause a moderate reduction in the absorption of erythromycin ethylsuccinate. There is some evidence that intravenous erythromycin can raise blood alcohol levels but the extent and the practical importance of this is unknown.

No action needed.

Alcohol + MAOIs ❌

Patients taking non-selective MAOIs can suffer a serious hypertensive reaction if they drink some beers, lagers or wines, including low-alcohol drinks, but apparently not spirits. However, this is a reaction to the tyramine content rather than the alcohol. The hypotensive adverse effects of the MAOIs may be exaggerated in a few patients by alcohol and they may experience dizziness and faintness after drinking relatively modest amounts.

Avoid tyramine-rich drinks and counsel patients on the possible response to alcohol.

Alcohol + Maprotiline ❓

Maprotiline can cause drowsiness and impair the ability to drive or handle other dangerous machinery, particularly during the first few days of treatment. This impairment may be increased by alcohol.

Patients should be warned that their usual response to alcohol may be greater than expected, and their ability to drive a car, or carry out any other tasks requiring alertness, may be impaired.

Alcohol + Methotrexate ❌

There is some inconclusive evidence to suggest that the consumption of alcohol may increase the risk of methotrexate-induced hepatic cirrhosis and fibrosis.

The manufacturers of methotrexate advise the avoidance of drugs, including alcohol, which have hepatotoxic potential. It is not clear whether moderate drinking poses a significant risk.

Alcohol + Methylphenidate ❌

Alcohol may increase methylphenidate levels and exacerbate some of its CNS effects.

The manufacturer recommends that alcohol should be avoided in those taking methylphenidate. Also, methylphenidate should be given cautiously to patients with a history of drug dependence or alcoholism because of its potential for abuse.

Alcohol + Metoclopramide ❓

There is some evidence to suggest that metoclopramide can increase the rate of absorption of alcohol, raise maximum blood alcohol levels, and possibly increase alcohol-related sedation.

At the risk of being over-cautious, warn all patients of the potential effects, and counsel against driving or undertaking other skilled tasks.

Alcohol + Metronidazole ❌

A disulfiram-like reaction has occurred in a few patients taking oral metronidazole who drank alcohol. There is one report of its occurrence when metronidazole was applied as a vaginal insert, and another when metronidazole was given intravenously. The interaction is alleged to occur with all other 5-nitroimidazoles (e.g. tinidazole).

This interaction has been extensively studied but it remains slightly controversial because the incidence has been reported as between 0 and 100%. Because of its unpredictability all patients given metronidazole should be warned what may happen if they drink alcohol. The reaction, when it occurs, normally seems to be more unpleasant and possibly frightening than serious, and usually requires no treatment, although rarely fatalities have occurred.

Alcohol + Mianserin ⚠

Mianserin can cause drowsiness and impair the ability to drive or handle other dangerous machinery, particularly during the first few days of treatment. This impairment may be increased by alcohol.

Patients should be warned that their usual response to alcohol may be greater than expected, and their ability to drive a car, or carry out any other tasks requiring alertness, may be impaired.

Alcohol + Mirtazapine ❌

The sedative effects of mirtazapine may be increased by alcohol.

The manufacturers advise against concurrent use. Patients should be warned that their usual response to alcohol may be greater than expected, and their ability to drive a car, or carry out any other tasks requiring alertness, may be impaired.

Alcohol + Nitrates ❓

Patients who take glyceryl trinitrate (nitroglycerin) and drink alcohol may feel faint and dizzy because of an increased susceptibility to postural hypotension. Consider also, antihypertensives, page 77.

The consumption of alcohol should not stop patients from using glyceryl trinitrate (nitroglycerin), but they should be warned of the possible effects and told what to do if they feel faint and dizzy (i.e. lie down, and to remain lying down until symptoms abate).

A

Alcohol + NSAIDs

Indometacin and Phenylbutazone ⚠

The skills related to driving are impaired by indometacin and phenylbutazone. Additive sedation occurs if patients drink while taking phenylbutazone, but this does not appear to occur with indometacin. See also Miscellaneous NSAIDs, below.

> The degree of impairment will depend on the individual patient. However, warn all patients of the potential effects, and counsel against driving or undertaking other skilled tasks.

Miscellaneous NSAIDs ❓

NSAIDs may increase the risk of gastrointestinal haemorrhage associated with alcohol, and a few isolated reports attribute acute renal failure to the acute excessive consumption of alcohol in patients taking NSAIDs.

> Serious problems seem rare. Concurrent use need not be avoided but be aware that there are some risks and these are increased in heavy drinkers.

Alcohol + Opioids ❓

The opioid analgesics can enhance the CNS depressant effects of alcohol, which has been fatal in some cases. The CNS depressant effects of alcohol are modestly increased by normal therapeutic doses of dextropropoxyphene (propoxyphene), but in deliberate suicidal overdosage the CNS depressant effects appear to be additive, and can be fatal. A single case report describes a fatality due to the combined CNS depressant effects of hydromorphone and alcohol. Alcohol has been associated with rapid release of hydromorphone and morphine from extended-release preparations, which could result in potentially fatal doses.

> The degree of impairment and/or sedation will depend on the individual patient, the opioid dose used and the amount of alcohol consumed. However, warn all patients of the potential effects, and with larger doses counsel against driving or undertaking other skilled tasks.

Alcohol + Paracetamol (Acetaminophen) ⚠

Many case reports describe severe liver damage, fatal in some instances, in some alcoholics and persistent heavy drinkers who take only moderate doses of paracetamol. However, controlled studies have found no association between alcoholism and paracetamol-induced hepatotoxicity. There is controversy about the use of paracetamol in alcoholics. Some consider standard therapeutic doses can be used, whereas others recommend the dose of paracetamol should be reduced, or paracetamol avoided. Occasional and moderate drinkers do not seem to be at any extra risk.

> There seems to be no way of identifying those alcoholics at risk. The combination need not be avoided, but caution patients against long-term regular use without close monitoring.

Alcohol + **Phenobarbital** ⚠

Moderate social drinking slightly affects the serum levels of phenobarbital, but no changes in the control of epilepsy seem to occur. Alcohol and the barbiturates are CNS depressants, which together can have additive and possibly even synergistic effects. Activities requiring alertness and good co-ordination, such as driving a car or handling other potentially dangerous machinery, can be made more difficult and more hazardous. Alcohol may also continue to interact the next day if the barbiturate has hangover effects.

Patients should be warned that their usual response to alcohol may be greater than expected, and their ability to drive a car, or carry out any other tasks requiring alertness, may be impaired.

Alcohol + **Phenytoin** ⚠

Chronic heavy drinking reduces serum phenytoin concentrations so that above average doses of phenytoin may be needed to maintain adequate levels. Moderate drinking appears to be safe in those taking phenytoin.

Although above average doses are likely to be needed in heavy drinkers be aware that patients with liver impairment usually need lower doses of phenytoin, so the picture may be more complicated.

Alcohol + **Pimecrolimus** ❓

Alcohol intolerance (moderate to severe facial flushing) and application site erythema have been reported rarely with pimecrolimus cream.

Patients should be warned of the possibility of a flushing reaction with alcohol, although the incidence of this reaction seems to be rare.

Alcohol + **Pregabalin** ❓

No clinically relevant pharmacokinetic interaction occurs between pregabalin and alcohol, and concurrent use does not appear to have a clinically important effect on respiration. However, the manufacturers suggest that pregabalin may potentiate the effects of alcohol.

Patients should be warned that their usual response to alcohol may be greater than expected, and their ability to drive a car, or carry out any other tasks requiring alertness, may be impaired.

Alcohol + **Reboxetine** ⚠

A study found that reboxetine does not effect cognitive or psychomotor function, and there is no interaction with alcohol.

No action needed, but note that as reboxetine has CNS effects the manufacturers say that patients should be cautioned if operating machinery or driving.

Alcohol + SSRIs ❓

Citalopram, escitalopram, fluoxetine, paroxetine, and sertraline do not appear to consistently and significantly interact with alcohol, but some modest interaction possibly occurs with fluvoxamine, which may cause impaired alertness and a slight 20% increase in fluvoxamine levels.

> Although no interaction has clearly been demonstrated (except perhaps with fluvoxamine) all the SSRIs can be sedating so some caution is warranted. The degree of impairment will depend on the individual patient. However, warn all patients of the potential effects, and counsel against driving or undertaking other skilled tasks.

Alcohol + Tacrolimus ⚠

Alcohol may cause facial flushing or skin erythema in patients using tacrolimus ointment. This reaction appears to be fairly common.

> Patients should be warned that alcohol may need to be avoided if flushing occurs.

Alcohol + Tetracyclines ✔

Doxycycline serum levels may fall below minimum therapeutic concentrations in alcoholic patients, but tetracycline is not affected. There is nothing to suggest that moderate amounts of alcohol have a clinically relevant effect on the serum levels of any tetracycline in non-alcoholic subjects.

> Information is limited, but the interaction between doxycycline and alcohol appears to be established and of clinical significance in alcoholics. One possible solution to the problem of enzyme induction is to give alcoholic subjects double the dose of doxycycline. Alternatively tetracycline could be used because it appears not to be affected. There is nothing to suggest that moderate or even occasional heavy drinking has a clinically relevant effect on any of the other tetracyclines in non-alcoholic subjects.

Alcohol + Tizanidine ❓

Sedation occurs in up to 50% of patients taking tizanidine; these effects may be additive with alcohol. Additive hypotensive effects also considered possible, see antihypertensives, page 77. Alcohol modestly increases tizanidine levels, which may enhance these effects.

> The degree of impairment will depend on the individual patient. However, warn all patients of the potential effects, and counsel against driving or undertaking other skilled tasks, and to sit or lie down if they become dizzy or faint.

Alcohol + Trazodone ❓

Trazodone can make driving or handling other dangerous machinery more hazardous, particularly during the first few days of treatment, and further impairment may occur with alcohol.

The degree of impairment will depend on the individual patient. However, warn all patients of the potential effects, and counsel against driving or undertaking other skilled tasks.

Alcohol + Tricyclics ❓

The ability to drive, handle dangerous machinery, or do other tasks requiring complex psychomotor skills may be impaired by amitriptyline, and to a lesser extent by doxepin, particularly during the first few days of treatment. This impairment is increased by alcohol. Amoxapine, clomipramine, desipramine, imipramine, and nortriptyline appear to interact with alcohol only minimally. Specific information about other tricyclic antidepressants appears to be lacking. There is also evidence that alcoholics may need larger doses of desipramine and imipramine to control depression.

Although an interaction has not been clearly demonstrated with all the tricyclic antidepressants some caution is warranted as they all have some sedative effects. The degree of impairment will depend on the individual patient. However, warn all patients of the potential effects, and counsel against driving or undertaking other skilled tasks. In addition some prescribers may feel it appropriate to offer further precautionary advice, because during the first 1 to 2 weeks of treatment many tricyclics (without alcohol) may temporarily impair the skills related to driving. Also be aware that alcoholic patients (without liver disease) may need higher doses of imipramine (possibly doubled) and desipramine to control depression, and if long-term abstinence is achieved the dosages may then eventually need to be reduced. Information about other tricyclics seems to be lacking.

Alcohol + Venlafaxine ❓

No important psychomotor interaction normally appears to occur between alcohol and venlafaxine in therapeutic doses. However, additive sedative effects are considered possible.

The manufacturers state that patients should be advised to avoid alcohol while taking venlafaxine.

Alcohol + Warfarin and other oral anticoagulants ❓

The effects of anticoagulants such as warfarin are unlikely to be changed in those with normal liver function who drink small or moderate amounts of alcohol, but heavy drinkers or patients with some liver disease may show considerable fluctuations in their prothrombin times when they drink alcohol.

Patients should be counselled about appropriate alcohol consumption when they start anticoagulant therapy.

A

Aliskiren

Aliskiren + **Diuretics**

Loop diuretics ⚠

Aliskiren reduces the plasma levels of furosemide by about 50%. Additive hypotensive effects likely when aliskiren is given with any diuretic, see antihypertensives, page 77.

The effects of furosemide may be reduced. Monitor blood pressure and/or disease control, and adjust the doses/treatment accordingly.

Potassium-sparing diuretics ⚠

Based on experience with the use of other substances that affect the renin-angiotensin system, the concurrent use of potassium-sparing diuretics and aliskiren may lead to increases in serum potassium. Additive hypotensive effects likely when aliskiren is given with any diuretic, see antihypertensives, page 77.

Monitor potassium levels and adjust treatment as necessary.

Allopurinol

Allopurinol + **Antidiabetics** ❓

Although allopurinol affects the half-life of chlorpropamide and tolbutamide, and a case of diabetic coma has been seen in a patient taking gliclazide and allopurinol, there appears to be little information to suggest that a clinically significant interaction usually occurs with sulphonylureas.

Bear these potential interactions in mind in case of an unexpected response to treatment.

Allopurinol + **Azathioprine** ⚠

The haematological effects of azathioprine are markedly increased by the concurrent use of allopurinol. Azathioprine is rapidly and extensively metabolised to mercapto-purine. Mercaptopurine is therefore expected to share the interactions of azathioprine.

The dosage of azathioprine or mercaptopurine should be reduced by two-thirds to three-quarters to minimise the risk of toxicity. Despite taking these precautions toxicity may still be seen and very close haematological monitoring is advisable if concurrent use is necessary.

Allopurinol + **Capecitabine** ❌

The activity of capecitabine is predicted to be decreased by allopurinol.

The UK manufacturers of capecitabine say that allopurinol should be avoided.

Allopurinol + **Carbamazepine** ⚠

There is some evidence to suggest that high-dose allopurinol (15 mg/kg or 600 mg daily) can gradually raise serum carbamazepine levels by about one-third. It appears that allopurinol 300 mg daily has no effect on carbamazepine levels.

This interaction may take weeks or months to develop. Warn patients taking high-dose allopurinol to monitor for indicators of carbamazepine toxicity, which include nausea, vomiting, ataxia and drowsiness. Monitor carbamazepine levels as necessary.

Allopurinol + **Ciclosporin (Cyclosporine)** ❓

In isolated cases markedly raised ciclosporin levels have occurred in patients given allopurinol. However, two clinical studies found a trend towards lower ciclosporin levels with low-dose allopurinol.

This interaction is unconfirmed and of uncertain clinical significance. There is insufficient evidence to recommend increased monitoring, but be aware of the potential for an interaction in case of an unexpected response to treatment.

Allopurinol + **Diuretics** ❓

The thiazide diuretics may increase the incidence of hypersensitivity reactions (rash, vasculitis, hepatitis, eosinophilia, progressive renal impairment) in patients taking allopurinol, especially in the presence of renal impairment.

The clinical significance of this interaction is unclear. Remember that thiazides can cause hyperuricaemia.

Allopurinol + **NRTIs** ⚠

Allopurinol increases didanosine absorption (69% rise in the maximum serum levels). In some patients the dosage of didanosine has been halved without the loss of antiviral efficacy.

If the dose of didanosine is not reduced, there is the potential for an increase in didanosine adverse effects. The UK manufacturer recommends close monitoring for adverse effects but the US manufacturer advises against concurrent use.

Allopurinol + **Penicillins** ❓

The incidence of skin rashes among those taking either ampicillin or amoxicillin is increased by allopurinol.

There would seem to be no strong reason for avoiding concurrent use, but prescribers should recognise that the development of a rash is by no means unusual. Whether this also occurs with penicillins other than ampicillin or amoxicillin is uncertain, but it does not seem to have been reported.

A

Allopurinol + **Phenytoin** ⚠

A case report describes phenytoin toxicity in a boy given allopurinol. Another study found raised phenytoin levels in 2 of 18 patients given allopurinol.

> The clinical importance of this interaction is probably small, but bear it in mind in case of an unexpected response to treatment. Indicators of phenytoin toxicity include blurred vision, nystagmus, ataxia or drowsiness.

Allopurinol + **Probenecid** ⚠

Probenecid appears to increase the renal excretion of the active metabolite of allopurinol, while allopurinol is thought to inhibit the metabolism of probenecid. Theoretically, the concurrent use of allopurinol and probenecid could lead to uric acid precipitation in the kidneys.

> The clinical significance of these interactions appears to be minimal. Nevertheless, the UK manufacturer of allopurinol recommends any reduction in efficacy should be assessed in each case. For allopurinol injection, the US manufacturer recommends a high urinary output of at least 2 litres daily, and the maintenance of neutral or slightly alkaline urine, to help prevent renal precipitation of urates.

Allopurinol + **Pyrazinamide** ❌

Allopurinol is unlikely to be effective against pyrazinamide-induced hyperuricaemia, and may exacerbate the situation.

> Note that pyrazinamide is contraindicated in hyperuricaemia and it should be stopped if gouty arthritis occurs.

Allopurinol + **Theophylline** ⚠

Evidence from clinical studies and a case report indicate that the effects of theophylline may be increased by allopurinol. It seems likely that aminophylline may interact similarly.

> Watch for symptoms of raised theophylline levels (headache, nausea, tremor). Consider monitoring theophylline levels, especially with high doses of allopurinol.

Allopurinol + **Warfarin and other oral anticoagulants** ⚠

Most patients taking oral anticoagulants with allopurinol do not develop an adverse interaction, but excessive hypoprothrombinaemia and bleeding can occur quite unpredictably in a few individuals. The interaction has only been reported with warfarin, phenprocoumon and dicoumarol, but it would be prudent to apply the same precautions with any coumarin.

> The clinical importance of this interaction is unknown, but bear it in mind when

using both drugs. Consider increasing the frequency of INR monitoring during the initial stages of concurrent use.

Alpha blockers

Alpha blockers + **Angiotensin II receptor antagonists** [?]

Severe first-dose hypotension, and synergistic hypotensive effects have occurred in patients given alpha blockers with *ACE inhibitors*. Angiotensin II receptor antagonists are predicted to interact similarly.

Acute hypotension (dizziness, fainting) sometimes occurs unpredictably with the first dose of some alpha blockers (particularly alfuzosin, prazosin and terazosin), and this can be exaggerated by other antihypertensives. Angiotensin II receptor antagonists would be expected to have a similar effect. Minimise the risk by starting with a low dose of alpha blocker, preferably given at bedtime, and escalate the dose slowly over a couple of weeks. Patients should be warned to lie down if symptoms such as dizziness, fatigue or sweating develop, and to remain lying down until symptoms abate.

Alpha blockers + **Azoles** [X]

Ketoconazole increases the AUC and maximum levels of alfuzosin (as a modified-release preparation) by 3.2-fold and 2.3-fold, respectively. Itraconazole would be expected to interact similarly.

The manufacturers cautiously contraindicate ketoconazole and itraconazole. If the concurrent use of these azoles is essential it would seem prudent to use the minimum dose of the alpha blocker and titrate as necessary, monitoring for adverse effects, particularly first-dose hypotension. The risks are likely to be greater in patients also taking other antihypertensives. Other alpha blockers do not appear to interact, and therefore they may be suitable alternatives.

Alpha blockers + **Beta blockers** [?]

The risk of first-dose hypotension with prazosin (resulting in dizziness or even fainting) is higher if the patient is already taking a beta blocker. This is likely to be true of other alpha blockers, particularly alfuzosin, bunazosin and terazosin. In a small study tamsulosin did not have any clinically relevant effects on blood pressure that was already well controlled by atenolol. Alpha blockers and beta blockers may be combined for additional lowering of blood pressure in patients with hypertension.

It is recommended that those already taking beta blockers should have the dose reduced to a maintenance dose and begin with a low-dose of an alpha blocker, with the first dose taken just before going to bed. They should also be warned about the possibility of postural hypotension and how to manage it (i.e. lay down, raise the legs, and get up slowly when recovered). Similarly, when adding a beta

A

blocker to an alpha blocker, it may be prudent to decrease the dose of the alpha blocker and re-titrate as necessary to achieve adequate blood pressure control.

Alpha blockers + Calcium-channel blockers ❓

Blood pressure may fall sharply when calcium-channel blockers are first given to patients already taking alpha blockers (particularly alfuzosin, prazosin, bunazosin and terazosin), and vice versa. In a small study, tamsulosin did not have any clinically relevant effects on blood pressure well controlled by nifedipine. Verapamil may increase the AUC of prazosin and terazosin. Alpha blockers and calcium-channel blockers may be combined for additional blood pressure lowering in patients with hypertension.

It is recommended that patients already taking calcium-channel blockers should have the dose reduced and start with a low-dose of alpha blocker, with the first dose taken just before going to bed. Caution should also be exercised when calcium-channel blockers are added to established alpha blocker therapy. Patients should also be warned about the possibility of postural hypotension and how to manage it (i.e. lay down, raise the legs, and get up slowly when recovered).

Alpha blockers + Ciclosporin (Cyclosporine) ⚠️

Preliminary studies show that prazosin causes a small reduction in the glomerular filtration rate of kidney transplant patients taking ciclosporin.

There would seem to be no strong reasons for totally avoiding prazosin in patients taking ciclosporin, but the authors of the report point out that the fall in glomerular filtration rate makes prazosin a less attractive antihypertensive.

Alpha blockers + Clonidine ❓

There is evidence that prazosin can reduce the antihypertensive effects of clonidine, whereas some other evidence suggests that this does not occur.

No action needed unless hypotension becomes excessive. If the combination of prazosin and clonidine is less effective than expected consider an interaction as the cause.

Alpha blockers + Digoxin ❓

A 60% rise in digoxin levels occurred over 3 days in one study when prazosin was also given. Clinical experience suggests this interaction is rare.

No action is usually need when prazosin is given with digoxin, although consider an interaction if adverse effects, such as bradycardia occur. Alfuzosin, doxazosin, tamsulosin and terazosin appear not to interact with digoxin.

Alpha blockers + Diuretics ❓

The use of an alpha blocker with a diuretic may result in an additive hypotensive effect, but aside from first-dose hypotension, this usually seems to be a beneficial interaction in patients with hypertension. An increased incidence of dizziness has been noted with the combination of terazosin and a diuretic. In patients with BPH, terazosin, with or without diuretics, had no additional antihypertensive effect in those with controlled blood pressure, but did reduce blood pressure in those with uncontrolled hypertension. Patients with congestive heart failure, who have had large doses of diuretics, should start prazosin treatment at the lowest dose.

No action needed unless hypotension becomes excessive.

Alpha blockers + H$_2$-receptor antagonists ✓

No important interaction occurs between cimetidine and alfuzosin, doxazosin, or tamsulosin.

No action needed. However, note that because tamsulosin levels are slightly raised the US manufacturers say that caution should be used, particularly with tamsulosin doses greater than 400 micrograms.

Alpha blockers + MAOIs

Indoramin ✗

The concurrent use of MAOIs is contraindicated by the manufacturers of indoramin based on a theoretical suggestion that the effects of noradrenaline (norepinephrine) may be potentiated. However, the pharmacology of these drugs suggests just the opposite, namely that hypotension is the more likely outcome. The manufacturers are not aware of any reported interactions between indoramin and MAOIs.

No action needed, but be aware that hypotension is a possibility.

Other Alpha blockers ❓

Both MAOIs and alpha blockers have hypotensive effects, which may be additive.

No action needed, but be aware that hypotension is a possibility if any alpha blocker is given with an MAOI.

Alpha blockers + NSAIDs ❓

Indometacin reduces the blood pressure lowering effects of prazosin in some individuals. Other alpha blockers appear not to interact with NSAIDs.

Consider monitoring blood pressure to ensure an adequate antihypertensive effect.

Alpha blockers + Phosphodiesterase type-5 inhibitors ⚠

Postural hypotension may occur with higher doses of sildenafil, tadalafil or vardenafil given at the same time as doxazosin or terazosin. It seems likely that this effect will

A

occur with most alpha blockers, although it is seen less frequently with modified-release alfuzosin and tamsulosin.

Patients should be stable on an alpha blocker before a phosphodiesterase type-5 inhibitor is started, and the lowest starting dose (e.g. sildenafil 25 mg) should be considered. The risk may also be minimised if administration is separated so that the peak levels of the two drugs do not coincide. Patients should be advised what to do if they develop postural hypotension (i.e. lay down, raise the legs and, when recovered, get up slowly).

Alpha blockers + **Protease inhibitors** ✖

Ketoconazole increases alfuzosin levels 2.3-fold. Protease inhibitors are predicted to interact similarly (CYP3A4 inhibition).

The manufacturers cautiously contraindicate potent CYP3A4 inhibitors (they name ritonavir). If concurrent use is essential it would seem prudent to use the minimum dose of the alpha blocker and titrate as necessary, monitoring for adverse effects, particularly first-dose hypotension. The risks are likely to be greater in patients also taking other antihypertensives. Other alpha blockers do not interact, and may therefore be suitable alternatives.

Alpha blockers + **SSRIs** ❓

Tamsulosin is extensively metabolised (mainly by CYP2D6 and CYP3A4). The US manufacturers therefore suggest that it should be used with caution in combination with inhibitors of CYP2D6 (e.g. fluoxetine, paroxetine), particularly at doses higher than 400 mg.

The clinical relevance of these predictions is unclear, but until more is known some caution seems prudent. If concurrent use is undertaken be aware that the effects of tamsulosin may be increased.

Amantadine

Amantadine + **Bupropion** ⚠

The manufacturer of bupropion says that limited clinical data suggests a higher incidence of undesirable effects (nausea, vomiting, excitement, restlessness, postural tremor) in patients also given amantadine.

Patients taking amantadine should be given small initial doses of bupropion, which are increased gradually. Good monitoring is advisable.

Amantadine + **Dopamine agonists** ⚠

The manufacturers of pramipexole predict that its clearance will be reduced by amantadine.

The clinical significance of this is uncertain, and there appear to be no reports of any adverse interactions. The manufacturers suggest a reduction of the pramipexole dose should be considered in patients taking amantadine.

Amfetamines

Amfetamines + **Atomoxetine** ⚠

The use of atomoxetine in patients taking amfetamines may lead to adverse effects, such as psychosis and movement disorders.

If both drugs are given, be aware that adverse CNS effects may develop, and consider reducing the doses or stopping one of the drugs should this occur.

Amfetamines + **Furazolidone** ⊗

The pressor responses to dexamfetamine in 4 hypertensive patients were increased 2- to 3-fold after 6 days of furazolidone use, and after 13 days they had increased by about 10-fold. Furazolidone has MAO-inhibitory activity, after 5 to 10 days of use, which is about equivalent to that of the non-selective MAOIs.

Concurrent use with amfetamines may be expected to result in a potentially serious rise in blood pressure and should therefore be avoided.

Amfetamines + **Guanethidine** ⊗

When hypertensive patients taking guanethidine were given single doses of dexamfetamine or metamfetamine, the hypotensive effects of the guanethidine were completely abolished, and in some instances the blood pressures rose higher than before treatment with the guanethidine.

Concurrent use should be avoided.

Amfetamines + **MAOIs** ⊗

The concurrent use of amfetamines and non-selective MAOIs can result in a potentially fatal hypertensive crisis.

Avoid concurrent use.

Amfetamines + **Moclobemide** ⊗

The concurrent use of ecstasy and moclobemide has resulted in fatalities, possibly as a result of the serotonin syndrome, page 392, although evidence is sparse.

It may be prudent to avoid the concurrent use of moclobemide and all amfetamines.

A

Amfetamines + **Protease inhibitors** ❓

An HIV-positive man taking ritonavir and saquinavir died after also taking metamfetamine and amyl nitrate. Toxicology reported extremely high metamfetamine levels, which were attributed to an interaction with ritonavir. A reaction similar to the serotonin syndrome and haemolytic anaemia has also been reported in patients taking ecstasy with ritonavir and metamfetamine with indinavir, respectively.

> Patients should be made aware of the additional potential risks of using amfetamines with ritonavir. Appropriate precautions, apart from avoidance, include a reduction of the usual dose of ecstasy to about 25%, taking breaks from dancing, checking that a medical team are on site, maintaining adequate hydration by avoiding alcohol, and replenishing fluids regularly.

Amfetamines + **SSRIs** ❓

Symptoms of schizophrenia occurred in one patient, and restlessness, agitation and hyperventilation occurred in another, after they took amfetamine with fluoxetine. A patient developed serotonin syndrome, page 392, when taking citalopram with dexamfetamine. Similar reactions have also been seen with ecstasy.

> The clinical significance of this interaction is unknown, but bear it in mind in case of an unexpected response to treatment.

Amfetamines + **Venlafaxine** ❓

An isolated case of serotonin syndrome, page 392, has been attributed to the concurrent use of dexamfetamine and venlafaxine.

> The clinical significance of this interaction is unknown, but bear it in mind in case of an unexpected response to treatment.

Aminoglutethimide

Aminoglutethimide + **Corticosteroids** ⚠️

The effects of dexamethasone can be reduced or abolished by aminoglutethimide.

> Doubling the dexamethasone dose has proven effective in some cases, although greater increases have been needed. Hydrocortisone is routinely given with aminoglutethimide without problem, and so may provide an alternative in some cases.

Aminoglutethimide + **Medroxyprogesterone** ⚠️

Aminoglutethimide reduces the plasma levels of medroxyprogesterone by at least half.

> It has been suggested that to achieve adequate plasma medroxyprogesterone acetate levels in breast cancer therapy (above 100 nanograms/mL) a daily dose of

800 mg of *Provera* is probably necessary in the presence of aminoglutethimide 125 or 250 mg twice daily. This is double the usual recommended dose of this preparation.

Aminoglutethimide + Tamoxifen ⚠

Aminoglutethimide markedly increases the clearance of tamoxifen and reduces its serum levels. Tamoxifen does not appear to affect aminoglutethimide levels.

Theoretically, the combination of an oestrogen antagonist such as tamoxifen and an aromatase inhibitor should provide additional benefit in the treatment of hormone-dependent cancers, however, no clinical studies have yet found this to be so. This interaction may partly explain this. It may be preferable to use these drugs sequentially rather than concurrently.

Aminoglutethimide + Theophylline ⚠

Aminoglutethimide increases theophylline clearance by almost 50% in some patients, but it is not known whether this results in a clinically relevant decrease in the effects of theophylline. Aminophylline would be expected to be similarly affected.

Monitor the effects and, if necessary, take theophylline levels. Increase the theophylline dosage accordingly.

Aminoglutethimide + Warfarin and other oral anticoagulants ⚠

Aminoglutethimide increases the clearance of warfarin: higher doses seem to have a greater effect, and up to 4-fold increases in the warfarin dosage have been needed. The effects of the interaction seem to develop over 14 days, and the interaction may persist for 2 weeks after aminoglutethimide is stopped. Similar effects have been seen with acenocoumarol.

Monitor the INR and adjust the anticoagulant dosage accordingly if aminoglutethimide is started or stopped. Information about other coumarins is generally lacking but it would seem prudent to apply the same precautions with any of them.

Aminoglycosides

The aminoglycosides are known to be nephrotoxic and many of their interactions occur as a result of this effect. Due to the number of known interactions with other nephrotoxic drugs (for examples see amphotericin, page 38, and ciclosporin, page 38), many manufacturers of other drugs with nephrotoxic effects caution concurrent use. It is advisable to monitor renal function in patients taking aminoglycosides, and it may be prudent to increase the frequency of this monitoring in patients taking other nephrotoxic drugs.

A

Aminoglycosides + **Amphotericin B** ❓

A number of patients developed nephrotoxicity, which was attributed to amphotericin B. Raised gentamicin or amikacin levels, without significant changes in creatinine, were seen in children treated with amphotericin B.

> Aminoglycosides are nephrotoxic and it is generally recommended that they should be avoided with other nephrotoxic drugs (such as amphotericin B). However, if concurrent use is essential it may be prudent to increase the renal function and drug level monitoring that is advised during aminoglycoside therapy.

Aminoglycosides + **Bisphosphonates** ⚠

Severe hypocalcaemia occurred in three patients given sodium clodronate when they were also given netilmicin or amikacin.

> If bisphosphonates are given with aminoglycosides, caution and close monitoring of calcium and magnesium levels has been advised. The renal loss of calcium and magnesium can continue for weeks after aminoglycosides are stopped, and bisphosphonates can also persist in bone for weeks. This means that the interaction is potentially possible whether the drugs are given concurrently or sequentially.

Aminoglycosides + **Ciclosporin (Cyclosporine)** ⚠

Nephrotoxicity is increased in some patients by the concurrent use of ciclosporin and amikacin, gentamicin or tobramycin. This interaction would be expected with all systemic aminoglycosides.

> The concurrent use of ciclosporin and aminoglycosides should only be undertaken if the clinical benefit outweighs the risk of renal damage. Close monitoring of renal function and aminoglycoside levels is required.

Aminoglycosides + **Digoxin** ⚠

The serum levels of digoxin can be increased (more than doubled) by the concurrent use of gentamicin in patients with congestive cardiac failure and diabetes.

> Patients should be monitored for signs of digoxin toxicity if gentamicin is given, especially those with diabetes or impaired renal function. Initially, checking pulse rate is probably adequate. There seems to be no information about other parenteral aminoglycosides. Consider also neomycin, page 224.

Aminoglycosides + **Diuretics**

Etacrynic acid ✖

The concurrent use of aminoglycosides and etacrynic acid should be avoided because their damaging actions on the ear can be additive. The intravenous use of etacrynic acid and renal impairment are additional causative factors. Even sequential use may not be safe, and the effects may be irreversible.

Avoid concurrent use. Other loop diuretics appear to be safer.

Other loop diuretics ⚠

Although *animal* studies suggest an interaction between loop diuretics such as furosemide and bumetanide and the aminoglycosides, the weight of clinical evidence suggests that they do not normally increase either the nephrotoxicity or ototoxicity associated with the aminoglycosides. It has been suggested that an interaction may occur if high-dose infusions of furosemide are used.

Increased monitoring (e.g. of renal function) would seem appropriate if high doses of furosemide are given. The same precautions would seem to be appropriate with other loop diuretics.

Aminoglycosides + NRTIs ⚠

The aminoglycosides are known to be nephrotoxic and many of their interactions occur as a result of this effect. Due to the number of known interactions with other nephrotoxic drugs (for examples see amphotericin, page 38, and ciclosporin, page 38), many manufacturers of other drugs with nephrotoxic effects, including tenofovir, caution concurrent use.

It is advisable to monitor renal function in patients taking aminoglycosides, and it may be prudent to increase the frequency of this monitoring in patients taking other nephrotoxic drugs.

Aminoglycosides + NSAIDs ⚠

Some reports claim that gentamicin and amikacin levels may be raised by indometacin, and that amikacin levels may be raised by ibuprofen lysine, when given to premature babies to treat patent ductus arteriosus, whereas others have not found an interaction.

Concurrent use should be closely monitored because of the toxicity that is associated with raised aminoglycoside levels. It has been suggested that the aminoglycoside dosage should be reduced before giving indometacin. It has also been suggested that the dose interval of amikacin should be increased by at least 6 to 8 hours if ibuprofen lysine is also given during the first days of life. The serum levels of the aminoglycosides and renal function should be well monitored during concurrent use. Other aminoglycosides possibly behave similarly. This interaction does not seem to have been studied in adults.

Aminoglycosides + Penicillins ⚠

A reduction in serum aminoglycoside levels can occur if aminoglycosides and penicillins are given together to patients with severe renal impairment. Carbenicillin, piperacillin and ticarcillin have been implicated with both gentamicin and tobramycin. Netilmicin appears not to interact with piperacillin. No interaction of

A

importance appears to occur either with intravenous aminoglycoside and penicillins in those with normal renal function, or between aminoglycosides and carbapenems.

In patients with renal impairment it has been recommended that the penicillin dosage should be adjusted according to renal function, and the serum levels of both antibacterials closely monitored. However, note that antibacterial inactivation can continue in the assay sample, and rapid assay is probably necessary. There would seem to be no reason for avoiding concurrent use in patients with normal renal function because no significant *in vivo* inactivation appears to occur. Moreover there is good clinical evidence that concurrent use is valuable, especially in the treatment of *Pseudomonas* infections. Consider also neomycin, page 338.

Aminoglycosides + Tacrolimus ⚠

The aminoglycosides are known to be nephrotoxic and many of their interactions occur as a result of this effect. Due to the number of known interactions with other nephrotoxic drugs (for examples see amphotericin, page 38, and ciclosporin, page 38), many manufacturers of other drugs with nephrotoxic effects, including tacrolimus, caution concurrent use.

It is advisable to monitor renal function in patients taking aminoglycosides, and it may be prudent to increase the frequency of this monitoring in patients taking other nephrotoxic drugs.

Aminoglycosides + Vancomycin ⚠

The nephrotoxicity of aminoglycosides appears to be potentiated by vancomycin.

Concurrent use is therapeutically useful, but the risk of increased nephrotoxicity should be borne in mind. Therapeutic drug monitoring and regular assessment of renal function is warranted.

Amiodarone

Note that amiodarone has a long half-life (25 to 100 days) so that interactions may occur for some time after amiodarone has been withdrawn.

Amiodarone + Beta blockers ❓

Hypotension, bradycardia, ventricular fibrillation and asystole have been seen in a few patients given amiodarone with propranolol, metoprolol or sotalol (for sotalol, see also drugs that prolong the QT interval, page 237). However, analysis of clinical studies suggests that the combination can be beneficial.

The concurrent use of beta blockers and amiodarone is not uncommon and may be therapeutically useful. However, concurrent use should be undertaken with caution and an appreciation of the potential adverse effects, especially with sotalol.

Amiodarone + **Calcium-channel blockers** ✖

Increased cardiac depressant effects (potentiation of negative chronotropic properties and conduction slowing effects) would be expected if amiodarone is given with diltiazem or verapamil. One case of sinus arrest and serious hypotension has been reported in a woman taking diltiazem with amiodarone.

It is advised that amiodarone should be avoided or used with caution with diltiazem or verapamil because cardiodepression may occur. Note that diltiazem has been used for rate control in patients developing postoperative atrial fibrillation despite the use of prophylactic amiodarone. There do not appear to be any reports of adverse effects attributed to the use of amiodarone with the dihydropyridine class of calcium-channel blockers (e.g. nifedipine), which typically have little or no negative inotropic activity at usual doses.

Amiodarone + **Ciclosporin (Cyclosporine)** ▲

Ciclosporin serum levels can be increased by amiodarone and nephrotoxicity has occurred as a result. Increased amiodarone levels and pulmonary toxicity have been reported in patients also given ciclosporin.

Ciclosporin levels and/or effects (e.g. on renal function) should be monitored as a matter of routine, but it may be prudent to increase monitoring if amiodarone is started or stopped. Adjust the dose of ciclosporin as necessary. The significance of the increase in amiodarone levels and the occurrence of pulmonary toxicity is unclear but bear these reports in mind in case of unexpected effects.

Amiodarone + **Colestyramine** ❓

Colestyramine appears to reduce the serum levels of amiodarone by about 50%.

Because amiodarone undergoes some enterohepatic recirculation, separating the doses may only minimise the interaction. Monitor for decreased amiodarone effects if colestyramine is started, and adjust the amiodarone dose as necessary, or consider an alternative to colestyramine.

Amiodarone + **Dextromethorphan** ▲

Amiodarone can modestly reduce the clearance of dextromethorphan.

The extent of the interaction is unlikely to be clinically relevant in patients taking dextromethorphan, since this drug has a wide therapeutic index and its dose is not individually titrated. Remember that dextromethorphan occurs in a considerable number of proprietary cough preparations.

Amiodarone + **Digoxin** ▲

Digoxin levels can be approximately doubled by amiodarone. Some individuals may show even greater increases. Digitalis toxicity will occur if the dosage of digoxin is not reduced appropriately.

The interaction occurs in most patients and is clearly evident after a few days but may take 4 weeks to fully develop. Reduce the digoxin dosage by between one-third to one-half initially and monitor digoxin levels. Further adjustment of the digoxin dosage may be needed after a week or two, and possibly a month or more depending on digoxin levels. Particular care is needed in children, who may show much larger rises in digoxin levels.

Amiodarone + Disopyramide ⊗

The QT interval prolonging effects are increased when disopyramide and amiodarone are used together (see drugs that prolong the QT interval, page 237, for a general discussion of QT prolongation).

Concurrent use should generally be avoided. If concurrent use is essential, the dose of disopyramide should be reduced by 30 to 50% several days after starting amiodarone. The continued need for disopyramide should be monitored, and withdrawal attempted if possible. If disopyramide is added to amiodarone, the initial dose of disopyramide should be about half of the usual recommended dose.

Amiodarone + Diuretics ⚠

Mild to moderate inhibitors of CYP3A4 (such as amiodarone) are predicted to increase eplerenone levels, which increases the risk of hyperkalaemia.

It is generally recommended that the dose of eplerenone should not exceed 25 mg daily in patients taking amiodarone. Note that hypokalaemia can exacerbate the QT-prolonging effects of amiodarone.

Amiodarone + Flecainide ⚠

Serum flecainide levels are increased by about 50% by amiodarone. An isolated report describes torsade de pointes in a patient taking amiodarone with flecainide.

Reduce the flecainide dosage by one-third to one-half if amiodarone is added and monitor for flecainide adverse effects. The interaction may take 2 weeks or more to develop fully.

Amiodarone + Grapefruit juice ⊗

Grapefruit juice appears to completely inhibit the metabolism of amiodarone to its major active metabolite, increases the AUC of amiodarone by 50% and increases the peak serum level by 84%, which may lead to toxicity. However, the effect of amiodarone on the PR and QTc intervals is apparently *decreased*, possibly due to reduced levels of the active metabolite.

Further study is needed. In the meantime, it may be prudent to suggest to patients that they avoid grapefruit juice.

Amiodarone + H$_2$-receptor antagonists ⚠

Cimetidine causes a modest rise in the serum levels of amiodarone in some patients.

Information seems to be limited to one study but this interaction may be clinically important in some patients. Be alert for amiodarone adverse effects.

Amiodarone + Levothyroxine ⚠

Patients taking levothyroxine for hypothyroidism may develop elevated levels of thyroid-stimulating hormone or overt hypothyroidism when also given amiodarone.

The manufacturer of amiodarone contraindicates its use in patients with evidence or a history of thyroid dysfunction and recommends thyroid function tests in all patients before starting amiodarone. Levothyroxine has been given to correct hypothyroidism induced by amiodarone. Close monitoring is required if amiodarone is given with levothyroxine.

Amiodarone + Lidocaine ❓

Isolated reports describe a seizure in a man taking lidocaine about 2 days after he started to take amiodarone, and sinoatrial arrest in another man with sick sinus syndrome who was given both drugs. There is conflicting evidence as to whether or not amiodarone affects the pharmacokinetics of lidocaine.

Careful monitoring is required if both drugs are used.

Amiodarone + Lithium ✖

Hypothyroidism developed very rapidly in 2 patients taking amiodarone when lithium was started.

Note that lithium has been tried for the treatment of amiodarone-induced hyperthyroidism, and regular monitoring of thyroid status is recommended throughout amiodarone treatment. Lithium therapy has rarely been associated with QT prolongation, and consequently the UK manufacturer of amiodarone contraindicates its combined use (see drugs that prolong the QT interval, page 237, for a general discussion of QT prolongation).

Amiodarone + Phenytoin ⚠

Serum phenytoin levels can be raised by amiodarone, markedly so in some individuals (4-fold rise reported). Amiodarone serum levels are reduced by phenytoin.

A 25 to 30% reduction in the phenytoin dose has been recommended for those taking 2 to 4 mg/kg daily, but it should be remembered that small alterations in phenytoin dose may result in a large change in phenytoin levels, as phenytoin kinetics are non-linear. The clinical significance of the effects on amiodarone are unclear.

A

Amiodarone + **Phosphodiesterase type-5 inhibitors** ⊗

Vardenafil slightly prolongs the QT interval (by 5 to 10 milliseconds). The manufacturers therefore contraindicate class III antiarrhythmics such as amiodarone. Consider also drugs that prolong the QT interval, page 237.

> Avoid concurrent use.

Amiodarone + **Procainamide** ⊗

The QT interval prolonging effects are increased when procainamide and amiodarone are used together (see drugs that prolong the QT interval, page 237, for a general discussion of QT prolongation). Amiodarone increases the levels of procainamide and its metabolite by 60% and 30%, respectively.

> Concurrent use should generally be avoided due to the QT prolonging effects of the combination. If the two drugs are considered essential, the dosage of procainamide may need to be reduced by 20 to 50%. Levels should be monitored where possible, and patients observed closely for adverse effects.

Amiodarone + **Protease inhibitors** ⊗

A rise in amiodarone levels of about 50% has been seen in a patient given indinavir. Other protease inhibitors would be expected to interact similarly.

> The concurrent use of amiodarone with a protease inhibitor is generally contraindicated. However, in the UK the exception is atazanavir, and in the US, caution and increased monitoring, including taking amiodarone levels, is recommended with amprenavir, atazanavir, fosamprenavir, and lopinavir.

Amiodarone + **Quinidine** ⊗

The QT interval prolonging effects of quinidine and amiodarone are increased when they are used together, and torsade de pointes has occurred (see drugs that prolong the QT interval, page 237, for a general discussion of QT prolongation). Quinidine levels can be increased by up to 40% by amiodarone.

> Concurrent use should generally be avoided due to the QT prolonging effects of the combination. If the two drugs are considered essential, the dosage of quinidine may need to be reduced by 30 to 50%. Levels should be monitored where possible. The QT interval on the ECG should also be monitored and patients observed closely for quinidine-related adverse effects.

Amiodarone + **Statins** ⊗

There is some evidence of a high incidence of myopathy when amiodarone is given with high doses of simvastatin. Rarely, cases of myopathy and rhabdomyolysis have been reported in patients taking this combination.

> It is generally recommended that the dose of simvastatin should not exceed

20 mg daily in patients taking amiodarone unless the clinical benefit is likely to outweigh the increased risk of myopathy and rhabdomyolysis. However, one manufacturer contraindicates the combination.

Amiodarone + **Warfarin and other oral anticoagulants** ⚠

The anticoagulant effects of warfarin, phenprocoumon and acenocoumarol are increased by amiodarone in most patients and bleeding may occur. The onset of this interaction may be slow (up to 2 weeks).

The dosage of warfarin and phenprocoumon should be reduced by one-third to two-thirds if amiodarone is added. The dosage of acenocoumarol should be reduced by between about 30 and 50%. However, these suggested reductions are only broad generalisations and individual patients may need more or less. The INR (or prothrombin times) should be very closely monitored both during and following treatment. One study advises weekly monitoring for the first 4 weeks of concurrent use.

Amphotericin B

See also drugs that prolong the QT interval, page 237, as QT-prolongation can be exacerbated by hypokalaemia, which is a common adverse effect of amphotericin. The renal toxicity of amphotericin B may be associated with sodium depletion.

Amphotericin B + **Azoles** ⚠

There is some clinical evidence that amphotericin B given with either itraconazole, ketoconazole or miconazole may possibly be less effective than amphotericin B given alone, and the adverse effects may be greater.

Despite extensive *in vitro* and *animal* data, it is not entirely clear whether or not azoles inhibit the efficacy of amphotericin B. Until more is known combined treatment should be limited to specific cases and the outcome should be very well monitored, being alert for a reduced antifungal response, or increasing LFTs.

Amphotericin B + **Ciclosporin (Cyclosporine)** ⚠

The risk of nephrotoxicity appears to be increased if ciclosporin is given with amphotericin B. Limited evidence suggests that liposomal amphotericin B (*AmBisome*) does not increase nephrotoxicity or hepatotoxicity when given to infants taking ciclosporin. Ciclosporin levels may be increased or decreased by amphotericin B.

It has been suggested that if amphotericin must be given, withholding ciclosporin until the serum level is less than about 150 nanograms/mL may be a means of decreasing renal toxicity without losing the immunosuppressive effect. The reports supporting a lack of significant nephrotoxicity all used liposomal

A

amphotericin, which would seem to suggest that, in patients taking ciclosporin, these formulations are advisable. Monitor both ciclosporin levels and renal function carefully on concurrent use.

Amphotericin B + Corticosteroids ⚠

Amphotericin B and corticosteroids can cause potassium loss and salt and water retention, which can have adverse effects on cardiac function.

Monitor electrolytes (especially potassium, which should be closely monitored in any patient taking amphotericin B) and fluid balance if amphotericin B is given with corticosteroids. The elderly would seem to be particularly at risk. Note that the renal toxicity of amphotericin B may be associated with sodium depletion.

Amphotericin B + Digoxin ⚠

Amphotericin B may cause hypokalaemia, which can be severe. Although there seem to be no reports of adverse interactions, it would be logical to expect that digitalis toxicity could develop in patients given both drugs if the potassium levels fall. Amiloride has been successfully used to counteract the potassium loss caused by amphotericin B.

Potassium levels should be monitored when amphotericin B is given, but extra care is needed in those taking digoxin. Supplement potassium or prevent its loss as appropriate.

Amphotericin B + Diuretics ⚠

Amphotericin B may cause hypokalaemia. Loop diuretics or thiazide and related diuretics increase the risk of hypokalaemia when given with amphotericin.

Potassium should be monitored closely on concurrent use, and serum levels adjusted accordingly.

Amphotericin B + Flucytosine ⚠

For some fungal infections the combination of flucytosine with amphotericin B may be more effective than flucytosine alone, but increased flucytosine toxicity may also occur.

Combined therapy is the recommended treatment for some systemic fungal infections. Nevertheless, flucytosine levels and renal function should be very closely monitored when the drugs are used concurrently.

Amphotericin B + NRTIs ⚠

Both tenofovir and amphotericin B are known to be nephrotoxic.

The manufacturers advise monitoring renal function at least weekly in those receiving both drugs.

Amphotericin B + **Pentamidine** ⚠

There is evidence that acute renal failure and electrolyte disturbances (e.g. hypomagnesaemia) may develop in patients taking amphotericin B if they are also given parenteral pentamidine: both drugs are known to be nephrotoxic. See also drugs that prolong the QT interval, page 237.

No interaction seems to occur when pentamidine is given by inhalation, probably because the serum levels achieved are low. Increased monitoring of renal function would be appropriate if both drugs are used.

Amphotericin B + **Tacrolimus** ⚠

Cases of nephrotoxicity have been seen when tacrolimus was given with amphotericin B.

Renal function should be monitored when either drug is used alone, but it may be prudent to increase the frequency of this monitoring on concurrent use.

Amphotericin B + **Vancomycin** ⚠

The risk of nephrotoxicity with vancomycin may possibly be increased if it is given with other drugs with similar nephrotoxic effects, such as amphotericin B.

There seems to be no direct evidence about this interaction. Even so, the general warning issued by the manufacturers to monitor carefully is a reasonable precaution.

Anastrozole

Anastrozole + **HRT** ✗

HRT would be expected to diminish the effects of anastrozole, so concurrent use is contraindicated.

Some information suggests that there need not be a complete restriction on their concurrent use, but this needs confirmation. Concurrent use should be avoided.

Angiotensin II receptor antagonists

Most angiotensin II receptor antagonist interactions are pharmacodynamic, that is, interactions that result in an alteration in drug effects rather than drug disposition, so in most cases interactions of individual drugs will be applicable to the group.

A

Angiotensin II receptor antagonists + Antidiabetics ✅

No clinically relevant pharmacokinetic interactions occur between glibenclamide (glyburide) and candesartan, telmisartan or valsartan, or between tolbutamide and irbesartan. Losartan and possibly eprosartan may reduce awareness of hypoglycaemic symptoms.

> The symptoms of hypoglycaemia may be reduced by losartan and possibly other angiotensin II receptor antagonists. Further study is needed to establish this interaction, but note that this is similar to the effect of ACE inhibitors, page 2.

Angiotensin II receptor antagonists + Aspirin ❓

Low-dose aspirin does not appear to affect the antihypertensive efficacy of losartan and would therefore not be expected to alter the effects of other angiotensin II receptor antagonists. High-dose aspirin does not appear to have been studied.

> No action needed if low-dose aspirin is used. Suspect an interaction with high-dose aspirin if the angiotensin-II receptor antagonist seem less effective or blood pressure control is erratic. Consider an alternative analgesic, but note that NSAIDs may also affect blood pressure control.

Angiotensin II receptor antagonists + Azoles ✅

Fluconazole reduces the conversion of losartan to its active metabolite and decreases the metabolism of irbesartan, but does not appear to influence the pharmacokinetics of eprosartan. Candesartan and valsartan also seem unlikely to interact with fluconazole. Itraconazole does not significantly affect the pharmacokinetics or antihypertensive effects of losartan. Ketoconazole does not affect the pharmacokinetics of eprosartan or losartan.

> Where an interaction was noted, the effects were modest, and no clinically significant effect is expected.

Angiotensin II receptor antagonists + Ciclosporin (Cyclosporine) ⚠

Studies have found no significant changes in renal function in patients taking ciclosporin with candesartan or losartan. There is a possible risk of hyperkalaemia if angiotensin II receptor antagonists are given with ciclosporin, as both drugs may raise potassium levels.

> Although renal failure has not been seen with this combination note that cases have occurred with ACE inhibitors, page 3. Monitor potassium levels more closely in the initial weeks of concurrent use.

Angiotensin II receptor antagonists + Digoxin ❓

A

Telmisartan may cause a 13% rise in trough serum digoxin levels and a 50% rise in peak serum levels.

> The small increase in the trough levels suggests that the dose of digoxin need not automatically be reduced when telmisartan is started, but consideration should be given to monitoring for digoxin adverse effects such as bradycardia, taking digoxin levels if necessary. Candesartan, eprosartan, irbesartan, losartan, and valsartan appear not to affect digoxin levels.

Angiotensin II receptor antagonists + Diuretics

Loop diuretics ⚠

Symptomatic hypotension may occur if an angiotensin II receptor antagonist is started in patients taking high-dose diuretics. Potassium levels may be either increased, decreased or not affected. There is no clinically significant pharmacokinetic interaction between valsartan and furosemide.

> It has been recommended that the dose of diuretic or angiotensin II receptor antagonist be reduced to begin with, to avoid hypotension. Initially monitor blood pressure and potassium levels.

Potassium-sparing diuretics ⚠

There is a risk of hyperkalaemia if angiotensin II receptor antagonists are given with amiloride, eplerenone, spironolactone or triamterene, particularly if other risk factors (such as advanced age, dose of spironolactone greater than 25 mg, reduced renal function and type II diabetes) are also present.

> Some manufacturers recommend that the combinations be used cautiously and that serum potassium should be monitored regularly. However, other manufacturers advise against concurrent use, which seems overly cautious, if adequate precautions are taken.

Thiazide diuretics ⚠

Symptomatic hypotension may occur if an angiotensin II receptor antagonist is started in a patient taking high-dose diuretics. Potassium levels may be either increased, decreased or not affected by the concurrent use of these drugs. No clinically relevant pharmacokinetic interactions appear to occur between candesartan, eprosartan, irbesartan, losartan, telmisartan or valsartan, and hydrochlorothiazide, although the bioavailability of hydrochlorothiazide may be modestly reduced.

> It has been recommended that the dose of diuretic or angiotensin II receptor antagonist be reduced to avoid hypotension. Initially monitor blood pressure and potassium levels.

Angiotensin II receptor antagonists + Epoetin ❓

Epoetin may cause hypertension and thereby reduce the effects of angiotensin II receptor antagonists. An additive hyperkalaemic effect is theoretically possible.

A

Blood pressure should be routinely monitored in patients treated with epoetin, but increased monitoring of potassium levels may be warranted.

Angiotensin II receptor antagonists + **Food** ✔

Food increases the bioavailability of eprosartan and losartan, slightly reduces the bioavailability of telmisartan, and modestly reduces the AUC of valsartan. Food appears to have little or no effect on the bioavailability of candesartan, irbesartan, or olmesartan.

None of these changes is likely to be clinically important. The UK manufacturer recommends that eprosartan is given with food, but the US manufacturer suggests that the interaction is not clinically significant.

Angiotensin II receptor antagonists + **Heparin** ⚠

An extensive review of the literature found that heparin (both unfractionated and low-molecular-weight heparins) and heparinoids inhibit the secretion of aldosterone, which can cause hyperkalaemia. This may be additive with the hyperkalaemic effects of angiotensin II receptor antagonists.

The CSM in the UK suggests that potassium should be measured in all patients with risk factors (renal impairment, diabetes mellitus, pre-existing acidosis and those taking potassium-sparing drugs) before starting heparin, and monitored regularly thereafter (every 4 days has been suggested).

Angiotensin II receptor antagonists + **Lithium** ⚠

Lithium toxicity has been seen in individual patients given candesartan, losartan, valsartan and possibly irbesartan. Other angiotensin II receptor antagonists would be expected to interact similarly. The risk of lithium toxicity would be expected to increase when risk factors such as advanced age, renal impairment, heart failure and volume depletion are also present.

Even though the interaction appears rare, patients should have their lithium levels monitored to avoid a potentially severe adverse interaction. The development of the interaction may be delayed (up to 7 weeks seen) so that weekly monitoring of lithium levels for several weeks has been advised. Patients taking lithium should be aware of the symptoms of lithium toxicity and told to immediately report them should they occur. This should be reinforced when they are given angiotensin II receptor antagonists.

Angiotensin II receptor antagonists +
Low-molecular-weight heparins ⚠

An extensive review of the literature found that heparin (both unfractionated and low-molecular-weight heparins) and heparinoids inhibit the secretion of aldosterone, which can cause hyperkalaemia. This may be additive with the hyperkalaemic effects of angiotensin II receptor antagonists.

The CSM in the UK suggests that potassium should be measured in all patients with risk factors (renal impairment, diabetes mellitus, pre-existing acidosis and those taking potassium-sparing drugs) before starting a low-molecular-weight heparin and monitored regularly thereafter (every 4 days has been suggested).

Angiotensin II receptor antagonists + NSAIDs ❓

Indometacin may attenuate the antihypertensive effect of losartan, valsartan, or other angiotensin II receptor antagonists. No clinically relevant pharmacokinetic interactions occur between telmisartan and ibuprofen or between valsartan and indometacin. The combination of an NSAID and angiotensin II receptor antagonist can increase the risk of renal impairment and hyperkalaemia.

Several manufacturers of angiotensin II receptor antagonists caution that, as with other antihypertensives, the effects on blood pressure may be attenuated by NSAIDs such as indometacin. Patients taking losartan, valsartan or other angiotensin II receptor antagonists, who require indometacin, should be monitored for alterations in blood pressure control. Other NSAIDs seem likely to interact similarly. Poor renal perfusion may increase the risk of renal failure if angiotensin II receptor antagonists are given with NSAIDs and so regular hydration of the patient and monitoring of renal function is recommended.

Angiotensin II receptor antagonists + Potassium ⚠

There is a risk of hyperkalaemia if angiotensin II receptor antagonists are given with potassium supplements or potassium-containing salt substitutes, particularly in those patients where other risk factors (such as advanced age, reduced renal function, and type II diabetes) are present.

Monitor potassium levels, adjusting supplementation as necessary.

Angiotensin II receptor antagonists + Rifampicin (Rifampin) ⚠

Rifampicin reduces the levels of the active metabolite of losartan and the blood pressure lowering effects of losartan.

This interaction is by no means established, but monitor the effects of concurrent use on blood pressure. Consider raising the losartan dose or using an alternative to losartan if problems occur. Note that theoretically irbesartan and possibly candesartan may also be affected.

Angiotensin II receptor antagonists + Tacrolimus ⚠

Candesartan and losartan do not affect the pharmacokinetics of tacrolimus. Concurrent use with angiotensin II receptor antagonists may increase the risk of developing hyperkalaemia and/or nephrotoxicity in those taking tacrolimus.

Both renal function and potassium levels should be monitored if angiotensin II receptor antagonists are given with tacrolimus.

A

Antacids

Antacids + Antihistamines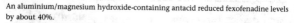

An aluminium/magnesium hydroxide-containing antacid reduced fexofenadine levels by about 40%.

> Although the clinical significance has not been assessed it is recommended that administration is separated by 2 hours.

Antacids + Antipsychotics

Antacids containing aluminium/magnesium hydroxide or magnesium trisilicate can reduce the urinary excretion of chlorpromazine by up to 45%. Similarly, an aluminium/magnesium hydroxide antacid reduced the absorption of sulpiride. *In vitro* studies suggest that this interaction may possibly also occur with other antacids and phenothiazines.

> The clinical importance of these interactions are not established, but it would seem reasonable to give chlorpromazine or sulpiride 2 to 3 hours after aluminium/magnesium hydroxide antacids to minimise any interaction.

Antacids + Aspirin

The serum salicylate concentrations of patients taking large doses of aspirin or other salicylates as anti-inflammatory drugs can be reduced to subtherapeutic levels by aluminium/magnesium hydroxide or sodium bicarbonate antacids.

> Care should be taken to monitor serum salicylate levels if any antacid is started or stopped in patients where the control of salicylate levels is critical. Probably of little importance with small or one-off doses of aspirin. Note that antacids may also increase the rate of absorption of aspirin given as enteric-coated tablets.

Antacids + Azoles

The gastrointestinal absorption of ketoconazole and itraconazole capsules is markedly reduced by antacids.

> Advise patients to take antacids not less than 2 to 3 hours before or after ketoconazole and not less than 1 hour before and 2 hours after itraconazole capsules. Monitor the effects to confirm that these azoles are effective. The absorption of fluconazole, itraconazole solution and posaconazole appears not to be significantly affected by antacids, so these azoles may be suitable alternatives.

Antacids + Bisphosphonates

The oral absorption of bisphosphonates is significantly reduced (90% reduction with clodronate) by aluminium/magnesium hydroxide and other antacids.

> Bisphosphonates should be prevented from coming into contact with antacids

(containing aluminium, bismuth, calcium, magnesium). Recommendations on the timing of administration of bisphosphonates in relation to food and other drugs varies. Alendronate and risedronate should be taken at least 30 minutes before taking the first *food or drink* of the day, clodronate should probably be taken at least 1 hour before or after antacids, ibandronate should be taken 1 hour before antacids, and etidronate and tiludronate should be taken at least 2 hours apart from antacids.

Antacids + **Cephalosporins**

Cefpodoxime 🔺

Aluminium/magnesium hydroxide has been shown to reduce the bioavailability of cefpodoxime proxetil by about 40%. Sodium bicarbonate and aluminium hydroxide seem to have similar effects.

It has been recommended that cefpodoxime is given at least 2 hours apart from antacids.

Other cephalosporins ✅

Aluminium/magnesium hydroxide reduced the AUC of a modified-release preparation of cefaclor by 18%, but this reduction is small and considered unlikely to be clinically important.

No action needed.

Antacids + **Chloroquine** 🔺

In a small study magnesium trisilicate reduced the AUC of chloroquine by 18.2%. Related *in vitro* studies found that the absorption of chloroquine was decreased as follows: magnesium trisilicate 31.3%, calcium carbonate 52% and gerdiga 36.1%. Gerdiga is a clay containing hydrated silicates with sodium and potassium carbonates and bicarbonates. It is used as an antacid and is similar to attapulgite. Hydroxychloroquine is predicted to interact like chloroquine.

The clinical significance of this reduction is unclear, but one way to minimise any possible effect on chloroquine absorption is to separate the dosages by at least 2 to 3 hours. Hydroxychloroquine should be given 4 hours before or after antacids.

Antacids + **Corticosteroids** 🔺

The absorption of prednisone can be reduced by large (60 mL) but not small doses of aluminium/magnesium hydroxide antacids. Prednisolone probably behaves similarly. Dexamethasone absorption is reduced by about 75% by magnesium trisilicate.

Some manufacturers of dexamethasone suggest that the doses of antacid should be separated as far as possible from the dexamethasone. In other similar antacid interactions 2 to 3 hours is usually sufficient. The manufacturers of deflazacort also issue a similar warning. It would seem prudent to follow this advice for large doses of antacid and any corticosteroid. Concurrent use should be monitored to confirm that the therapeutic response is adequate.

A

Antacids + Digoxin

Antacids ✓

Although some studies suggest that antacids can reduce the bioavailability of digoxin, there is other evidence suggesting that no clinically relevant interaction occurs.

Separating the dosages by 1 to 2 hours to minimise admixture is effective with many other drugs that interact with antacids. However, unless further information becomes available it seems unlikely that separating administration is necessary, although it may be worth bearing in mind if, on rare occasions, a patient seems to experience an interaction.

Calcium ⚠

In two cases the concurrent use of intravenous calcium and digoxin resulted in fatal arrhythmias. This seems to be the only direct clinical evidence of a serious adverse interaction, although there is plenty of less direct evidence that an interaction is possible.

Intravenous calcium should be avoided in patients taking digoxin. If that is not possible, it has been suggested that it should be given slowly or only in small amounts in order to avoid transient high serum calcium levels.

Antacids + Dipyridamole ❓

The effective disintegration, dissolution and eventual absorption of dipyridamole in tablet or suspension form depends upon having a low pH in the stomach. Drugs that raise the gastric pH are expected to reduce the bioavailability of dipyridamole.

The clinical significance of this possible interaction is unknown. Note that Modified-release preparations of dipyridamole (that are buffered) do not appear to be affected. For other preparations, consider separating the dosing by 2 to 3 hours, as this minimises other absorption interactions with antacids.

Antacids + Diuretics ⚠

Hypercalcaemia and possibly metabolic alkalosis can develop in patients given large amounts of calcium (with or without high doses of vitamin D) if they are also given thiazide diuretics, which can reduce the urinary excretion of calcium.

This interaction is unlikely to be of importance in patients taking occasional calcium e.g. in antacids. Consider monitoring calcium levels in those given a thiazide and a calcium supplement or large amounts of calcium antacids regularly.

Antacids + Enteral feeds ⚠

Aluminium-containing antacids can interact with high-protein liquid enteral feeds (in enteral or nasogastric tubes) within the oesophagus to produce an obstructive plug (a bezoar).

It has been suggested that if an antacid is needed, it should be given some time after the nutrients, and the tube should be vigorously flushed beforehand.

Antacids + **Ethambutol** ✔

Both aluminium hydroxide and aluminium/magnesium hydroxide can cause a small reduction in the absorption of ethambutol (e.g. AUC decreased by 10%) in some patients.

The reduction in absorption is generally small and variable, and it seems doubtful if it will have a significant effect on the treatment of tuberculosis. However, the US manufacturer suggests that aluminium hydroxide-containing antacids should not be taken until 4 hours after a dose of ethambutol.

Antacids + **Fibrates** ⚠

Antacids (aluminium hydroxide, aluminium magnesium silica hydrate) reduced the maximum plasma gemfibrozil levels by about 50 to 70% in one study. More study is needed to confirm these findings.

It has been suggested that gemfibrozil should be given 1 to 2 hours before antacids.

Antacids + **Gabapentin** ⚠

An aluminium/magnesium hydroxide antacid given with or 2 hours after gabapentin reduced its bioavailability by about 20%. When the antacid was given 2 hours before gabapentin, the bioavailability was reduced by about 10%.

These small changes are unlikely to be of clinical importance. However, the manufacturer recommends that gabapentin is taken about 2 hours after aluminium/magnesium-containing antacids.

Antacids + **Iron** ⚠

The absorption of iron and the expected haematological response can be reduced by the concurrent use of antacids (sodium bicarbonate, calcium carbonate, aluminium/magnesium hydroxide, magnesium trisilicate).

Separate the administration of iron preparations and antacids as much as possible to avoid admixture in the gut. Note that separating the dosing by 2 to 3 hours minimises other absorption interactions with antacids.

Antacids + **Isoniazid** ✔

The absorption of isoniazid is modestly reduced by aluminium hydroxide (about 25%), less so by magaldrate, and not affected by aluminium/magnesium hydroxide tablets or didanosine chewable tablets (formulated with an antacid buffer).

The clinical importance of the modest reductions in isoniazid levels is uncertain, but it is likely to be small.

Antacids + **Levodopa** ✔

Antacids do not appear to interact significantly with immediate release levodopa, but

A

they may reduce the bioavailability of modified release preparations of levodopa (e.g. *Madopar CR*).

> Concurrent use need not be avoided with standard preparations. With modified-release preparations it would seem advisable to avoid concurrent administration (2 to 3 hours is usually enough in other similar situations). The outcome should be monitored.

Antacids + Levothyroxine ⚠

A few reports describe reduced levothyroxine effects in patients given aluminium/magnesium-containing antacids. The efficacy of levothyroxine can also be reduced by the concurrent use of calcium carbonate.

> The general importance of the interaction with aluminium/magnesium-containing antacids is not known, but be alert for the need to increase the levothyroxine dosage in any patient given antacids. With calcium carbonate, the mean reduction in the absorption of levothyroxine is quite small, but some individuals can experience a clinically important effect. The cautious approach would be to advise all patients to separate the dosages by at least 4 hours.

Antacids + Lithium ⚠

The ingestion of marked amounts of sodium can prevent the establishment or maintenance of adequate serum lithium levels.

> Warn patients not to take non-prescription antacids or urinary alkalinisers without first seeking informed advice. Sodium bicarbonate comes in various guises and disguises e.g. Alka-Seltzer (55.8%), *Andrews Salts* (22.6%), Eno (46.4%), *Jaap's Health Salts* (21.3%), or Peptac (28.8%). Substantial amounts of sodium also occur in some urinary alkalinising agents (e.g. *Citralka*, *Citravescent*). An antacid containing aluminium/magnesium hydroxide with simeticone has been found to have no effect on the bioavailability of lithium carbonate, and so antacids of this type may be suitable alternatives.

Antacids + Macrolides ⚠

Aluminium/magnesium hydroxide antacids may reduce the peak levels of azithromycin.

> It is suggested that azithromycin should not be given at the same time as antacids, but should be taken at least 1 hour before or 2 hours after.

Antacids + Mexiletine ✗

Large changes in urinary pH caused by the concurrent use of alkalinising drugs such as sodium bicarbonate can, in some patients, have a marked effect on the plasma levels of mexiletine.

> The effect does not appear to be predictable. The UK manufacturer of mexiletine recommends that concurrent use should be avoided.

Antacids + **Mycophenolate** ⚠

An aluminium/magnesium hydroxide antacid reduced the AUC of mycophenolate by about 20% in one study, but the clinical relevance of this is uncertain.

> The US manufacturer says that aluminium/magnesium antacids can be used in patients taking mycophenolate, but that they should not be given simultaneously. With many other antacid interactions, a 2 to 3 hour separation is usually sufficient to avoid an interaction.

Antacids + **NNRTIs** ⚠

When delavirdine was given 10 minutes after an antacid (type and dose not stated) the maximum serum levels of delavirdine were reduced by 57%.

> The manufacturer of delavirdine recommends separating administration by at least one hour. Note that aluminium/magnesium antacids do not interact to a clinically relevant extent with efavirenz or nevirapine.

Antacids + **NRTIs** ⚠

Aluminium/magnesium hydroxide caused a 25% reduction in the bioavailability of zalcitabine. The changes are moderate and of uncertain clinical importance.

> The manufacturer of zalcitabine recommends that it should not be taken at the same time as aluminium/magnesium-containing antacids. A separation of 2 to 3 hours is usually sufficient with other similar interactions.

Antacids + **NSAIDs**
Diflunisal ⚠

Antacids containing aluminium with or without magnesium can reduce the absorption of diflunisal by up to 40%, but no important interaction occurs if food is taken at the same time. Magnesium hydroxide can increase the rate of diflunisal absorption, which may improve the onset of analgesia.

> If diflunisal is taken with or after food as advised, it appears that this interaction should have little clinical relevance.

Other NSAIDs ✓

Studies have shown that antacids have no clinically significant effect on the pharmacokinetics of azapropazone, celecoxib, dexketoprofen, diclofenac, etodolac, etoricoxib, ibuprofen, indometacin, flurbiprofen, ketoprofen, ketorolac, lornoxicam, lumiracoxib, mefenamic acid, meloxicam, metamizole, nabumetone, piroxicam, sulindac, tenoxicam, tolfenamic acid, or tolmetin. The rate of absorption of some of these NSAIDs is moderately affected by antacids, which may affect the onset of analgesia. However, if NSAIDs are taken after food, as recommended, these effects are unlikely to be clinically significant.

> No action needed.

Antacids + **Penicillamine** ⚠

The absorption of penicillamine can be reduced by 30 to 40% if antacids containing aluminium/magnesium hydroxide are taken concurrently.

> For maximal absorption separate administration. A separation of 2 to 3 hours is usually sufficient with other similar interactions. Note that sodium bicarbonate does not appear to interact to a clinically significant extent.

Antacids + **Phenytoin** ❓

Some, but not all studies have shown that antacids (containing aluminium, calcium or magnesium) do not usually interact to a clinically relevant extent with phenytoin. However, in some instances antacids have reduced phenytoin serum levels and this may have been responsible for some loss of seizure control in a few patients.

> Concurrent use need not be avoided but if there is any hint that an epileptic patient is being affected by this interaction, separating the dosages by 2 to 3 hours may minimise the effects.

Antacids + **Proguanil** ⚠

The bioavailability of proguanil was reduced by almost two-thirds by magnesium trisilicate. Other antacids, such as those containing aluminium, may interact similarly.

> The clinical significance of this reduction is unclear, but one way to minimise any possible effect is to separate the dosages by at least 2 to 3 hours.

Antacids + **Protease inhibitors** ⚠

Drugs that increase gastric pH are predicted to reduce the plasma levels of atazanavir, and possibly also amprenavir. Tipranavir levels are decreased by up to 30% by antacids (containing aluminium/magnesium hydroxide).

> The manufacturers of atazanavir recommend that it should be given 2 hours before or one hour after buffered medicinal products. This would include didanosine buffered tablets and antacids. The manufacturer of amprenavir recommends that it should not be given within one hour of antacids, and the manufacturer of tipranavir recommends that it should not be given within 2 hours of antacids.

Antacids + **Proton pump inhibitors**

Antacids may cause a slight reduction in the bioavailability of lansoprazole, but this is not considered clinically relevant.

> The manufacturer recommends that antacids should not be taken within one hour of lansoprazole.

Antacids + **Quinidine** ❓

Large rises in urinary pH due to the concurrent use of some antacids (such as sodium bicarbonate) can cause the retention of quinidine, which could lead to toxicity, but there seems to be only one case on record of an adverse interaction (with aluminium/magnesium hydroxide). Aluminium hydroxide appears not to interact.

> It is difficult to predict which antacids, if any, are likely to interact. Monitor the effects if drugs that can markedly change urinary pH are started or stopped. Adjust the quinidine dosage as necessary.

Antacids + Quinolones ⚠

The serum levels of many of the quinolones can be reduced by aluminium/magnesium antacids. Calcium compounds interact to a lesser extent, and bismuth compounds only minimally.

> As a very broad rule-of-thumb, the quinolones should be taken at least 2 hours before and not less than 4 to 6 hours after aluminium/magnesium antacids. The interaction with calcium compounds is variable, and some quinolones may not interact, but in the absence of direct information a 2-hour separation errs on the side of caution. The interaction with bismuth is minimal and no action is likely to be needed. The H_2-receptor antagonists and the proton pump inhibitors do not interact and may therefore be suitable alternatives.

Antacids + Rifampicin (Rifampin) ❓

The absorption of rifampicin can be reduced up to about one-third by antacids, but the clinical importance of this does not appear to have been assessed.

> If antacids are given it would be prudent to be alert for any evidence that treatment is less effective than expected. The US manufacturers advise giving rifampicin one hour before antacids.

Antacids + Statins

Rosuvastatin ⚠

The bioavailability of rosuvastatin is reduced by antacids but the clinical significance of this is uncertain.

> No interaction occurs with rosuvastatin when the doses are separated by 2 hours. The manufacturers of rosuvastatin recommend that it is not given within 2 to 3 hours of antacids.

Other statins ✓

Aluminium/magnesium hydroxide antacids cause a moderate reduction in the bioavailability of atorvastatin and pravastatin, but this does not appear to reduce their lipid-lowering efficacy.

> No action needed.

A

Antacids + **Strontium** ⚠

Aluminium/magnesium hydroxide slightly reduces the absorption of strontium ranelate (AUC decreased by 20 to 25%) if given with or 2 hours before strontium, but not when given 2 hours after strontium. Calcium reduces the bioavailability of strontium ranelate by about 60 to 70%.

Antacids should be taken 2 hours after strontium ranelate. However, because it is also recommended that strontium ranelate is taken at bedtime, the manufacturers say that if this dosing interval is impractical, concurrent intake is acceptable. For calcium preparations administration should be separated by 2 hours.

Antacids + **Tetracyclines** ⚠

The serum levels and therefore the therapeutic effectiveness of the tetracyclines can be markedly reduced or even abolished by antacids containing aluminium, bismuth, calcium or magnesium. Other antacids, such as sodium bicarbonate, may also reduce the bioavailability of some tetracyclines. Even intravenous doxycycline levels can be reduced by antacids.

As a general rule none of the aluminium, bismuth, calcium or magnesium-containing antacids should be given at the same time as the tetracycline antibacterials. If they must be used, separate the dosages by 2 to 3 hours or more, to prevent their admixture in the gut. This also applies to quinapril formulations containing substantial quantities of magnesium (such as *Accupro*), although the interaction is less pronounced, and didanosine tablets formulated with antacids. H_2-receptor antagonists do not interact, and they may therefore be a suitable alternative.

Antacids + **Zinc** ⚠

Calcium (either as the carbonate or the citrate) reduces the AUC of zinc by up to 80%.

The clinical importance of this interaction is unknown, but it would seem prudent to separate the administration of zinc and calcium. Note that separating the dosing by 2 to 3 hours minimises other absorption interactions with antacids.

Antidiabetics

Antidiabetics + **Antidiabetics** ⚠

Pioglitazone and rosiglitazone may cause fluid retention and peripheral oedema, which can worsen or cause heart failure. There is evidence that the incidence of these effects is higher when pioglitazone or rosiglitazone are combined with insulin. The incidence of hypoglycaemia may also be increased on concurrent use.

Concurrent use need not be avoided, but some caution is warranted. It is suggested that low doses are used initially and that the combination should not be used in patients with moderate to severe heart failure. If symptoms and signs suggest congestive heart failure, the American Heart Association and American Diabetes

Association recommend that a dosage change and temporary or permanent discontinuance of the thiazolidinedione should be considered. If there is no evidence of heart failure, they suggest that the thiazolidinedione may be continued, with consideration of dosage reduction or addition of diuretics, and with continued observation of the oedema. Note that, in the UK rosiglitazone is contraindicated with insulin, whereas the combined metformin/rosiglitazone preparation is not. In the US pioglitazone and rosiglitazone are licenced for use with insulin.

Antidiabetics + **Antipsychotics** ⚠️

Chlorpromazine may raise blood glucose levels, particularly in daily doses of 100 mg or more, and disturb the control of diabetes (incidence of hyperglycaemia is about 25%). Smaller chlorpromazine doses of 50 to 70 mg daily do not appear to cause hyperglycaemia. Clozapine, olanzapine and risperidone are associated with an increased risk of glucose intolerance.

Increases in the dosage requirements of the antidiabetic should be anticipated during concurrent use. Increased blood glucose monitoring is recommended with chlorpromazine, clozapine, olanzapine and risperidone.

Antidiabetics + **Aprepitant** ⚠️

Aprepitant reduces the AUC of tolbutamide by about 25%. Fosaprepitant is a prodrug of aprepitant and would be expected to interact similarly.

As the clinical relevance of this reduction has not been assessed the manufacturer advises caution, but changes of this magnitude are rarely clinically significant.

Antidiabetics + **Aspirin** ❓

Aspirin and other salicylates can lower blood glucose levels, but small analgesic doses do not normally have an adverse effect on patients taking antidiabetics. Large doses of salicylates may have a more significant effect.

No action is needed with low-dose aspirin or with small analgesic doses, but it may be prudent to increase monitoring of blood glucose levels during the initial use of large doses of aspirin or salicylates.

Antidiabetics + **Azoles**

Fluconazole ❓

Fluconazole normally appears not to affect the diabetic control of most patients taking sulphonylureas, but isolated reports describe hypoglycaemic coma and aggressive behaviour following concurrent use. Fluconazole may cause marked increases in plasma levels of glimepiride, but the significance of this is unclear. Nateglinide plasma levels may also be increased by fluconazole, but this did not affect the control of blood glucose levels.

There is no reason to avoid concurrent use but warn patients to report any unexpected changes in blood glucose levels.

A

Itraconazole ⚠

Itraconazole appears not to affect diabetic control in most patients, but there are occasional reports of hypoglycaemia or hyperglycaemia associated with its use. Itraconazole caused modest increases in repaglinide and nateglinide levels, but without affecting the control of blood glucose levels. Itraconazole has no effect on pioglitazone pharmacokinetics.

No action is normally needed but warn patients to report any unexpected changes in blood glucose levels.

Ketoconazole ⚠

Ketoconazole increases the blood glucose lowering effects of tolbutamide in healthy subjects and possibly increases the effects of rosiglitazone and pioglitazone.

If ketoconazole is added to tolbutamide, patients should be warned to be alert for any evidence of increased hypoglycaemia; adjust the tolbutamide dose as necessary. It may be prudent to increase the frequency of blood glucose monitoring if ketoconazole is given with rosiglitazone or pioglitazone.

Miconazole ❓

Hypoglycaemia has been seen in a few diabetics taking tolbutamide, glibenclamide (glyburide) or gliclazide when they were given miconazole.

Concurrent use should be monitored and the dosage of the sulphonylurea reduced if necessary. Warn patients to report any unexpected changes in blood glucose levels.

Posaconazole ❓

Posaconazole slightly enhanced the blood glucose lowering effects of glipizide in healthy subjects, but did not affect single-dose tolbutamide metabolism.

No action is normally needed but warn patients to report any unexpected changes in blood glucose levels.

Voriconazole ⚠

The manufacturers of voriconazole predict that it may raise the levels of the sulphonylureas, and hypoglycaemia may result.

Until more is known careful monitoring of blood glucose is advisable during concurrent use.

Antidiabetics + Beta blockers ⚠

In diabetics using insulin, the normal rise in blood sugar in response to hypoglycaemia may be impaired by propranolol, but serious and severe hypoglycaemia (sometimes accompanied by an increase in blood pressure) seems rare. Other beta blockers normally interact to a lesser extent or not at all. The blood glucose lowering effects of sulphonylureas may possibly be reduced by beta blockers. Be aware that in the presence of beta blockers some of the familiar warning signs of hypoglycaemia may not occur.

Monitor the effects of concurrent use well, avoid the non-selective beta blockers where possible, and check for any evidence that the dosage of the antidiabetic needs some adjustment. Warn all patients that some of the normal premonitory signs of a hypoglycaemic attack may not appear, in particular tachycardia and tremors, whereas the hunger, irritability and nausea signs may be unaffected, and sweating may even be increased.

Antidiabetics + Bosentan ❌

There appears to be an increased risk of liver toxicity if bosentan is used with glibenclamide (glyburide). Glibenclamide (glyburide) modestly reduces the plasma levels of bosentan, and bosentan reduces the plasma levels of glibenclamide (glyburide).

The manufacturers suggest the combination should be avoided.

Antidiabetics + Calcium-channel blockers ✅

Calcium-channel blockers are known to have effects on insulin secretion and glucose regulation, but significant disturbances in the control of diabetes appear to be rare.

No particular precautions normally seem to be necessary, but bear the potential for interaction in mind if the control of diabetes seems unusually difficult.

Antidiabetics + Chloramphenicol ⚠️

The blood glucose lowering effects of tolbutamide and chlorpropamide may be increased by chloramphenicol and acute hypoglycaemia can occur. Other sulphonylureas are often predicted to interact similarly, but there does not seem to be any direct evidence of this.

An increased blood glucose lowering effect should be expected if both drugs are given but few patients experience a severe effect. Monitor concurrent use carefully and reduce the dosage of the sulphonylurea as necessary. No interaction would be expected with topical chloramphenicol because the systemic absorption is likely to be small.

Antidiabetics + Ciclosporin (Cyclosporine) ❓

Some preliminary evidence suggests that glibenclamide (glyburide) can raise serum ciclosporin levels to a moderate extent. Glipizide caused about a 2-fold increase in ciclosporin levels in 2 patients, but no change was noted in a study. Ciclosporin increased repaglinide bioavailability in one study, but another suggested that this did not affect blood glucose levels.

These interactions are unconfirmed, but note that one of the rare adverse effects of ciclosporin is hyperglycaemia. There is insufficient evidence to generally recommend increased monitoring, but be aware of the potential for an interaction with the sulphonylureas if ciclosporin levels are unexpectedly raised, and with repaglinide if blood glucose levels become undesirably lowered.

Antidiabetics + **Clonidine** ❓

Clonidine may possibly suppress the signs and symptoms of hypoglycaemia in diabetics. Marked hyperglycaemia occurred in a child using insulin when clonidine was given. However, the effect of clonidine on carbohydrate metabolism appears to be variable, as other reports have described both increases and decreases in blood glucose levels.

Warn all patients that some of the normal premonitory signs of hypoglycaemia may not appear. Suspect an interaction if disturbances in the control of diabetes occur in patients given clonidine.

Antidiabetics + **Colestyramine**

Acarbose ⚠

Colestyramine may enhance the effect of acarbose, and a rebound effect may occur if both drugs are stopped at the same time.

The clinical importance of the effects of colestyramine on acarbose in diabetics is uncertain, but some care seems appropriate. It may be worth increasing the blood glucose monitoring if concurrent use is started or stopped.

Glipizide ⚠

The absorption of glipizide may be reduced by about 30% if it is taken at the same time as colestyramine.

It has been suggested that glipizide should be taken 1 to 2 hours before colestyramine, but this may only be partially effective because glipizide may undergo some enterohepatic recirculation.

Antidiabetics + **Contraceptives** ❓

Some women may require small increases or decreases in their dosage of antidiabetic while taking oral contraceptives, but it is unusual for the control of diabetes to be seriously disturbed.

Routine monitoring should be adequate to detect any interaction as the effects seem to be gradual. However, note that occasionally severe disturbances in control do occur. Irrespective of diabetic control, hormonal contraceptives should be used with caution in patients with diabetes because of the increased risk of arterial disease.

Antidiabetics + **Corticosteroids** ⚠

Corticosteroids with glucocorticoid (hyperglycaemic) activity oppose the blood glucose lowering effects of the antidiabetics. Significant hyperglycaemia has been seen with systemic corticosteroids, and in cases with inhaled corticosteroids or high-potency topical corticosteroids.

It would seem prudent to increase blood glucose monitoring when a corticosteroid is started and adjust the antidiabetic treatment accordingly. Routine monitoring of local corticosteroids appears over-cautious, but be aware that isolated cases of hyperglycaemia have been reported.

Antidiabetics + **Co-trimoxazole** ❓

Occasionally and unpredictably acute hypoglycaemia has occurred in patients given various sulfonylureas and co-trimoxazole, although pharmacokinetic studies have not established an interaction. In high doses, co-trimoxazole alone may rarely cause hypoglycaemia. See also trimethoprim, page 73, for its effects on repaglinide and rosiglitazone.

> The general importance of this interaction is uncertain. It may be prudent to increase blood glucose monitoring in diabetics taking high-dose co-trimoxazole.

Antidiabetics + **Digoxin** ⚠

Some but not all studies have found that digoxin plasma levels can be markedly reduced by acarbose.

> Just why there is an inconsistency between these reports is not understood but it would clearly be prudent to consider monitoring digoxin for any evidence of a reduced effect (e.g. check heart rate), taking levels as necessary.

Antidiabetics + **Disopyramide** ⚠

Disopyramide occasionally causes hypoglycaemia, which may be severe. Isolated reports describe severe hypoglycaemia when disopyramide was given to diabetic patients.

> Patients at particular risk of hypoglycaemia are the elderly, the malnourished and diabetics. Impaired renal function or cardiac function may also be predisposing factors. It has been suggested that blood glucose levels should be closely monitored and the disopyramide stopped if problems arise.

Antidiabetics + **Diuretics**

Loop diuretics ✅

The control of diabetes is not usually significantly disturbed by etacrynic acid, furosemide, or torasemide, although there are a few reports showing that etacrynic acid and furosemide can sometimes raise blood glucose levels.

> No action needed.

Thiazide diuretics ⚠

By raising blood glucose levels, the thiazide and related diuretics can reduce the effects of the antidiabetics and impair the control of diabetes. However, this effect appears to be dose-related, and is less frequent at the low doses now commonly used for hypertension. Hyponatraemia has rarely been reported with chlorpropamide combined with a thiazide and potassium-sparing diuretic.

> This interaction is of only moderate practical importance. Recent guidelines on the treatment of hypertension in diabetes recommend the use of thiazides.

A

However, if higher doses are used, increased monitoring of diabetic control would seem prudent.

Antidiabetics + **Fibrates**

Sulphonylureas or Insulin ❓

The effects of the sulphonylureas can be enhanced by clofibrate in some patients, and a reduction in the dosage of the antidiabetics may be necessary. Hypoglycaemia has been reported with bezafibrate, ciprofibrate, fenofibrate and gemfibrozil in patients receiving sulphonylureas. Gemfibrozil has both increased and decreased the dosage requirements of insulin and various sulfonylurea antidiabetics.

There would seem to be no good reason for avoiding the concurrent use of sulphonylureas and fibrates, but be aware that the dosage of the antidiabetic may need adjustment. Patients should be warned that excessive hypoglycaemia occurs occasionally and unpredictably.

Nateglinide ⚠️

Only a modest pharmacokinetic interaction occurs between gemfibrozil and nateglinide.

The manufacturer of nateglinide recommends particular caution, but this seems a very wary approach.

Pioglitazone or Rosiglitazone ⚠️

Gemfibrozil causes large increases in the AUCs of pioglitazone and rosiglitazone.

The clinical relevance of this interaction has not been assessed. Until further experience is gained, caution is warranted. Consider an increased frequency of blood glucose monitoring when the combination is first started.

Repaglinide ✖️

The combination of gemfibrozil and repaglinide results in a marked pharmacokinetic interaction that can result in serious hypoglycaemia.

On the basis of studies and reports of serious hypoglycaemic episodes with gemfibrozil and repaglinide, the European Medicines Agency contraindicate concurrent use.

Antidiabetics + **H₂-receptor antagonists**

Metformin ⚠️

Cimetidine appears to reduce the clearance of metformin, and may have contributed to a case of metformin-associated lactic acidosis.

It has been suggested that the dosage of metformin may need to be reduced if cimetidine is used, bearing in mind the possibility of lactic acidosis if levels become too high.

A

Miglitol ⚠

Miglitol decreases the AUC of ranitidine by 60%.

The clinical significance of this effect is unknown. It may be prudent to monitor for ranitidine efficacy.

Sulphonylureas ❓

Cimetidine and ranitidine generally cause no clinically important changes in the pharmacokinetics or pharmacodynamics of the sulphonylureas, although isolated cases of raised sulphonylurea levels and hypoglycaemia have been seen.

The evidence suggests that most diabetics do not experience any marked changes in their diabetic control if they are given cimetidine. However, a warning that cimetidine may rarely and unpredictably cause hypoglycaemia may be helpful when cimetidine is first started.

Antidiabetics + Herbal medicines or Dietary supplements

Glucosamine +/- Chondroitin ❓

In a controlled study glucosamine with chondroitin had no effect on the glycaemic control of patients taking oral antidiabetics, but one report notes that unexpected increases in blood glucose levels have occurred.

It may be prudent to increase monitoring of blood glucose if glucosamine supplements are taken. Also, if glucose control unexpectedly deteriorates, bear in mind the possibility of self-medication with supplements such as glucosamine.

Karela (Momordica charantia) ❓

The blood glucose lowering effects of chlorpropamide and other antidiabetics can be increased by karela.

Karela is used to flavour foods such as curries, and also used as a herbal medicine for the treatment of diabetes mellitus. Health professionals should therefore be aware that patients may possibly be using karela as well as more orthodox drugs to control their diabetes. Irregular consumption of karela as part of the diet could possibly contribute to unexplained fluctuations in diabetic control.

St John's wort (Hypericum perforatum) ✔

St John's wort decreased the AUC of rosiglitazone (modest decrease of about 25%).

The clinical relevance of the modest reduction in rosiglitazone levels has not been assessed, but it would seem unlikely to be important.

Antidiabetics + HRT ❓

Some women may require small increases or decreases in their dosage of antidiabetic while taking HRT, but it is unusual for the control of diabetes to be seriously disturbed.

A

Routine monitoring should be adequate to detect any interaction as the effects seem to be gradual. However, note that occasionally severe disturbances in control do occur.

Antidiabetics + Ketotifen ⊗

The concurrent use of biguanides (e.g. metformin) and ketotifen appears to be well tolerated, but a fall in the number of platelets has been seen in one study in patients taking the combination.

The clinical importance of this is uncertain. The manufacturers recommend that concurrent use should be avoided until the effect is explained.

Antidiabetics + Lanreotide ⚠

Lanreotide may affect glucose levels in diabetic patients.

The manufacturer of lanreotide recommends that blood glucose levels should be checked in diabetic patients to determine whether antidiabetic treatment needs to be adjusted. This seems prudent.

Antidiabetics + Leflunomide ⚠

The active metabolite of leflunomide (A771726) has been shown by *in vitro* studies to be an inhibitor of CYP2C9, which is concerned with the metabolism of tolbutamide. The manufacturers advise caution if leflunomide is given with tolbutamide as increased tolbutamide levels may result.

It may be prudent to monitor blood glucose levels on concurrent use.

Antidiabetics + Macrolides

Sulphonylureas ❓

Isolated cases of hypoglycaemia have been described in patients taking glibenclamide (glyburide) or glipizide with clarithromycin or erythromycin. A study in healthy subjects found that hypoglycaemia may occur if tolbutamide is given with clarithromycin.

The general importance of these isolated cases is uncertain, but some caution may be warranted on concurrent use.

Repaglinide ⚠

A pharmacokinetic study suggests that clarithromycin may enhance the effects of repaglinide (40% increase in AUC).

Until more is known it may be prudent to increase blood glucose monitoring on concurrent use.

Antidiabetics + MAOIs ⚠

The blood glucose lowering effects of insulin and the oral antidiabetics can be increased by MAOIs. This may improve the control of blood glucose levels in most diabetics, but in a few it may cause undesirable hypoglycaemia.

It may be prudent to increase blood glucose monitoring on concurrent use.

Antidiabetics + Neomycin ⚠

Neomycin alone can reduce postprandial blood glucose levels, and may enhance the reduction in postprandial glucose levels associated with acarbose. Neomycin also appears to increase the unpleasant gastrointestinal adverse effects (flatulence, cramps and diarrhoea) of acarbose.

The manufacturers suggest that if these adverse effects are severe the dosage of acarbose should be reduced.

Antidiabetics + Nicotinic acid (Niacin) ❓

Nicotinic acid causes deterioration in glucose tolerance, which may be dose-related, and can result in the need for dose adjustment of a patient's antidiabetic drugs. Nevertheless, its beneficial effects on lipids may outweigh its effects on glucose tolerance in some diabetics.

Diabetic control should be closely monitored, recognising that some adjustment of the antidiabetic drugs may be needed.

Antidiabetics + NSAIDs

Azapropazone or Phenylbutazone ✗

Although in general NSAIDs do not appear to interact with antidiabetics (see below) azapropazone and particularly phenylbutazone seem to cause a consistent lowering of blood glucose levels (probably by inhibiting the metabolism of the sulphonylureas), which has resulted in severe hypoglycaemia in a number of cases.

Concurrent use with phenylbutazone should be well monitored and a reduction in the dosage of the sulphonylurea may be necessary to avoid excessive hypoglycaemia. The manufacturers of azapropazone say that the concurrent use of sulphonylureas is not recommended.

Pioglitazone or Rosiglitazone ❓

The risk of fluid retention with pioglitazone or rosiglitazone is increased by NSAIDs.

Caution is appropriate, and patients should be monitored for signs of heart failure.

Antidiabetics, general ❓

No adverse interaction normally occurs between most NSAIDs and antidiabetics, although in some isolated cases hypoglycaemia has occurred.

No action needed, but be aware that NSAIDs may rarely and unpredictably cause hypoglycaemia.

Antidiabetics + **Octreotide** ⚠

Octreotide decreases insulin resistance so that the dosage of insulin used by diabetics can be reduced. Octreotide appears to have no benefits in those with intact insulin reserves (type 2 diabetes). In addition, octreotide has been reported to reduce sulphonylurea-induced hypoglycaemia.

If octreotide is used, anticipate the need to reduce the insulin dosage (studies suggest by up to 50%). Octreotide may affect insulin secretion, and therefore glucose tolerance, and so it would certainly be prudent to monitor the effects of giving octreotide with any of the oral antidiabetics.

Antidiabetics + **Orlistat**

Acarbose ✕

The manufacturers of orlistat recommend avoiding the concurrent use of acarbose because of a lack of interaction studies.

Avoid concurrent use.

Other antidiabetics ⚠

Orlistat improved glycaemic control, which resulted in the need to reduce the dose of glibenclamide (glyburide) or glipizide in almost half of the patients in one study. In other studies, orlistat reduced the dose requirement for metformin and insulin.

Monitor the outcome of concurrent use on blood sugar levels and adjust the antidiabetic treatment accordingly.

Antidiabetics + **Pancreatic enzymes** ⚠

The manufacturers of acarbose and miglitol reasonably suggest that digestive enzyme preparations (such as amylase, pancreatin) would be expected to reduce the effects of these antidiabetics.

The manufacturers advise avoiding concurrent use.

Antidiabetics + **Phenytoin** ❓

Large and toxic doses of phenytoin have been observed to cause hyperglycaemia, but normal therapeutic doses do not usually affect the control of diabetes. Two isolated cases of phenytoin toxicity have been attributed to the use of tolazamide or tolbutamide.

No interaction of clinical importance normally occurs and so no special precautions would seem to be necessary.

Antidiabetics + Probenecid ⚠

The clearance of chlorpropamide is prolonged by probenecid, but the clinical importance of this is uncertain.

Monitor the effect of concurrent use on blood glucose levels and adjust the sulphonylurea dose if necessary. Tolbutamide appears not to interact with probenecid, and so may be a suitable alternative.

Antidiabetics + Quinolones ❓

A number of reports describe severe hypoglycaemia in diabetic patients taking gatifloxacin with various antidiabetics including some sulphonylureas, insulin, metformin, pioglitazone, repaglinide, rosiglitazone, and voglibose. Isolated cases describe hypoglycaemia in diabetic patients taking glibenclamide (glyburide) with ciprofloxacin, levofloxacin, or norfloxacin.

Studies have shown that gatifloxacin may cause hypoglycaemia and hyperglycaemia with at least a 10-fold higher incidence than other quinolones. Studies using ciprofloxacin and levofloxacin with glibenclamide (glyburide) suggest plasma glucose levels are not usually affected to a clinically relevant extent Therefore in general these interactions seem unlikely to be clinically significant, although increased blood glucose monitoring may be prudent if gatifloxacin is given to diabetics.

Antidiabetics + Rifabutin ⚠

The manufacturers and the CSM in the UK warn that rifabutin may also possibly reduce the effects of oral antidiabetics, although this is likely to be to at lesser extent than rifampicin. Rifampicin has the following effects:

● reduces the levels and blood glucose lowering effects of tolbutamide, gliclazide, chlorpropamide (single case) and glibenclamide (glyburide), and to a lesser extent glimepiride, glipizide and glymidine.
● reduces the AUC and effects of repaglinide, and possibly nateglinide.
● reduces the AUCs of pioglitazone and rosiglitazone by about 50%, which could be clinically relevant.

Monitor the outcome of concurrent use on blood sugar levels and adjust the antidiabetic treatment accordingly. In many cases an increase in the dose of the antidiabetic may possibly be needed.

Antidiabetics + Rifampicin (Rifampin) ⚠

Rifampicin reduces the levels and blood glucose lowering effects of tolbutamide, gliclazide, chlorpropamide (single case) and glibenclamide (glyburide), and to a lesser extent glimepiride, glipizide and glymidine. Rifampicin also reduces the AUC and effects of repaglinide, and possibly nateglinide. Rifampicin reduces the AUCs of pioglitazone and rosiglitazone by about 50%, which could be clinically relevant.

Monitor the outcome of concurrent use on blood sugar levels and adjust the antidiabetic treatment accordingly. In many cases an increase in the dose of the antidiabetic seems likely to be needed.

A

Antidiabetics + SSRIs 🔲

Hypoglycaemia has occurred in patients with diabetes when they were given fluoxetine or sertraline, and a loss of hypoglycaemic awareness has also been reported with fluoxetine. Conversely, two isolated reports describe hyperglycaemia in patients given fluvoxamine or sertraline.

There would seem to be little reason for avoiding concurrent use of fluoxetine, fluvoxamine or sertraline with sulphonylureas, but the cautious may want to increase blood glucose monitoring. The manufacturers of the SSRIs warn that dosages of insulin or oral antidiabetics may need adjustment during concurrent use, but the available evidence suggests that this is rare.

Antidiabetics + Statins ✅

One study reported an increased incidence of adverse effects when repaglinide was given with simvastatin, and there is a possibility of increased liver and muscle effects when pioglitazone or rosiglitazone are used with atorvastatin.

As yet there is insufficient evidence to recommend special precautions when the statins are used with any antidiabetic drug. No clinically relevant adverse interactions appear to have been reported between statins and sulphonylureas. The use of statins in patients with diabetes is known to be beneficial for both primary and secondary prevention of cardiovascular events.

Antidiabetics + Sulfinpyrazone ✅

Sulfinpyrazone has no effect on the insulin requirements of diabetics, nor does it affect the diabetic control of patients taking glibenclamide (glyburide). Sulfinpyrazone reduces the clearance of tolbutamide, but as yet there appear to be no case reports of this interaction. Sulfinpyrazone modestly increased the AUC of nateglinide, but this is unlikely to be clinically relevant.

No action needed.

Antidiabetics + Sulfonamides 🔲

The blood glucose lowering effects of some of the sulphonylureas are increased by some, but not all, sulfonamides. The sulfonamides now available appear less likely to interact. Nevertheless, occasionally and unpredictably acute hypoglycaemia has occurred.

The general importance of this interaction is uncertain.

Antidiabetics + Tibolone ⚠️

Tibolone may slightly impair glucose tolerance and therefore possibly reduce the effects of antidiabetics.

The manufacturers of tibolone say that patients with diabetes should be closely supervised. Initially, increased monitoring of blood glucose levels would seem adequate.

Antidiabetics + **Tricyclics** ❓

Interactions between antidiabetics and tricyclic antidepressants appear to be rare, but isolated cases of hypoglycaemia have been recorded in patients taking insulin or sulphonylureas with a tricyclic.

These cases seem unlikely to be of general importance.

Antidiabetics + **Trimethoprim**

Repaglinide ❌

In one study trimethoprim increased the AUC of single-dose repaglinide by about 60% without changing its blood glucose lowering effects.

The UK manufacturers advise that concurrent use should be avoided as the effect of larger doses of both drugs are unknown. However, the US manufacturers suggest that repaglinide dosage adjustments may be necessary. If both drugs are used it would seem prudent to increase the frequency of blood glucose monitoring until the effects are known.

Rosiglitazone ✔

Trimethoprim appears to increase the AUC of rosiglitazone by about one-third.

This interaction is not expected to be clinically significant.

Sulphonylureas ✔

Trimethoprim does not appear to significantly affect the pharmacokinetics of tolbutamide. Consider also co-trimoxazole, page 65, which may interact.

No action needed.

Antidiabetics + **Warfarin and other oral anticoagulants** ✔

Although isolated cases of interactions (raised prothrombin times, bleeding or hypoglycaemia) have been seen in patients taking anticoagulants and acarbose, metformin or sulphonylureas, in general no important interaction appears to occur. A decrease in prothrombin time has also been seen with acarbose or metformin.

The isolated cases of bleeding are not expected to represent a general interaction. No interaction has been seen between the oral anticoagulants and miglitol, nateglinide, pioglitazone, repaglinide, rosiglitazone, or voglibose.

Antihistamines

No specific interaction studies have been performed with antihistamine eye drops. However, interactions are not anticipated since very little drug is expected to reach the

A

systemic circulation. Note also that the sedative antihistamines may cause additive sedation with any other CNS depressant drug.

Antihistamines + Aprepitant ❌

Aprepitant can increase the levels of CYP3A4 substrates in the short-term, then reduce them within 2 weeks of concurrent use. Terfenadine and astemizole are metabolised by CYP3A4 and therefore their levels would be expected to be increased by aprepitant. This may increase the risk of life-threatening arrhythmias. Fosaprepitant, a prodrug of aprepitant, would be expected to interact similarly.

> The manufacturers of aprepitant contraindicate concurrent use, and advise caution for the 2 weeks following the use of aprepitant.

Antihistamines + Azoles

Astemizole, Mizolastine or Terfenadine ❌

Some of the azoles raise astemizole and terfenadine levels, which may increase the risk of serious life-threatening arrhythmias. Cases of torsade de pointes have been reported when astemizole is given with ketoconazole, and when terfenadine is given with itraconazole or ketoconazole. An arrhythmia has also been reported in a patient taking terfenadine and using topical oxiconazole. Ketoconazole raises mizolastine levels, which caused a small increase in the QT interval in one study.

> The manufacturers of astemizole, mizolastine and terfenadine contraindicate the concurrent use of azoles and the manufacturer of terfenadine extends this contraindication to the concurrent use of topical azoles.

Other antihistamines ✓

Ketoconazole very markedly raised ebastine levels and markedly raised loratadine levels. In one study, this was associated with a small increase in the QT interval for both antihistamines, but there was no obvious alteration in the adverse event profile. Ketoconazole markedly raised the plasma levels of fexofenadine, and modestly raised those of desloratadine and emedastine, but these changes had no effect on the QT interval, or on adverse events. The combinations may therefore be assumed to be safe in terms of cardiac effects.

> The manufacturer of ebastine advises against the use of itraconazole or ketoconazole. However, in general these changes are not expected to have a clinically relevant effect, although some caution may be warranted. Azelastine, cetirizine, levocabastine and levocetirizine do not appear to interact with ketoconazole and may therefore be suitable alternatives.

Antihistamines + Benzodiazepines ✓

Benzodiazepines impair psychomotor performance, but neither ebastine nor mizolastine (both non-sedating antihistamines) further impair this. An enhanced sedative effect would be expected if known sedative antihistamines are given with benzodiazepines.

> No action is needed if ebastine or mizolastine are taken with benzodiazepines. However, warn all patients taking sedating antihistamines of the potential effects,

and counsel against driving or undertaking other skilled tasks. The degree of impairment will depend on the individual patient.

Antihistamines + Betahistine ❓

A single report describes the re-emergence of labyrinthine symptoms in a patient taking betahistine with terfenadine. This interaction had been predicted on theoretical grounds because betahistine is an analogue of histamine. Betahistine may therefore oppose the effects of all antihistamines.

The use of antihistamines should be carefully considered in patients taking betahistine.

Antihistamines + Grapefruit juice ✖

Grapefruit juice causes terfenadine to accumulate in the body, increasing the risk of serious cardiotoxicity (prolongation of the QTc interval) and the possibility of torsade de pointes arrhythmia. Consider drugs that prolong the QT interval, page 237.

Concurrent use is contraindicated.

Antihistamines + H₂-receptor antagonists ✔

Cimetidine moderately raises hydroxyzine levels and considerably raises loratadine levels, but this is not thought to be of clinical significance. The manufacturer of mizolastine recommends caution if cimetidine is taken concurrently because it might increase mizolastine levels and prolong the QT interval. This is a cautious approach since a link between mizolastine and cardiac arrhythmias has not been proven.

No action needed.

Antihistamines + Herbal medicines or Dietary supplements ❓

One study found that St John's wort increased the clearance of fexofenadine by 1.6-fold, whereas another study found no clinically relevant effect.

If fexofenadine is less effective in a patient taking regular St John's wort, consider this interaction as a possible cause.

Antihistamines + Macrolides ✖

Erythromycin causes terfenadine and astemizole to accumulate in a few individuals, which can prolong the QT interval and lead to life-threatening torsade de pointes arrhythmias. Cases of torsade de pointes have been reported for astemizole with erythromycin, and terfenadine with erythromycin. Other macrolides are believed to interact similarly, with the exception of azithromycin and possibly dirithromycin. Erythromycin modestly raises mizolastine levels, although this has no effect on the QT interval. Erythromycin markedly raises ebastine levels, which caused a modest

A

prolongation of the QT interval in one study. Consider also drugs that prolong the QT interval, page 237.

The manufacturers of astemizole, ebastine, mizolastine and terfenadine contraindicate their use with all macrolides, with the isolated exception of astemizole with azithromycin. The manufacturer of terfenadine extends this contraindication to the concurrent use of topical macrolides. Azelastine, cetirizine, desloratadine, fexofenadine and intranasal levocabastine may be suitable non-interacting alternatives. Note that the macrolides differ in the likely extent of their interaction, see macrolides, page 310.

Antihistamines + MAOIs

Antihistamines, general ✅

The alleged interaction between MAOIs and most antihistamines appears to be based on a single animal study, and is probably more theoretical than real. The exception seems to be cyproheptadine and promethazine (see below).

The UK manufacturers of most of the sedating antihistamines (alimemazine, brompheniramine, chlorphenamine, diphenhydramine) state that MAOIs may intensify the antimuscarinic effect of antihistamines, and many contraindicate or caution concurrent use.

Cyproheptadine ❌

Isolated reports describe delayed hallucinations in a patient taking phenelzine and cyproheptadine, and the rapid re-emergence of depression when cyproheptadine was given to two other patients taking brofaromine or phenelzine.

It would be prudent to monitor for a reduction in efficacy or an adverse response if cyproheptadine is given with any MAOI or RIMA. The manufacturer of cyproheptadine contraindicates concurrent use with MAOIs, however, there appears to be no reason why cyproheptadine cannot be used to treat serotonin syndrome occurring in a patient taking an MAOI.

Promethazine ❌

Promethazine is a phenothiazine antihistamine. Rarely, cases of neuroleptic malignant syndrome or extrapyramidal symptoms have been seen when phenothiazines have been given with MAOIs.

The UK manufacturer contraindicates the use of promethazine both with and for 14 days after stopping treatment with an MAOI, whereas the US manufacturer advises caution.

Antihistamines + Protease inhibitors

Astemizole or Terfenadine ❌

Nelfinavir markedly increases terfenadine levels, which is expected to increase the risk of QT prolongation and torsade de pointes arrhythmias. Other protease inhibitors are predicted to interact similarly with both terfenadine and astemizole.

Concurrent use is contraindicated.

Other antihistamines ✅

Cetirizine and fexofenadine levels are raised by ritonavir, but this is not expected to be clinically significant.

No action needed.

Antihistamines + **Rifampicin (Rifampin)** ❓

Rifampicin increases the oral clearance of fexofenadine, by more than 5-fold in some cases, but the clinical significance of this is unclear.

Until more is known it would seem prudent to monitor the efficacy of fexofenadine if it is given with rifampicin.

Antihistamines + **SSRIs** ❌

Two isolated reports provide some evidence of cardiotoxicity, which was attributed to the concurrent use of terfenadine and fluoxetine, although other evidence suggests that an interaction is unlikely. Terfenadine does not appear to interact with paroxetine or sertraline. Nevertheless, the manufacturers of both astemizole and terfenadine contraindicate the concurrent use of SSRIs.

Avoid concurrent use.

Antihistamines + **Zafirlukast** ⚠️

Terfenadine reduced the mean maximum serum levels of zafirlukast by about 70% and reduced its AUC by about 60% in one study. Terfenadine serum levels remained unchanged and no ECG alterations occurred.

The reduction in zafirlukast serum levels would be expected to reduce its antiasthmatic effects, but this needs clinical assessment. The combination need not be avoided but be alert for a reduced response.

Antihypertensives

The hypotensive effect of antihypertensives can be enhanced by other antihypertensives, as would be expected. Although first-dose hypotension' (dizziness, lightheadedness, fainting) can occur with some combinations (e.g. see ACE inhibitors, page 1 and alpha blockers, page 31), the additive effects are usually clinically useful. Perhaps of more concern is the use of antihypertensives with drugs that have hypotension as an adverse effect, where the effects may not be anticipated or deliberately sought. The situation with alcohol is slightly more complex. Chronic moderate to heavy drinking raises blood pressure and reduces, to some extent, the effectiveness of antihypertensive drugs. A few patients taking antihypertensives may experience postural hypotension, dizziness and fainting shortly after having an alcoholic drink. See also alpha blockers, page 14, beta blockers, page 16 and calcium-channel blockers, page 17, for more specific information on these individual groups. Patients with hypertension who are moderate to heavy drinkers should be encouraged to reduce their intake of alcohol. It may then become possible to reduce the dosage of the antihypertensive. It should be noted that epidemiological studies show that regular light to moderate alcohol consumption is associated with a *lower* risk of cardiovascular disease. Drugs where hypotension is the main effect include:

- ACE inhibitors
- Aliskiren
- Alpha blockers
- Angiotensin II receptor antagonists
- Beta blockers
- Calcium-channel blockers
- Clonidine
- Diazoxide
- Diuretics
- Guanethidine
- Hydralazine
- Methyldopa
- Minoxidil
- Moxonidine
- Nitrates
- Nitroprusside

Drugs where hypotension is a significant adverse effect include:

- Alcohol
- Aldesleukin
- Alprostadil
- Antipsychotics
- Dopamine agonists (e.g. apomorphine, bromocriptine, pergolide)
- Levodopa
- MAOIs
- Moxisylyte
- Nicorandil
- Tizanidine

Antimuscarinics

Remember that other drugs, (e.g. clozapine, nefopam, tricyclic antidepressants) have antimuscarinic adverse effects, and therefore may interact similarly.

Antimuscarinics + Antimuscarinics ❓

Additive antimuscarinic effects can develop if two or more drugs with antimuscarinic effects are used together. The easily recognised and common peripheral antimuscarinic effects are blurred vision, dry mouth, constipation, difficulty in urination, reduced sweating and tachycardia. Central effects include confusion, disorientation, visual hallucinations, agitation, irritability, delirium, memory problems, belligerence and even aggressiveness. Problems are most likely to arise in patients with particular physical conditions such as glaucoma, prostatic hypertrophy or constipation, in whom antimuscarinic drugs should be used with caution, if at all. It has been pointed out that the antimuscarinic adverse effects can mimic the effects of normal ageing. Consider also antipsychotics, below.

> Concurrent use need not be avoided but some caution is warranted, especially in the disease states mentioned.

Antimuscarinics + **Antipsychotics** ❓

Antipsychotics and antimuscarinics are often given together advantageously and uneventfully, but occasionally serious and even life-threatening interactions occur. These include heat-stroke in hot and humid conditions, severe constipation, adynamic ileus, and atropine-like psychoses. Antimuscarinics used to counteract the extrapyramidal adverse effects of antipsychotics may also reduce or abolish their therapeutic effects. See also antimuscarinics, page 78, as many antipsychotics also have antimuscarinic adverse effects.

> These drugs have been widely used together with apparent advantage and often without problems. However, be aware that an unspectacular low-grade antimuscarinic toxicity can easily go undetected, particularly in the elderly. Also note that serious problems can sometimes develop, particularly if high doses are used. Consider:
>
> - warning patients (particularly those on high doses) to minimise outdoor exposure and/or exercise in hot and humid climates.
> - being alert for severe constipation and for the development of complete gut stasis, which can be fatal.
> - that the symptoms of central antimuscarinic psychosis can be confused with the basic psychotic symptoms of the patient.
> - withdrawal of one or more of the drugs, or a dosage reduction and/or appropriate symptomatic treatment if any of these interactions occur.

Some antipsychotics and antimuscarinics prolong the QT interval. For interactions resulting from additive effects on the QT interval see drugs that prolong the QT interval, page 237. Remember that many drugs have antimuscarinic adverse effects (e.g. tricyclics, page 91).

Antimuscarinics + **Donepezil** ⚠

The effects of donepezil are expected to oppose the actions of drugs with antimuscarinic effects, and in turn to be opposed by antimuscarinics. However, in practice two cases describe confusional states resulting from the concurrent use of anticholinesterases and drugs with antimuscarinic effects, which is the opposite effect to that expected.

> Whether this interaction is of real practical importance awaits confirmation. Monitor concurrent use for an increase in adverse effects.

Antimuscarinics + **Galantamine** ⚠

The effects of galantamine are expected to oppose the actions of drugs with antimuscarinic effects, and in turn to be opposed by antimuscarinics. However, in practice two cases describe confusional states resulting from the concurrent use of

A

anticholinesterases and drugs with antimuscarinic effects, which is the opposite effect to that expected.

> Whether this interaction is of real practical importance awaits confirmation. Monitor concurrent use for an increase in adverse effects.

Antimuscarinics + Levodopa ⚠

Antimuscarinics may modestly reduce the rate and possibly the extent of levodopa absorption. One case describes levodopa toxicity, which occurred after the withdrawal of an antimuscarinic.

> Concurrent use is of established benefit. The presence of a dopa-decarboxylase inhibitor would be expected to minimise the effects of any interaction. There is certainly no need to avoid concurrent use, but it would be prudent to be alert for any evidence of a reduced levodopa response if antimuscarinics are added, or for levodopa toxicity if they are withdrawn.

Antimuscarinics + MAOIs ✓

Some manufacturers of older irreversible non-selective MAOIs and antimuscarinics issue cautions about the possibility of increased antimuscarinic effects in the presence of MAOIs. This seems to be a theoretical prediction. No adverse interactions between the MAOIs and antimuscarinics have been reported.

> Bear this possible interaction in mind on concurrent use.

Antimuscarinics + Nitrates ❓

Drugs with antimuscarinic effects, such as the tricyclic antidepressants and disopyramide, depress salivation and many patients complain of having a dry mouth. In theory sublingual glyceryl trinitrate (nitroglycerin) tablets will dissolve less readily under the tongue in these patients, thereby reducing their absorption and effects. However, no formal studies seem to have been done to confirm that this actually happens.

> A possible alternative is to use a glyceryl trinitrate (nitroglycerin) spray in patients who suffer from dry mouth.

Antimuscarinics + Rivastigmine ⚠

The effects of rivastigmine are expected to oppose the actions of drugs with antimuscarinic effects, and in turn to be opposed by antimuscarinics. However, in practice two cases describe confusional states resulting from the concurrent use of anticholinesterases and drugs with antimuscarinic effects, which is the opposite effect to that expected.

> Whether this interaction is of real practical importance awaits confirmation. Monitor concurrent use for an increase in adverse effects.

Antimuscarinics + SSRIs ❓

Several patients have developed delirium when given fluoxetine, paroxetine or sertraline with benzatropine, in the presence of perphenazine or haloperidol. Concurrent use in other patients has been uneventful.

The general clinical importance of this interaction is uncertain, but be alert for evidence of confusion and possible delirium in patients given SSRIs with benzatropine, particularly if they are also taking other drugs with antimuscarinic actions.

Antimuscarinics + Tacrine ⚠️

The effects of tacrine are expected to oppose the actions of drugs with antimuscarinic effects, and in turn to be opposed by antimuscarinics. However, in practice two cases describe confusional states resulting from the concurrent use of anticholinesterases and drugs with antimuscarinic effects, which is the opposite effect to that expected.

Whether this interaction is of real practical importance awaits confirmation. Monitor concurrent use for an increase in adverse effects.

Antipsychotics

Antipsychotics + Antipsychotics

Clozapine ❓

The concurrent use of clozapine and risperidone can be effective and well tolerated but isolated reports describe a rise in serum clozapine levels when risperidone was added, and another describes the development of atrial ectopics. Dystonia has been seen when clozapine was replaced by risperidone.

The raised clozapine levels and other adverse reactions seem to be isolated cases and therefore of doubtful general significance.

Quetiapine ⚠️

Thioridazine moderately reduces quetiapine levels and a case report describes a seizure in a patient taking olanzapine and quetiapine.

Concurrent use need not be avoided. The case highlights the importance of considering seizure potential when prescribing multiple antipsychotic medications.

Other antipsychotics ✖️

Additive QT-prolonging effects likely with some antipsychotic combinations, see drugs that prolong the QT interval, page 237.

A

Antipsychotics + **Apomorphine** ❌

Centrally-acting dopamine antagonists (such as the antipsychotics, including prochlorperazine used at an antiemetic dose) may antagonise the effects of apomorphine. However, note that clozapine may be used to reduce the symptoms of neuropsychiatric complications of Parkinson's disease. Additive hypotensive effects are also possible, see antihypertensives, page 77.

Concurrent use should be avoided, or monitored closely to ensure apomorphine remains effective. Note that prochlorperazine has been used safely in patients taking apomorphine for erectile dysfunction.

Antipsychotics + **Aprepitant** ❌

Aprepitant inhibits the enzymes involved in the metabolism of pimozide, and is therefore expected to raise pimozide levels, which may result in potentially fatal torsade de pointes arrhythmias. Fosaprepitant, a prodrug of aprepitant, would be expected to interact similarly.

Concurrent use is contraindicated. Caution is needed in the 2 weeks after aprepitant is stopped as there may be some residual enzyme inhibiting activity.

Antipsychotics + **Azoles**

Pimozide and Sertindole ❌

Ketoconazole and itraconazole are predicted to raise the levels of pimozide and sertindole, which could lead to potentially fatal torsade de pointes arrhythmias.

The concurrent use of azoles with pimozide or sertindole is contraindicated.

Other antipsychotics ⚠

The levels of some antipsychotics may be raised by azole antifungals:

- Aripiprazole levels are predicted to be increased by itraconazole and ketoconazole.
- Haloperidol levels are raised by 30% or more by itraconazole, but there was wide variation between subjects. Adverse neurological effects were seen in some subjects.
- Quetiapine levels are increased 6-fold by ketoconazole. Other azole antifungals are predicted to interact similarly.
- Risperidone levels were raised by about 80% by itraconazole in one study. Ketoconazole would be expected to interact similarly.

Monitor for signs of adverse antipsychotic effects if these azoles are given, and consider reducing the dose as necessary. The manufacturers of aripiprazole suggest halving its dose if itraconazole or ketoconazole are given.

Antipsychotics + **Benzodiazepines**

Antipsychotics, general ⚠

Additive sedative effects would be expected when antipsychotics are given with benzodiazepines. Concurrent use has resulted in severe hypotension, respiratory depression and, in rare cases, the neuroleptic malignant syndrome. Rarely, fatal hypotension and respiratory arrest have been reported when clozapine was given with benzodiazepines.

Be aware of these potential adverse effects, but note that concurrent use is common and most often uneventful.

Olanzapine ⚠

Excessive sedation may occur if parenteral benzodiazepines are given with intramuscular olanzapine.

Parenteral benzodiazepines should not be given until at least one hour after intramuscular olanzapine. If a parenteral benzodiazepine has already been given, intramuscular olanzapine should be given with care and the patient should be closely monitored for sedation and cardiorespiratory depression.

Antipsychotics + Beta blockers

Sotalol ✗

Additive QT-prolonging effects likely, see drugs that prolong the QT interval, page 237.

Concurrent use should generally be avoided.

Beta blockers, general ❓

The concurrent use of chlorpromazine and propranolol can result in a marked rise in the plasma levels of both drugs. Propranolol also markedly increases plasma thioridazine levels. Additive hypotensive effects are also possible, see antihypertensives, page 77.

Monitor the outcome of concurrent use, adjusting the doses of both drugs as necessary.

Antipsychotics + Bupropion ⚠

Bupropion is predicted to inhibit the metabolism of haloperidol, risperidone, and thioridazine.

The manufacturers recommend that if any of these drugs are added to treatment with bupropion, they should be given in doses at the lower end of the range. If bupropion is added to existing treatment, decreased dosages of the antipsychotics should be considered. However, there appear to be no reports of problems with the concurrent use of any of these drugs. Note that both bupropion and antipsychotics can lower the seizure threshold. A maximum dose of 150 mg of bupropion should be considered for patients prescribed other drugs that may lower the convulsive threshold.

Antipsychotics + Buspirone ❓

Two studies found that buspirone can cause a rise in plasma haloperidol levels, while another found that no interaction occurred.

A

There would seem to be no reason for avoiding concurrent use. However, be aware that some patients seem to experience large rises in haloperidol levels, so consider this interaction if the effects of haloperidol seem excessive.

Antipsychotics + **Calcium-channel blockers** ⊗

Diltiazem, nifedipine, and verapamil reduce the clearance of sertindole by about 20%. Additive hypotensive effects possible, see antihypertensives, page 77.

Concurrent use of these calcium-channel blockers is contraindicated as raised sertindole levels may prolong the QT interval.

Antipsychotics + **Carbamazepine** ⚠

Clozapine, haloperidol and risperidone plasma levels can be roughly halved by carbamazepine. Aripiprazole, bromperidol, fluphenazine, olanzapine, quetiapine, sertindole, and tiotixene levels are also reduced by carbamazepine. An increase in the serum levels of carbamazepine or its epoxide metabolite (which is thought to cause some of the adverse effects of carbamazepine) has been reported in patients given loxapine, haloperidol, quetiapine, risperidone, or chlorpromazine with amoxapine. Toxicity has occurred. Isolated cases of Stevens-Johnson syndrome and the neuroleptic malignant syndrome have occurred in patients taking antipsychotics with carbamazepine.

Monitor carbamazepine levels if loxapine, haloperidol, quetiapine, risperidone, or chlorpromazine are given. Also monitor concurrent use to ensure that the antipsychotics remain effective, (especially risperidone, clozapine and haloperidol). The manufacturers recommend using double the dose of aripiprazole in patients taking carbamazepine. The risk of Stevens-Johnson syndrome seems to be highest during the first 2 weeks of treatment and appears to be mostly confined to the first 8 weeks of treatment. Also note that the combination of clozapine and carbamazepine is predicted to increase agranulocytosis and one case of fatal pancytopenia has been reported. It is also important to consider the seizure potential when prescribing antipsychotic medications.

Antipsychotics + **Darifenacin** ⚠

Darifenacin increases the levels of CYP2D6 substrates such as the tricyclics (imipramine AUC increased by 70%). The manufacturers therefore advise caution with other CYP2D6 substrates, and specifically name thioridazine.

If the combination is used it would be prudent to closely monitor for thioridazine adverse effects, and consider the possibility of ventricular arrhythmias.

Antipsychotics + **Dopamine agonists** ⚠

Centrally-acting dopamine antagonists (such as the antipsychotics, including prochlorperazine used at an antiemetic dose) are expected to oppose the effects of the dopamine agonists.

Concurrent use should be avoided, or monitored closely to ensure that the dopamine agonist remains effective. Additive hypotensive effects possible, see antihypertensives, page 77.

Antipsychotics + **Duloxetine** ✖

Duloxetine is predicted to inhibit the metabolism of thioridazine.

In the US concurrent use is contraindicated. If the combination is used it would be prudent to closely monitor for thioridazine adverse effects, and consider the possibility of ventricular arrhythmias.

Antipsychotics + **Grapefruit juice** ✖

The manufacturers predict that grapefruit juice will, like other CYP3A4 inhibitors, raise pimozide levels. This may lead to potentially life-threatening torsade de pointes arrhythmias.

Concurrent use is contraindicated.

Antipsychotics + **Guanethidine** ❓

Large doses of chlorpromazine may reduce or even abolish the antihypertensive effects of guanethidine. The antihypertensive effects of guanethidine can be reduced by haloperidol and thiothixene. However, in some patients the hypotensive effect of chlorpromazine may predominate. Note also, that the antipsychotics can cause postural hypotension.

Increases or decreases in blood pressure may occur as a result of concurrent use. Monitor blood pressure adjusting the guanethidine dose as necessary.

Antipsychotics + **H₂-receptor antagonists**

Antipsychotics, general ⚠

One study found that chlorpromazine levels are reduced by cimetidine, while another study suggested that chlorpromazine levels can be increased. A single case report describes clozapine toxicity when cimetidine, but not ranitidine, was also taken.

The clinical significance of these interactions is unclear.

Sertindole ✖

Cimetidine is predicted to increase sertindole levels (by inhibiting CYP3A4), which may result in potentially fatal torsade de pointes arrhythmias.

The manufacturers contraindicate concurrent use.

Antipsychotics + **Herbal medicines or Dietary supplements**

Evening primrose oil ❓

Although seizures have occurred in a few schizophrenics taking phenothiazines with evening primrose oil, no adverse effects were seen in others, and there appears to be no

A

firm evidence that evening primrose oil should be avoided by epileptic patients.

No action needed; it seems likely that the phenothiazine, rather than the evening primrose oil caused this adverse reaction.

St John's wort (Hypericum perforatum) ⚠

The manufacturers of aripiprazole say that St John's wort may be expected to reduce its levels.

The manufacturers recommend using double the dose of aripiprazole, then titrating to effect.

Antipsychotics + Levodopa ⊗

Centrally-acting dopamine antagonists (such as the antipsychotics, including prochlorperazine used at an antiemetic dose) may antagonise the effects of levodopa. However, note that clozapine may be used to reduce the symptoms of neuropsychiatric complications of Parkinson's disease. Additive hypotensive effects possible, see antihypertensives, page 77.

Concurrent use should be avoided, or monitored closely, to ensure levodopa remains effective.

Antipsychotics + Lithium ⚠

Chlorpromazine levels can be reduced to subtherapeutic concentrations by lithium, and one study suggested that lithium may reduce olanzapine plasma levels. Lithium may increase amisulpride levels. The development of severe extrapyramidal adverse effects or severe neurotoxicity has been seen in one or more patients given lithium with amoxapine, chlorpromazine, chlorprothixene, clopenthixol, clozapine, flupentixol, fluphenazine, haloperidol, levomepromazine, loxapine, mesoridazine, molindone, olanzapine, perphenazine, prochlorperazine, risperidone, sulpiride, thioridazine, tiotixene, trifluoperazine or zuclopenthixol. Sleep-walking has been described in some patients taking chlorpromazine-like drugs and lithium. Additive QT-prolonging effects also possible, see drugs that prolong the QT interval, page 237.

Monitor the outcome of concurrent use being aware that on occasion dosage adjustments may be needed to manage adverse effects. Withdraw one or both drugs if severe neurotoxicity occurs.

Antipsychotics + Macrolides

Potential interactions ⚠

A study in healthy subjects found no evidence of an interaction between clozapine and erythromycin, but three case reports describe clozapine toxicity (seizures in one patient, drowsiness, incoordination and incontinence in another, and neutropenia in the third) when the patients also took erythromycin. Quetiapine levels are increased by erythromycin.

The clinical importance of these interactions is uncertain, but bear them in mind in case of an unexpected response to treatment. The manufacturers suggest that lower quetiapine doses should be considered if macrolides are given. Note that not all macrolides would be expected to interact, see macrolides, page 310.

Serious interactions ❌

Clarithromycin can increase the levels of pimozide, which is believed to increase its serious cardiotoxicity. The manufacturers predict that other macrolides will interact similarly, but note that not all macrolides would be expected to interact, see macrolides, page 310. Erythromycin slightly raises the levels of sertindole, and concurrent use increases the incidence of adverse effects (diarrhoea, abdominal pain, dizziness) but no ECG changes appear to occur.

The concurrent use of macrolides is contraindicated with pimozide and sertindole because of the risks of QT interval prolongation. Consider also drugs that prolong the QT interval, page 237.

Antipsychotics + NNRTIs ⚠

Efavirenz and nevirapine are potent inhibitors of CYP3A4 and are predicted increase the metabolism of aripiprazole.

The manufacturers recommend using double the dose of aripiprazole, then titrating to effect.

Antipsychotics + NSAIDs ⚠

Profound drowsiness and confusion have been described in patients given haloperidol and indometacin.

Evidence of this interaction appears to be very limited, but the incidence (6 out of 20) is high. If concurrent use is thought appropriate, warn patients to be alert for this effect.

Antipsychotics + Opioids ⚠

Pethidine (meperidine) and chlorpromazine can be used together to enhance analgesia and for premedication before anaesthesia, but increased respiratory depression, sedation, CNS toxicity and hypotension can also occur. Similar effects would be expected with other phenothiazines and opioids.

The combination need not be avoided, but care obviously needs to be taken. The US manufacturer suggests that the dose of pethidine (meperidine) should be proportionally reduced (usually by 25 to 50%) when it is given with phenothiazines. Note that additive QT-prolonging effects are possible with methadone, see drugs that prolong the QT interval, page 237.

Antipsychotics + Phenobarbital ⚠

Haloperidol plasma levels, and possibly clozapine levels, are roughly halved by phenobarbital. Aripiprazole, chlorpromazine and possibly thioridazine levels are also reduced by phenobarbital. The plasma levels of quetiapine are predicted to be reduced by barbiturates.

Monitor concurrent use to ensure that the antipsychotics remain effective. The manufacturers of aripiprazole suggest doubling its dose. It is also important to consider the seizure potential when prescribing antipsychotic medications.

A

Antipsychotics + **Phenytoin** ⚠

Clozapine and haloperidol serum levels are expected to be halved by phenytoin. Aripiprazole and sertindole levels are also significantly reduced by phenytoin. The clearance of quetiapine is increased by phenytoin. The serum levels of phenytoin can be raised or lowered by the use of chlorpromazine, prochlorperazine or thioridazine. Fosphenytoin, a prodrug of phenytoin, may interact similarly.

Monitor phenytoin levels if chlorpromazine, prochlorperazine or thioridazine are given. The manufacturers of aripiprazole suggest doubling its dose. Also monitor concurrent use to ensure that the antipsychotics remain effective. It is also important to consider the seizure potential when prescribing antipsychotic medications.

Antipsychotics + **Protease inhibitors**

Aripiprazole ⚠

Aripiprazole is metabolised by CYP3A4, which is strongly inhibited by the protease inhibitors. Increased aripiprazole levels are therefore expected.

Caution and monitoring are recommended. The manufacturers suggest that the dose of aripiprazole should be halved.

Clozapine ✖

Clozapine levels are predicted to be raised by ritonavir, resulting in serious haematological toxicity.

Concurrent use is therefore contraindicated.

Olanzapine ⚠

Olanzapine levels are roughly halved by ritonavir. As this interaction appears to occur because of CYP1A2 inhibition other protease inhibitors would not be expected to interact.

If concurrent use is necessary monitor olanzapine efficacy and increase the dose if necessary.

Pimozide ✖

Pimozide is metabolised by CYP3A4, which is inhibited by the protease inhibitors. Raised pimozide levels, which increase the risk of potentially fatal arrhythmias, would be expected.

Concurrent use is contraindicated.

Quetiapine ⚠

Quetiapine levels are increased 6-fold by ketoconazole, a potent inhibitor of CYP3A4. Protease inhibitors are also inhibitors of CYP3A4 and are therefore predicted to interact similarly.

Monitor for signs of adverse antipsychotic effects if a protease inhibitor is also given, and consider reducing the dose as necessary.

Risperidone ⚠

Neuroleptic malignant syndrome occurred in one patient and extrapyramidal adverse effects in another given risperidone with indinavir and ritonavir.

Concurrent use need not be avoided, but be aware that these adverse effects may occur.

Sertindole ⊗

Sertindole levels are predicted to be raised by the protease inhibitors (inhibition of CYP3A4), which may lead to potentially life-threatening torsade de pointes arrhythmias.

Concurrent use is contraindicated.

Antipsychotics + **Quinidine** ⊗

Quinidine appears to double aripiprazole and haloperidol levels. Additive QT-prolonging effects likely, see drugs that prolong the QT interval, page 237.

It may be prudent to avoid the combination. However, if quinidine is given with haloperidol be alert for increased haloperidol adverse effects. The manufacturers of aripiprazole suggest halving its dose.

Antipsychotics + **Quinolones** ⚠

An isolated report describes the development of agitation in an elderly man taking clozapine, tentatively attributed to elevated serum levels caused by an interaction with ciprofloxacin. A study supports this observation. Ciprofloxacin may inhibit olanzapine metabolism, which may result in increased adverse effects. Additive QT-prolonging effects are possible with gatifloxacin, levofloxacin, moxifloxacin, and particularly sparfloxacin, and with the antipsychotics, see drugs that prolong the QT interval, page 237.

Monitor the outcome of concurrent use closely for clozapine adverse effects. The manufacturers of olanzapine recommend a reduced dose. Other quinolones may also interact, see quinolones, page 382.

Antipsychotics + **Rifabutin** ⚠

Rifabutin is predicted to reduce aripiprazole levels.

The manufacturers recommend using double the dose of aripiprazole then titrating to effect. Remember to readjust the dose if rifabutin is stopped.

Antipsychotics + **Rifampicin (Rifampin)** ⚠

Rifampicin is predicted to decrease aripiprazole and quetiapine levels. An isolated report describes a marked fall in the serum levels of a patient taking clozapine when he was given rifampicin. Haloperidol levels appear to be decreased by rifampicin.

Be alert for the need to use an increased dosage of these antipsychotics in the presence of rifampicin. The manufacturers recommend that the dose of aripiprazole should be doubled.

Antipsychotics + **SSRIs**

Pimozide ✕

Pimozide levels are expected to be increased by fluoxetine, fluvoxamine, paroxetine, or sertraline. The use of SSRIs and pimozide has also led to extrapyramidal adverse effects, oculogyric crises and sedation in rare cases.

Raised pimozide levels can cause torsade de pointes arrhythmias, which can be fatal. The manufacturers of pimozide contraindicate its use with SSRIs.

Thioridazine ✕

Thioridazine levels are expected to be increased by fluoxetine, fluvoxamine (225% rise seen), paroxetine, and possibly escitalopram.

The US manufacturers of fluoxetine, fluvoxamine, and paroxetine, contraindicate the concurrent use of as raised levels increase the risk of QT prolongation, see drugs that prolong the QT interval, page 237. The use of thioridazine is also contraindicated for 5 weeks after fluoxetine has been stopped. It has been suggested that the dose of thioridazine may need to be reduced when it is given with escitalopram.

Other antipsychotics ⚠

On the whole no significant adverse interactions appear to occur between most antipsychotics and the SSRIs. However, a number of case reports describe extrapyramidal adverse effects and serotonin syndrome following the use of fluoxetine or paroxetine with an antipsychotic. The levels of some antipsychotics are raised by SSRIs:

- Aripiprazole levels are predicted to be raised by fluoxetine and paroxetine.
- Clozapine and olanzapine levels are raised by fluoxetine, paroxetine, sertraline and possibly citalopram: particularly large increases can occur with fluvoxamine. Toxicity has been seen in some patients.
- Haloperidol levels raised by 20 to 30% by fluoxetine and by 20 to 60% by fluvoxamine.
- Perphenazine levels possibly raised by fluoxetine and paroxetine, which increased extrapyramidal adverse effects in a few cases.
- Risperidone levels raised by fluvoxamine, fluoxetine and paroxetine.
- Sertindole levels are raised 2- to 3-fold by fluoxetine and paroxetine.
- Zotepine levels are raised by fluoxetine (amount unstated).

Where antipsychotic levels are raised monitor the outcome of concurrent use and adjust the doses as necessary. Some have suggested that the antipsychotic dose should be re-evaluated before the SSRI is started. The manufacturers of sertindole suggest that low maintenance doses of sertindole are used and that ECG monitoring is necessary as sertindole can prolong the QT interval. The manufacturers recommend halving the dose of aripiprazole. Note that both groups of drugs lower the seizure threshold.

Antipsychotics + Sucralfate ⚠

Sucralfate can reduce the absorption of sulpiride by about 40%.

Separating dosing by 2 hours appears to minimise this interaction.

Antipsychotics + Tricyclics ❓

Studies and case reports have described increased tricyclic antidepressant levels with phenothiazines. There is currently evidence for this interaction between:

● chlorpromazine and imipramine
● flupentixol and imipramine or desipramine
● fluphenazine and imipramine
● haloperidol and desipramine
● levomepromazine and nortriptyline
● perphenazine and amitriptyline, imipramine, desipramine or nortriptyline
● thioridazine and desipramine, imipramine or nortriptyline

Further, antipsychotic levels may be raised or their clearance reduced by the tricyclics, and this has been seen with:

● doxepin or nortriptyline and tiotixene
● amitriptyline, imipramine or nortriptyline and chlorpromazine

The concurrent use of antipsychotics and tricyclics has also resulted in extrapyramidal reactions and seizures (both groups of drugs lower the seizure threshold). Despite these reactions these drugs are widely used in combination, and a number of fixed-dose combinations have been marketed. Also note that additive QT-prolonging effects are possible with certain combinations, see drugs that prolong the QT interval, page 237.

No action is needed but bear the interaction in mind in case of problems. Additive antimuscarinic adverse effects are also possible. See antimuscarinics, page 78.

Antipsychotics + Valproate ⚠

Sodium valproate can apparently lower serum clozapine and olanzapine levels. The combination of olanzapine and valproate appears to increase the risk of hepatic injury in children.

Monitor the levels of clozapine and adjust the dose as necessary. With olanzapine, it has been suggested that liver enzymes should be monitored every 3 to 4 months for the first year of treatment, thereafter monitoring every 6 months if no adverse effects are detected.

Antipsychotics + Venlafaxine ⚠

Venlafaxine can almost double haloperidol levels. Adverse effects resulting from this interaction have been seen in practice. A retrospective study found that venlafaxine caused a 27% increase in olanzapine levels. The concurrent use of aripiprazole with venlafaxine has led to adverse effects such as the neuroleptic malignant syndrome and extrapyramidal symptoms.

Monitor the outcome closely, being alert for the need to reduce the haloperidol dosage. The clinical significance of the raised olanzapine levels is unclear. Be aware

A

of the possibility of an interaction between aripiprazole and venlafaxine if adverse effects become troublesome.

Apomorphine

Apomorphine + **Metoclopramide** ❌

Metoclopramide is a centrally-acting dopamine antagonist and can oppose the effects of apomorphine, and also worsen Parkinson's disease.

Concurrent use should generally be avoided. Domperidone is the antiemetic of choice in Parkinson's disease.

Aprepitant

Fosaprepitant is a prodrug of aprepitant, and therefore has the potential to interact similarly.

Aprepitant + **Azoles** ⚠

Ketoconazole increases the AUC of aprepitant 5-fold. The manufacturer recommends caution when aprepitant is used with ketoconazole or other strong inhibitors of CYP3A4, such as itraconazole. Fosaprepitant, a prodrug of aprepitant, would be expected to interact similarly.

The lowest dose of aprepitant may be appropriate. Counsel patients about adverse effects (e.g. hiccups, fatigue, constipation, headache).

Aprepitant + **Benzodiazepines** ⚠

Aprepitant inhibits the metabolism of midazolam and doubles the levels of oral midazolam after 5 days of concurrent use. A few days after aprepitant treatment is stopped a transient slight reduction in midazolam plasma levels may occur. Other benzodiazepines metabolised by CYP3A4 (alprazolam, triazolam) would be expected to interact similarly. Aprepitant appears to have less effect on *intravenous* midazolam. Fosaprepitant, a prodrug of aprepitant, would be expected to interact similarly.

Aprepitant may be expected to increase the drowsiness and length of sedation and amnesia in patients given midazolam (and possibly alprazolam or triazolam). Consider reducing the midazolam dose and monitor the outcome of concurrent use carefully.

Aprepitant + **Calcium-channel blockers** ⚠

The concurrent use of aprepitant and diltiazem appears to increase the levels of both drugs by almost 2-fold, although this did not result in any significant cardiovascular effects. Fosaprepitant, a prodrug of aprepitant, would be expected to interact similarly.

The clinical relevance of this interaction is uncertain, however the lowest dose of aprepitant may be appropriate. Be alert for the adverse effects of both drugs.

Aprepitant + Carbamazepine ⊗

Rifampicin, a potent inducer of CYP3A4, reduces the AUC of aprepitant by 91%; reduced efficacy would be expected. Carbamazepine, another potent inducer of CYP3A4, is predicted to interact similarly, both with aprepitant, and its prodrug fosaprepitant.

The UK manufacturer recommends that concurrent use should be avoided.

Aprepitant + Contraceptives ⚠

Aprepitant reduces the levels of ethinylestradiol and norethisterone (given as a combined hormonal contraceptive). Greater effects were seen in another study when dexamethasone was also given with aprepitant. Fosaprepitant, a prodrug of aprepitant, would be expected to interact similarly.

Although the effects of these reduced contraceptive steroid levels on ovulation were not assessed, it is likely that they could result in reduced efficacy. The manufacturer recommends that alternative or additional contraceptive methods should be used during aprepitant therapy and for 2 months (UK advice) or one month (US advice) after the last dose of aprepitant. For general advice on the use of enzyme inducers and contraceptives, see contraceptives, page 199.

Aprepitant + Corticosteroids ⚠

In the short-term, aprepitant increases the AUC of dexamethasone (by about 60%) and methylprednisolone (by up to 2.5-fold). Fosaprepitant, a prodrug of aprepitant, would be expected to interact similarly.

The manufacturer recommends that the usual dose of dexamethasone should be reduced by about 50% when given with aprepitant. In clinical studies a dexamethasone regimen of 12 mg on day one and 8 mg on days 2 to 4 was used, and this is the recommended regimen. They also recommend that the usual dose of intravenous methylprednisolone is reduced by 25%, and the usual oral dose by 50%, in the presence of aprepitant. However, the manufacturer also notes that during continuous treatment with methylprednisolone, levels would be expected to decrease over the following 2 weeks.

Aprepitant + Ergot derivatives ⊗

Aprepitant can increase the levels of the ergot derivatives in the short-term, then reduce them within 2 weeks. Ergotism could occur. Fosaprepitant, a prodrug of aprepitant, would be expected to interact similarly.

The effect may persist for 2 weeks after aprepitant is stopped. Avoid the combination where possible. Concurrent use needs close monitoring.

A

Aprepitant + Herbal medicines or Dietary supplements ✗

Rifampicin, a potent inducer of CYP3A4, reduces the AUC of aprepitant by 91%; reduced efficacy would be expected. St John's wort, another inducer of CYP3A4, is predicted to interact similarly, both with aprepitant, and its prodrug fosaprepitant.

The UK manufacturer recommends that concurrent use should be avoided.

Aprepitant + HRT ❓

Aprepitant reduces the levels of ethinylestradiol and norethisterone (given as a combined hormonal contraceptive). Greater effects were seen in another study when dexamethasone was also given with aprepitant. The hormones in HRT are similar to those used in hormonal contraceptives, and so may be affected by enzyme-inducing drugs in the same way. Note that fosaprepitant, a prodrug of aprepitant, would also be expected to reduce HRT levels.

Consider the possibility of reduced HRT efficacy.

Aprepitant + Macrolides ⚠

Ketoconazole, a potent CYP3A4 inhibitor, increases the AUC of aprepitant 5-fold. The manufacturer recommends caution when aprepitant is used with any potent inhibitor of CYP3A4, (such as clarithromycin and telithromycin). Fosaprepitant, a prodrug of aprepitant, would also be expected to interact with the macrolides in this way.

The lowest dose of aprepitant may be appropriate. Counsel patients about adverse effects (e.g. hiccups, fatigue, constipation, headache). Other macrolides may also interact, although it seems unlikely that they all will, see macrolides, page 310.

Aprepitant + Phenobarbital ✗

Rifampicin, a potent inducer of CYP3A4, reduces the AUC of aprepitant (and probably its prodrug fosaprepitant) by 91%; reduced efficacy would be expected. Phenobarbital (and therefore probably primidone), another potent inducer of CYP3A4, is predicted to interact similarly.

The UK manufacturer recommends that concurrent use should be avoided.

Aprepitant + Phenytoin ✗

The manufacturers say that aprepitant should not be used with phenytoin as the levels of aprepitant and its efficacy are expected to be reduced. Phenytoin levels may also be reduced. Fosaprepitant, a prodrug of aprepitant, would be expected to interact similarly.

Avoid concurrent use. If both drugs are given monitor aprepitant efficacy and phenytoin levels carefully.

Aprepitant + **Protease inhibitors** ⚠

Ketoconazole increases the AUC of aprepitant 5-fold. The manufacturer recommends caution when aprepitant is used with any potent inhibitor of CYP3A4, such as the protease inhibitors ritonavir and nelfinavir. Fosaprepitant, a prodrug of aprepitant, would also be expected to interact with the protease inhibitors in this way.

The lowest dose of aprepitant may be appropriate. Counsel patients about adverse effects (e.g. hiccups, fatigue, constipation, headache).

Aprepitant + **Rifampicin (Rifampin)** ❌

Rifampicin reduced the AUC of aprepitant by 91%, and reduced efficacy would be expected. Fosaprepitant, a prodrug of aprepitant, would be expected to interact similarly.

The UK manufacturer recommends that concurrent use should be avoided.

Aprepitant + **Warfarin and other oral anticoagulants** ⚠

Aprepitant modestly reduces warfarin levels and slightly decreases the INR in healthy subjects. Fosaprepitant, a prodrug of aprepitant, would be expected to interact similarly.

The manufacturer recommends that the INR should be monitored closely for 2 weeks, particularly 7 to 10 days after each 3-day course of aprepitant. They also recommend similar caution with acenocoumarol.

Aspirin

Aspirin + **Contraceptives** ✔

Hormonal contraceptives lower aspirin levels. A few early reports suggest that the very occasional failure of copper IUDs to prevent pregnancy may have been due to an interaction with aspirin, but there is insufficient evidence to warrant avoiding the combination.

No action needed.

Aspirin + **Corticosteroids** ❓

Serum salicylate levels are reduced by corticosteroids, and therefore salicylate levels may rise, possibly to toxic concentrations, if the corticosteroid is withdrawn without salicylate dosage adjustment. Concurrent use increases the risk of gastrointestinal bleeding and ulceration.

Patients taking high-dose salicylates should be monitored to ensure that the levels

A

remain adequate when corticosteroids are added and do not become excessive if they are withdrawn.

Aspirin + **Diuretics**

Loop diuretics ✓

Aspirin may reduce the diuretic effect of bumetanide, furosemide, and piretanide, and the combination of aspirin and furosemide may increase the risk of acute renal failure and salicylate toxicity. The risk of ototoxicity with high doses of salicylates may theoretically be increased by loop diuretics..

The clinical significance of this interaction is unclear. However, aspirin should be avoided in patients with recurrent hospital admissions for worsening heart failure. Be aware that renal impairment and otoxicity are a possibility in patients receiving high dose of salicylates, and consider increasing monitoring for these effects.

Spironolactone ❓

Although studies in healthy subjects have found that the spironolactone-induced loss of sodium in the urine is reduced, a study in hypertensive patients showed that the blood pressure lowering effects of spironolactone were not affected by aspirin.

Concurrent use need not be avoided, but if the diuretic response to spironolactone is less than expected, consider this interaction as a cause.

Aspirin + **Food** ✓

Food delays the absorption of aspirin but does not affect the overall amount absorbed.

Avoid food if rapid analgesia is needed. Otherwise aspirin is better taken with or after food to minimise gastric irritation.

Aspirin + **Gold** ⚠

A study in rheumatoid patients given aspirin suggested that the concurrent use of gold can increase aspirin-induced hepatotoxicity. However, concurrent treatment was more effective than aspirin alone.

Other analgesics, such as fenoprofen appear safer than aspirin (in analgesic doses) so it is probably wise to consider an alternative analgesic.

Aspirin + **Heparin** ❓

Although the concurrent use of aspirin and heparin is effective in the prevention of post-operative thromboembolism, the risk of bleeding in patients receiving heparin is increased almost 2.5-fold by the use of aspirin.

Unless specifically indicated, such as in unstable angina, it may be prudent to avoid the combined use of aspirin with heparin because of the likely increased risk of bleeding. Patients should be monitored closely for signs of bleeding.

Aspirin + **Herbal medicines or Dietary supplements**

Ginkgo biloba ❓

An isolated report describes spontaneous bleeding from the iris associated with the use of aspirin 325 mg daily with a *Ginkgo biloba* extract.

> The evidence is too slim to forbid patients from taking aspirin and *Ginkgo biloba* concurrently, but some do recommend caution. This seems prudent as caution is generally recommended with antiplatelet drugs, and bleeding has been seen with the use of *Ginkgo biloba* alone Medical professionals should be aware of the possibility of increased bleeding tendency with *Ginkgo biloba*.

Tamarindus indica ⚠

Tamarindus indica fruit extract caused a 3-fold increase in the serum levels of aspirin.

> The clinical relevance of this interaction is unknown, but large rises in the aspirin levels may result in toxicity. It therefore seems unlikely to be a problem with low-dose aspirin.

Aspirin + **Kaolin** ✔

Kaolin-pectin causes a small reduction in the absorption of aspirin, which is not clinically relevant.

> No action needed.

Aspirin + **Low-molecular-weight heparins** ❓

Although the concurrent use of aspirin and heparin is effective in the prevention of post-operative thromboembolism, the risk of bleeding in patients receiving heparin is increased almost 2.5-fold by the use of aspirin. Cases of retroperitoneal and spinal haematoma have been reported with concurrent use of low-molecular-weight heparins (e.g. enoxaparin) and aspirin.

> Unless specifically indicated, such as in unstable angina, it may be prudent to avoid the combined use of aspirin with LMWHs because of the likely increased risk of bleeding. Patients should be monitored closely for signs of bleeding.

Aspirin + **Methotrexate** ⚠

Analgesic-dose aspirin slightly reduces the clearance of methotrexate. Concurrent use may increase the incidence of toxicity (pancytopenia, pneumonitis).

> Regular antiplatelet-dose aspirin in patients stabilised on methotrexate seems unlikely to cause a significant problem. With analgesic-dose aspirin the risks are likely to be lowest in those taking low-dose methotrexate for psoriasis or rheumatoid arthritis. Patients should be counselled regarding non-prescription aspirin use. Patients should be told to report any sign or symptom suggestive of infection, particularly sore throat (which might possibly indicate that white cell counts have fallen) or dyspnoea or cough (suggestive of pulmonary toxicity).

A

Aspirin + Metoclopramide ✅

Although some studies have found that metoclopramide increases the rate of aspirin absorption, others have found no change, and the clinical efficacy of aspirin seems unaltered.

> No action needed.

Aspirin + Mifepristone ❓

Theoretically NSAIDs (including aspirin) might reduce the efficacy of mifepristone, and combined use is often not recommended. However, evidence from two studies with naproxen and diclofenac suggests no reduction in mifepristone efficacy.

> Because of theoretical concerns of antagonistic effects, NSAID analgesics have been avoided in protocols for medical abortion. However, the limited available evidence suggests that this might not be necessary.

Aspirin + NSAIDs ❓

There is some evidence that non-selective NSAIDs such as ibuprofen antagonise the antiplatelet effects of low-dose aspirin but that coxibs do not. However, some NSAIDs (particularly coxibs) are also associated with an increased thrombotic/cardiovascular risk. Some epidemiological studies have shown that non-selective NSAIDs reduce the cardioprotective effects of low-dose aspirin. Combined use of NSAIDs (including coxibs) and aspirin, even in low-dose, increases the risk of gastrointestinal bleeds.

> The evidence suggesting antagonism of antiplatelet effects is currently insufficient to recommend a change in practice. The CSM in the UK has advised that the combination of a non-aspirin NSAID and low-dose aspirin should be used only if absolutely necessary, and patients taking long-term aspirin should be reminded to avoid NSAIDs, including those bought without prescription. If antiplatelet dose aspirin is used with NSAIDs, gastroprotection (e.g. a PPI) should be considered, especially when other risk factors (e.g. corticosteroids) are present. There is no clinical rationale for the combined use of anti-inflammatory/analgesic doses of aspirin and NSAIDs, and such use should be avoided.

Aspirin + Phenytoin ✅

No clinically significant interaction appears to occur between phenytoin and aspirin even though aspirin can displace phenytoin from its protein binding sites.

> No action needed.

Aspirin + Probenecid ⚠️

The uricosuric effects of high doses of aspirin or other salicylates and probenecid are paradoxically mutually antagonistic.

> Regular dosing with substantial amounts of salicylates should be avoided, but small very occasional analgesic doses probably do not matter. Serum salicylate levels of 50 to 100 mg/L are necessary before this interaction occurs. Antiplatelet-dose aspirin seems unlikely to interact.

Aspirin + Quinidine ❓

A patient and two healthy subjects given quinidine with aspirin showed a 2- to 3-fold increase in bleeding times. The patient developed petechiae and gastrointestinal bleeding.

This interaction appears to result from the additive effects of the two drugs. Be aware of the potential for this interaction if the combination is used. However, significant interactions seem rare.

Aspirin + SSRIs ❓

The SSRIs may increase the risk of upper gastrointestinal bleeding and the risk appears to be further increased by concurrent aspirin. The overall evidence for an increased risk of bleeding when giving an SSRI with antiplatelet-dose aspirin is conflicting, with some studies demonstrating an increased risk and others suggesting no additional antiplatelet effect occurs.

The manufacturers of the SSRIs warn that patients should be cautioned about the concurrent use of aspirin. Alternatives such as paracetamol (acetaminophen), or less gastrotoxic NSAIDs such as ibuprofen may be considered, but if the combination of an SSRI and NSAID cannot be avoided, prescribing of gastro-protective drugs (such as proton pump inhibitors) should be considered, especially in elderly patients or those with a history of gastrointestinal bleeding.

Aspirin + Sulfinpyrazone ⚠

The uricosuric effects of the salicylates and sulfinpyrazone are paradoxically mutually antagonistic.

Concurrent use for uricosuria should be avoided. Analgesic doses of aspirin as low as 700 mg can cause an appreciable fall in uric acid excretion but the effects of antiplatelet-dose aspirin are probably of little practical importance.

Aspirin + Valproate ❓

Sodium valproate toxicity developed in several patients given large and repeated doses of aspirin and one elderly patient given low-dose aspirin.

Any interaction seems rare. Consider advising patients to monitor for indicators of valproate toxicity (nausea, vomiting, dizziness).

Aspirin + Vitamin C ✓

Aspirin appears to reduce the absorption of vitamin C by about one-third.

The clinical importance of this interaction is unclear, however it has been suggested that normal physiological requirements of vitamin C (30 to 60 mg ascorbic acid daily) may need to be increased to 100 to 200 mg daily.

Aspirin + **Warfarin and other oral anticoagulants** ⚠

High doses of aspirin (4 g daily or more) can increase prothrombin times. It also damages the stomach wall, which increases the risks of bleeding. Low-dose aspirin (75 to 325 mg daily) increases the risk of bleeding when given with warfarin by about 1.5- to 2.5-fold, although, in most studies the absolute risks have been small. Increased warfarin effects have been seen when the salicylates methyl salicylate or trolamine salicylate, were used on the skin.

It is usual to avoid normal analgesic and anti-inflammatory doses of aspirin while taking any anticoagulant. Patients should be told that many non-prescription analgesic, antipyretic, cold and influenza preparations may contain substantial amounts of aspirin. Warn them that it may be listed as acetylsalicylic acid. Paracetamol (acetaminophen) is a safer analgesic substitute. Low-dose aspirin appears to interact to a lesser extent, and where problems are seen it still appears that the benefits of use sometimes outweigh the risks. Any interaction with topical salicylates seems likely to be rare.

Aspirin + **Zafirlukast** ✔

Aspirin 650 mg four times daily increases plasma zafirlukast levels by 45%.

The clinical importance of this interaction awaits assessment but the manufacturers do not recommend an alteration in the zafirlukast dosage.

Atomoxetine

Atomoxetine + **MAOIs** ✖

The manufacturer notes that other drugs that affect brain monoamine levels (like atomoxetine) have caused serious reactions (serotonin syndrome, page 392, neuroleptic malignant syndrome) when taken with MAOIs.

The manufacturer contraindicates the use of atomoxetine during and for 2 weeks after stopping an MAOI.

Atomoxetine + **Mirtazapine** ⚠

Atomoxetine is a sympathomimetic that acts as a noradrenaline reuptake inhibitor. The manufacturers therefore predict that it may have additive or synergistic pharmacological effects with other drugs that affect noradrenaline, such as mirtazapine.

The manufacturer recommends caution. Be aware that additive effects are possible and monitor e.g. somnolence or agitation, as appropriate.

Atomoxetine + **Nasal decongestants** ⚠

Atomoxetine is a sympathomimetic that acts as a noradrenaline reuptake inhibitor. The manufacturers therefore predict that it may have additive or synergistic pharmacological effects with other drugs that affect noradrenaline, such as pseudoephedrine.

> The manufacturer recommends caution. Be aware that additive effects are possible and monitor e.g. somnolence or agitation, as appropriate.

Atomoxetine + Quinidine ⚠

Paroxetine increases the AUC and levels of atomoxetine by 6.5-fold and 3.5-fold, respectively by inhibiting its metabolism by CYP2D6. Quinidine, also a CYP2D6 inhibitor, is expected to interact similarly.

> The atomoxetine dose should be titrated slowly with the dose increased only if symptoms fail to improve and if the initial dose is well tolerated. The UK manufacturers say that the initial dose should be maintained for a minimum of 7 days before considering an increase.

Atomoxetine + Salbutamol (Albuterol) and related bronchodilators ⚠

Atomoxetine potentiated the increase in heart rate and blood pressure caused by salbutamol infusions in one study, but another study found no adverse interaction.

> The manufacturers recommend caution when atomoxetine is given to patients receiving intravenous, oral, or high-dose nebulised salbutamol or other beta$_2$ agonists. Monitor heart rate and blood pressure carefully in the initial stages of combined use.

Atomoxetine + SSRIs ⚠

Paroxetine increases the AUC and levels of atomoxetine by 6.5-fold and 3.5-fold, respectively. Fluoxetine interacts similarly.

> The atomoxetine dose should be titrated slowly. The UK manufacturers say that the initial dose should be maintained for a minimum of 7 days before considering an increase.

Atomoxetine + Terbinafine ⚠

Paroxetine increases the AUC and levels of atomoxetine by 6.5-fold and 3.5-fold, respectively by inhibiting its metabolism by CYP2D6. Terbinafine, also a CYP2D6 inhibitor, is expected to interact similarly.

> The atomoxetine dose should be titrated slowly with the dose increased only if symptoms fail to improve and if the initial dose is well tolerated. The UK manufacturers say that the initial dose should be maintained for a minimum of 7 days before considering an increase.

Atomoxetine + Tricyclics ⚠

Atomoxetine is a sympathomimetic that acts as a noradrenaline reuptake inhibitor.

A

The manufacturers therefore predict that it may have additive or synergistic pharmacological effects with other drugs that affect noradrenaline, such as imipramine, and other tricyclics.

The manufacturer recommends caution. Be aware that additive effects are possible and monitor e.g. somnolence or agitation, as appropriate.

Atomoxetine + Venlafaxine ⚠

Atomoxetine is a sympathomimetic that acts as a noradrenaline reuptake inhibitor. The manufacturers therefore predict that it may have additive or synergistic pharmacological effects with other drugs that affect noradrenaline, such as venlafaxine.

The manufacturer recommends caution. Be aware that additive effects are possible and monitor e.g. somnolence or agitation, as appropriate.

Atovaquone

Atovaquone + Food ⚠

Taking atovaquone (tablets or suspension) with fatty food markedly increases its AUC by 2- to 3-fold.

Atovaquone/proguanil tablets should be taken with food or an enteral supplement, and atovaquone suspension should be taken with food. Monitor patients who are unable to tolerate taking atovaquone with food for treatment failure; consider intravenous treatment in the case of Pneumocystis pneumonia.

Atovaquone + Metoclopramide ❓

Metoclopramide appears to halve the levels of atovaquone.

It has been suggested that metoclopramide should be given only if other antiemetics are unavailable, and, if it is used, that parasitaemia should be closely monitored.

Atovaquone + NRTIs ⚠

Atovaquone inhibits the glucuronidation of zidovudine, but this only resulted in a small 25% decrease in its clearance in one study, and no significant pharmacokinetic changes in another.

The increased plasma levels of zidovudine are unlikely to be clinically significant. Nevertheless, the manufacturers recommend regular monitoring for zidovudine-associated adverse effects, particularly if atovaquone suspension is used, as this achieves higher atovaquone levels.

Atovaquone + **Protease inhibitors** ⚠

Atovaquone decreases the minimum serum levels of indinavir by almost 25%.

The manufacturers recommend caution because of the potential risk of indinavir treatment failure. However, the effect on indinavir was small, and indinavir is usually used with other antiretrovirals, which might modify the interaction.

Atovaquone + **Rifabutin** ❓

In one study the concurrent use of atovaquone and rifabutin resulted in a 34% decrease in the AUC of atovaquone and a small 19% decrease in rifabutin levels.

It has been suggested that no atovaquone dosage adjustment is needed. However, in the UK, the manufacturer of atovaquone still considers that rifabutin use could result in subtherapeutic atovaquone levels and so they advise against the use of this combination.

Atovaquone + **Rifampicin (Rifampin)** ⚠

Rifampicin reduces serum atovaquone levels by about 50% whereas atovaquone modestly raises serum rifampicin levels.

The combination should be avoided because of the likelihood of sub-therapeutic atovaquone levels.

Atovaquone + **Tetracyclines** ⚠

Tetracycline reduces the plasma levels of atovaquone by about 40%.

The manufacturers suggest that parasitaemia should be closely monitored in patients taking atovaquone/proguanil and tetracycline. In the UK, they also say that tetracycline should be given with caution to patients taking atovaquone for Pneumocystis pneumonia.

Azathioprine

Azathioprine is rapidly and extensively metabolised to mercaptopurine. Mercaptopurine is therefore expected to share the interactions of azathioprine.

Azathioprine + **Balsalazide** ⚠

The haematological toxicity of azathioprine and mercaptopurine may be increased by 5-aminosalicylates, although balsalazide may be less likely to interact.

Full blood counts should be monitored if azathioprine or mercaptopurine is used. If any abnormalities arise, consider this interaction as a possible cause.

A

Azathioprine + **Co-trimoxazole** ⚠

There is some evidence that the risk of haematological toxicity may be increased in renal transplant patients taking azathioprine if they are also given co-trimoxazole or trimethoprim, particularly if both drugs are taken for extended periods. However, other evidence suggests that the drugs may be used together safely, and the combination is commonly used in practice. Azathioprine is rapidly and extensively metabolised to mercaptopurine. Mercaptopurine is therefore expected to interact similarly.

Full blood count should be monitored if azathioprine or mercaptopurine is used. If any abnormalities arise, consider this interaction as a possible cause.

Azathioprine + **Leflunomide** ✖

The manufacturers say that the concurrent use of leflunomide and azathioprine has not yet been studied but it would be expected to increase the risk of serious adverse reactions (haematological toxicity or hepatotoxicity). Azathioprine is rapidly and extensively metabolised to mercaptopurine. Mercaptopurine is therefore expected to interact similarly.

The manufacturers advise avoiding concurrent use. As the active metabolite of leflunomide has a long half-life of 1 to 4 weeks, a washout with colestyramine or activated charcoal should be given if patients are to be switched to other DMARDs.

Azathioprine + **Mesalazine (Mesalamine)** ⚠

The haematological toxicity of azathioprine and mercaptopurine may be increased by mesalazine.

Full blood counts should be monitored if azathioprine or mercaptopurine is used. If any abnormalities arise, consider this interaction as a possible cause.

Azathioprine + **Mycophenolate** ✖

The manufacturers have recommended that mycophenolate should not be given with azathioprine because they say that concurrent use has not been studied and both drugs have the potential to cause bone marrow suppression. Azathioprine is rapidly and extensively metabolised to mercaptopurine. Mercaptopurine is therefore expected to interact similarly.

Avoid concurrent use.

Azathioprine + **Olsalazine** ⚠

The haematological toxicity of azathioprine and mercaptopurine may be increased by olsalazine.

Full blood counts should be monitored if azathioprine or mercaptopurine is used. If any abnormalities arise, consider this interaction as a possible cause.

Azathioprine + Sulfasalazine ⚠️

The haematological toxicity of azathioprine and mercaptopurine may be increased by sulfasalazine.

> Full blood counts should be monitored if azathioprine or mercaptopurine is used. If any abnormalities arise, consider this interaction as a possible cause.

Azathioprine + Sulfonamides ⚠️

There is some evidence that the risk of haematological toxicity may be increased in renal transplant patients taking azathioprine if they are also given co-trimoxazole (which contains the sulfonamide, sulfamethoxazole), particularly if both drugs are taken for extended periods. However, other evidence suggests that the drugs may be used together safely, and the combination is commonly used in practice. Azathioprine is rapidly and extensively metabolised to mercaptopurine. Mercaptopurine is therefore expected to interact similarly.

> Full blood count should be monitored if azathioprine or mercaptopurine is used. If any abnormalities arise, consider this interaction as a possible cause.

Azathioprine + Trimethoprim ⚠️

There is some evidence that the risk of haematological toxicity may be increased in renal transplant patients taking azathioprine if they are also given trimethoprim, particularly if both drugs are taken for extended periods. However, other evidence suggests that the drugs may be used together safely, and the combination is commonly used in practice. Azathioprine is rapidly and extensively metabolised to mercaptopurine. Mercaptopurine is therefore expected to interact similarly.

> Full blood count should be monitored if azathioprine or mercaptopurine is used. If any abnormalities arise, consider this interaction as a possible cause.

Azathioprine + Vaccines ⚠️

The immune response of the body is suppressed by cytotoxic antineoplastics. The effectiveness of vaccines may be poor and generalised infection may occur in patients immunised with live vaccines. In one study the antibody response to pneumococcal vaccination was reduced by 60% in patients receiving antineoplastics, and suboptimal responses to influenza and measles vaccines have been reported.

> Extreme care should be taken when considering vaccinating immunosuppressed patients, especially with live vaccines, which should generally be avoided. Monitor the immune response to other types of vaccine. Consider whether vaccination can be carried out before or after azathioprine or mercaptopurine use.

Azathioprine + Warfarin and other oral anticoagulants ⚠️

Azathioprine appears to increase warfarin requirements, and cases of bleeding have occurred when azathioprine is stopped. Dose increases of up to 4-fold have been needed. Mercaptopurine appears to interact similarly with acenocoumarol.

A

Monitor the anticoagulant effect if azathioprine or mercaptopurine is added or withdrawn and adjust the warfarin dose as necessary. Similar precautions would seem necessary with any coumarin.

Azoles

The azole antifungals are potent enzyme inhibitors, but they do not all affect the same isoenzymes. This explains their differing interaction profiles.

- Fluconazole is a potent inhibitor of CYP2C9 and CYP2C19, and generally only inhibits CYP3A4 at high doses (greater than 200 mg daily). Interactions are less likely with single doses used for genital candidiasis than with longer term use.
- Itraconazole and its major metabolite, hydroxy-itraconazole, are potent inhibitors of CYP3A4.
- Ketoconazole is a potent inhibitor of CYP3A4.
- Miconazole is a potent inhibitor of CYP2C9.
- Posaconazole is an inhibitor of CYP3A4.
- Voriconazole is an inhibitor of CYP2C9, CYP2C19 and CYP3A4.

A number of other azole antifungals are only used topically in the form of skin creams or intravaginal preparations, and are not usually been associated with drug interactions, presumably because their systemic absorption is so low. Fluconazole, ketoconazole and voriconazole have been associated with prolongation of the QT interval, although generally not to a clinically relevant extent. However, they may also raise the levels of other drugs that prolong the QT interval, and these combinations are often contraindicated.

Azoles + **Benzodiazepines**

Midazolam and Triazolam A

Fluconazole, itraconazole, and ketoconazole very markedly increase the bioavailability of oral midazolam and triazolam (AUCs increased by 3.5-fold to about 15-fold), thereby increasing and prolonging their sedative and amnesic effects.

Expect increased and prolonged sedation. It may be prudent to reduce the dose of midazolam or triazolam by at least 50% with fluconazole and by 75% with itraconazole or ketoconazole. Other azoles are likely to interact similarly.

Other benzodiazepines A

The effects of the benzodiazepines may be increased and prolonged by azole antifungals. Moderate interactions have been seen between alprazolam and itraconazole or ketoconazole, brotizolam and itraconazole, or zolpidem and ketoconazole.

The deepness of sleep and its duration may be increased. Monitor the outcome of concurrent use and consider decreasing the benzodiazepine or zolpidem dose.

Azoles + Bexarotene ❓

The manufacturers say that, in theory, itraconazole and ketoconazole may possibly raise bexarotene levels.

This interaction does not appear to have been studied in patients, so the clinical importance of these predictions are unknown.

Azoles + Bosentan ❌

Ketoconazole increases bosentan levels 2-fold, but the clinical significance of this is unclear. Fluconazole and voriconazole are predicted to have a greater effect.

As elevated bosentan levels are associated with an increased risk of liver toxicity the manufacturers do not recommend the concurrent use of azoles (particularly fluconazole). If the combination is used it may be prudent to monitor liver function closely. The manufacturers suggest that no dosage adjustment is likely to be required if ketoconazole were to be used with bosentan.

Azoles + Buspirone ⚠

The plasma levels of buspirone are markedly increased by itraconazole (13-fold). Ketoconazole is predicted to interact similarly.

The manufacturers recommend reducing the buspirone dose to 2.5 mg either daily or twice daily if these azoles are used.

Azoles + Busulfan ⚠

Itraconazole reduces the clearance of busulfan by a modest 20%. There is some limited evidence that ketoconazole may increase the risk of hepatic veno-occlusive disease in those given high-dose busulfan.

Although the rise in levels is only moderate, it would be prudent to monitor for busulfan toxicity. Fluconazole appears not to interact, and so may be a useful alternative.

Azoles + Calcium-channel blockers

Felodipine, Lercanidipine or Nisoldipine ❌

Itraconazole (and therefore probably ketoconazole) can markedly raise the serum levels of felodipine (by up to about 8-fold), which increases its adverse effects, in particular ankle and leg swelling. Ketoconazole raises the levels of lercanidipine and nisoldipine (peak plasma levels increased by roughly 10-fold).

Concurrent use is contraindicated.

Other calcium-channel blockers ❌

A few case reports suggest that isradipine and nifedipine can interact similarly with itraconazole, and that fluconazole can also interact with nifedipine. The manufacturers of nimodipine predict that the azoles will increase nimodipine levels.

A

Monitor the outcome of concurrent use, being prepared to reduce the dose of calcium-channel blocker as necessary.

Azoles + **Carbamazepine**

Fluconazole, Ketoconazole, or Miconazole ⚠

Carbamazepine toxicity has been caused by fluconazole and miconazole, and carbamazepine levels may be raised by 30% by ketoconazole.

Evidence is limited. Nevertheless, monitor for signs of carbamazepine toxicity, which may present as nausea, vomiting, ataxia or drowsiness. Consider monitoring carbamazepine levels and adjust the dose if necessary.

Itraconazole, Posaconazole, or Voriconazole ✖

Carbamazepine, either alone or when given with phenobarbital or phenytoin, has been shown to decrease itraconazole levels resulting in treatment failure. Carbamazepine is predicted to decrease posaconazole and voriconazole levels.

Concurrent use should be avoided unless the benefits are expected to outweigh the risks, although note that the use of voriconazole is specifically contraindicated. If concurrent use is necessary it seems likely that the antifungal dose will need to be increased. It would seem prudent to use other alternatives wherever possible or monitor efficacy very closely.

Azoles + **Ciclosporin (Cyclosporine)**

Posaconazole ⚠

Three heart transplant patients required ciclosporin dose reductions of about 15 to 30% when posaconazole was added. The manufacturers also report cases of ciclosporin toxicity which resulted in significant adverse effects, including nephrotoxicity and one case of fatal leukoencephalopathy.

The manufacturers suggest that the dose of ciclosporin should be reduced by about 25% when posaconazole is started, with careful monitoring of ciclosporin levels and further dose adjustment as needed.

Voriconazole ⚠

Voriconazole increases the AUC of ciclosporin in stable renal transplant patients by between about 1.7- and 2.5-fold.

The dose of ciclosporin should be halved when initiating voriconazole, and ciclosporin levels should be carefully monitored during treatment. The ciclosporin dose should be increased again when voriconazole is withdrawn.

Other azoles ⚠

Ciclosporin levels may be increased by some azole antifungals. The effects seem variable and may be affected by dose, ethnicity and gender. The azoles implicated are fluconazole (up to 2-fold increase in ciclosporin levels), itraconazole (ciclosporin dose reductions of about 80% needed), ketoconazole (ciclosporin dose reductions of up to

85% needed), and miconazole (65% rise in ciclosporin levels). However, many patients may not be affected.

Ciclosporin levels and/or effects (e.g. on renal function) should be monitored as a matter of routine, but it may be prudent to increase monitoring if these azoles are stopped, started, or if the doses are altered.

Azoles + Cilostazol ⚠

Ketoconazole increases the AUC of cilostazol by more than 2-fold. Itraconazole is predicted to interact similarly. Fluconazole and miconazole may also interact, but probably to a lesser extent.

The US manufacturers suggest halving the dose of cilostazol in the presence of itraconazole or ketoconazole. However, the UK manufacturers contraindicate the concurrent use of CYP3A4 inhibitors (which could be taken to mean all of the azoles).

Azoles + Cinacalcet ⚠

Ketoconazole raises cinacalcet levels 2-fold and increased the incidence of cinacalcet adverse effects. Itraconazole and voriconazole are predicted to interact similarly.

It may be prudent to monitor parathyroid hormone and serum calcium more frequently if any of these azoles is started or stopped.

Azoles + Co-artemether ✅

Ketoconazole doubled the AUC of artemether and lumefantrine in one study. However, this is within is within the range of inter-individual variability and no changes in ECG parameters or increases in adverse events were reported.

This increase is unlikely to be clinically relevant, and no dosage adjustment is necessary when co-artemether is used with ketoconazole.

Azoles + Contraceptives ✅

There are isolated reports of breakthrough bleeding and failure of combined oral contraceptives with fluconazole, itraconazole and ketoconazole. Conversely, both fluconazole and itraconazole have been shown to modestly *increase* serum levels of contraceptive steroids.

Although anecdotal reports suggest that these antifungals can rarely make hormonal contraception less reliable, the pharmacokinetic data suggest that, if anything, an *enhanced* effect of the combined hormonal contraceptives is likely. Note that, of all the drugs proven to decrease the efficacy of combined hormonal contraceptives, all have also been shown to decrease the steroid levels. Furthermore, the manufacturers do not advise any special precautions when taking oral contraceptives and azoles. However, some consider that the data warrant consideration being given to the use of additional contraceptive measures. The theoretical teratogenic risk from these azoles may have a bearing on this.

A

Azoles + **Corticosteroids** ⚠

There is some evidence that itraconazole can increase the levels and/or effects of the active metabolite of ciclesonide, oral deflazacort, dexamethasone, methylprednisolone, and to a lesser extent, prednisolone and prednisone, as well as inhaled budesonide and fluticasone. Similarly, ketoconazole reduces the metabolism and clearance of methylprednisolone, increases the serum levels of the active metabolite of ciclesonide, modestly increases the systemic effect of inhaled budesonide and possibly inhaled fluticasone, and markedly increases the AUC of oral budesonide.

> Dose reductions of up to 50% have been recommended if ketoconazole is given with methylprednisolone, but it would seem prudent to monitor the outcome of concurrent use of any of the combinations and adjust the dose according to the patients' response. Be alert for evidence of adrenal suppression (e.g. moonface, flushing, increased bruising and acne). The concurrent use of oral budesonide and ketoconazole is not recommended by the manufacturers. The manufacturers of ciclesonide suggest that the concurrent use of ketoconazole or itraconazole should be avoided unless the benefits outweigh the risks.

Azoles + **Cyclophosphamide** ⚠

Fluconazole and itraconazole inhibit the metabolism of cyclophosphamide. There is some evidence that, compared with fluconazole, itraconazole might increase cyclophosphamide toxicity.

> Until more is known it may be prudent to encourage caution when azoles are used in patients taking cyclophosphamide (other than therapies established in randomised clinical studies) being alert for unexpected toxicity.

Azoles + **Darifenacin**

Fluconazole ⚠

Fluconazole almost doubles darifenacin levels.

> The UK manufacturers recommend that the dose of darifenacin is limited to 7.5 mg daily. The US manufacturers suggest that no dosage adjustment is needed.

Itraconazole and Ketoconazole ❌

Ketoconazole markedly increases the AUC of darifenacin by up to 10-fold. Itraconazole is predicted to interact similarly.

> The UK manufacturers contraindicate concurrent use with potent CYP3A4 inhibitors whereas the US manufacturers recommend that the daily dose of darifenacin is limited to 7.5 mg daily. It may be prudent to assess adverse effects in these patients, and withdraw the drug if it is not tolerated.

Azoles + **Digoxin** ⚠

Itraconazole can cause a marked increase in digoxin levels (usually doubled, but a 6-fold increase was seen in one case). Toxicity may occur unless the digoxin dosage is suitably reduced. Voriconazole and posaconazole may interact similarly.

Monitor concurrent use for digoxin toxicity (e.g. bradycardia or nausea), taking digoxin levels as necessary. Adjust the dose accordingly. Note that, based on the interaction with itraconazole, the manufacturer of posaconazole advises monitoring digoxin levels.

Azoles + Diuretics

Eplerenone with Fluconazole 🛆

Fluconazole increases the AUC of eplerenone by 2.2-fold.

The dose of eplerenone should not exceed 25 mg. Monitor for an increase in dose-related adverse effects such as hyperkalaemia.

Eplerenone with Itraconazole or Ketoconazole ✕

Ketoconazole increases the AUC of eplerenone by 5.4-fold. Itraconazole is predicted to interact similarly.

Concurrent use of either itraconazole or ketoconazole is contraindicated.

Hydrochlorothiazide with Fluconazole ✔

A very brief report describes a 40% increase in fluconazole serum levels in a small group of healthy subjects also given hydrochlorothiazide.

It has been suggested that the fluconazole dose need not be altered, but bear this interaction in mind in case of an unexpected response to treatment.

Azoles + Donepezil ✔

Ketoconazole raises the maximum serum levels and AUC of donepezil by about 25%, which was not considered to be clinically relevant.

Despite this finding the manufacturer recommends that donepezil should be used with ketoconazole or itraconazole with care.

Azoles + Dopamine agonists ❓

Two patients taking cabergoline had improvements in their Parkinson's disease symptoms while taking itraconazole. In one case a 300% increase in cabergoline levels occurred, and the other patient reduced the dose of her medications without adversely affecting disease control.

It would be prudent to monitor toxicity and efficacy in any patient taking cabergoline with itraconazole, or similar potent inhibitors of CYP3A4 such as ketoconazole.

Azoles + Dutasteride 🛆

Potent CYP3A4 inhibitors (itraconazole, ketoconazole) may cause a clinically significant rise in dutasteride levels.

A

The manufacturers suggest reducing the dosing frequency if increased dutasteride adverse effects occur.

Azoles + **Ergot derivatives** ✖

Ketoconazole, itraconazole, posaconazole and voriconazole may increase the levels of ergot derivatives such as ergotamine, dihydroergotamine, and methysergide, which may result in ergotism. Other azoles, such as fluconazole, may interact similarly, although to a lesser extent.

The UK manufacturers of various ergot derivatives contraindicate use with all azole antifungals. The US manufacturers of ergotamine and dihydroergotamine advise caution with fluconazole and clotrimazole, which are moderate CYP3A4 inhibitors. Any patient taking an ergot derivative with an azole should be closely monitored for signs of ergotism.

Azoles + **Food** ❓

Some foods increase the absorption of itraconazole capsules or tablets, but appears to decrease the bioavailability of itraconazole solution. Studies with ketoconazole have shown little effect of food on absorption although one found a decrease. Food increases the bioavailability of posaconazole suspension. The bioavailability of voriconazole is modestly reduced by food.

Itraconazole capsules are best taken with or after food, whereas the acidic solution should be taken at least 1 hour before food. Similarly, posaconazole should be taken with food. A confusing and conflicting picture is presented by the studies with ketoconazole; however, one manufacturer of ketoconazole says that it should always be taken with meals. The manufacturers of voriconazole recommend that it should be taken at least one hour before or at least one to two hours after a meal. Food does not appear to affect fluconazole capsules. Cola drinks may increase itraconazole and ketoconazole bioavailability, see H$_2$-receptor antagonists, below, and proton pump inhibitors, page 120.

Azoles + **Galantamine** ⚠

Ketoconazole increases the bioavailability of galantamine by 30%, which is predicted to increase galantamine adverse effects (e.g. nausea and vomiting).

A clinically significant interaction is not expected, however a decrease in the galantamine maintenance dose should be considered in patients who develop galantamine adverse effects.

Azoles + **H$_2$-receptor antagonists** ⚠

H$_2$-receptor antagonists reduce the absorption of itraconazole (AUC reduced by about 50%), ketoconazole (AUC reduced by 60% and even 95% in some reports) and posaconazole (AUC reduced by about 40%).

The manufacturers recommend that if H$_2$-receptor antagonists are used, itracona-zole and ketoconazole should be given with an acidic drink (such as cola), which increase their bioavailability. Posaconazole may also be given with an acidic drink to improve its bioavailability with H$_2$-receptor antagonists. However, the manufacturers currently recommend avoiding concurrent use. Fluconazole and voriconazole do not appear to interact and may therefore be suitable alternatives in some cases.

Azoles + Herbal medicines or Dietary supplements ❌

Two weeks of treatment with St John's wort (*Hypericum perforatum*) halved the levels of a single dose of voriconazole.

Patients requiring voriconazole should be asked about current or recent use of St John's wort, since they may be at risk of treatment failure. Monitor carefully. The manufacturers contraindicate concurrent use.

Azoles + Imatinib ❓

Ketoconazole increases the AUC of imatinib by 40%. Voriconazole increased imatinib levels 2-fold in one patient. The manufacturers of imatinib predict that itraconazole will interact similarly.

Caution is warranted on concurrent use, being alert for increased imatinib adverse effects.

Azoles + Isoniazid ⚠

Ketoconazole levels can be reduced by 50 to 80% by *rifampicin* (*rifampin*), and there seems to be a modest additional effect when isoniazid is also given.

Monitor efficacy closely and consider increasing the dose of ketoconazole if required. It may be prudent to consider an alternative antifungal.

Azoles + Leflunomide ⚠

A woman developed fatal hepatotoxicity after taking itraconazole with leflunomide.

The general importance of this case is unknown but it highlights the need to follow the recommended hepatic monitoring for leflunomide.

Azoles + Macrolides ⚠

Although some pharmacokinetic interactions occur between the azoles and macrolides, most do not appear to be of clinical significance. However, clarithromycin appears to almost double itraconazole levels, and ketoconazole may almost double telithromycin levels.

Monitor the effects of concurrent use of these azoles with clarithromycin or telithromycin. Consider either reducing the dose of the affected drug if adverse effects occur or using a different combination.

A

Azoles + Mefloquine ⚠

Ketoconazole increases the AUC of mefloquine by 79%. Itraconazole may interact similarly.

The clinical relevance of this is uncertain, but it may be prudent to exercise caution on concurrent use in case of an increase in adverse events.

Azoles + Mirtazapine ⚠

Ketoconazole is reported to increase the peak plasma levels and AUC of mirtazapine by about 30% and 45%, respectively.

The manufacturers of mirtazapine advise caution on concurrent use with itraconazole or ketoconazole. Monitor for adverse effects (e.g. oedema, sedation).

Azoles + NNRTIs

Delavirdine with Ketoconazole ⚠

Ketoconazole appears to raise the serum levels of delavirdine by 50%.

The clinical significance of this interaction is unclear. Monitor concurrent use for delavirdine adverse effects.

Delavirdine with Posaconazole ⚠

Any interaction between posaconazole and the NNRTIs is not established but the manufacturers reasonably predict that NNRTI levels may be increased.

Monitor for delavirdine adverse effects.

Delavirdine with Voriconazole ⚠

Voriconazole is predicted to increase delavirdine levels, and delavirdine is predicted to increase voriconazole levels.

The manufacturers suggest that patients be carefully monitored for evidence of drug toxicity and/or loss of efficacy during concurrent use.

Efavirenz with Itraconazole ⚠

Efavirenz decreased the maximum plasma levels and the AUC of itraconazole by 37% and 39%, respectively. The pharmacokinetics of efavirenz were not affected by itraconazole.

The manufacturers of efavirenz say that alternatives to itraconazole should be considered. If there are no appropriate alternatives, it might be prudent to increase the dose of itraconazole, with increased monitoring for efficacy and toxicity of the combination.

Efavirenz with Ketoconazole ⚠

Efavirenz is predicted to interact in the same way as nevirapine with ketoconazole, below.

Efavirenz with Posaconazole ⚠

Any interaction between posaconazole and the NNRTIs is not established but the manufacturers reasonably predict that NNRTI levels may be increased.

Monitor for efavirenz adverse effects.

Efavirenz with Voriconazole ⚠

Efavirenz decreases voriconazole levels, and voriconazole increases efavirenz levels.

The manufacturers contraindicate concurrent use unless the doses of both drugs are adjusted. The recommendation is to double the usual dose of voriconazole to 400 mg twice daily, and to halve the usual efavirenz dose to 300 mg once daily.

Nevirapine with Fluconazole ⚠

Fluconazole appears to double the exposure to nevirapine.

Caution is warranted. Monitor the effects of nevirapine carefully.

Nevirapine with Itraconazole ⚠

Nevirapine is expected to reduce itraconazole levels.

Monitor itraconazole efficacy carefully and anticipate the need to increase the dose.

Nevirapine with Ketoconazole ⚠

Ketoconazole raises nevirapine plasma levels by 15 to 28% and nevirapine lowers the ketoconazole AUC by about 72%.

The manufacturers of nevirapine suggest that ketoconazole should be avoided.

Nevirapine with Posaconazole ⚠

Any interaction between posaconazole and the NNRTIs is not established but the manufacturers reasonably predict that NNRTI levels may be increased.

Monitor for nevirapine adverse effects.

Nevirapine with Voriconazole ⚠

Voriconazole is predicted to increase levels of nevirapine whereas nevirapine is predicted to decrease voriconazole levels.

The manufacturers suggest that patients be carefully monitored for evidence of drug toxicity and/or loss of efficacy during concurrent use.

Azoles + NRTIs

Didanosine ⚠

Itraconazole levels may become undetectable if buffered didanosine is taken at the same time. In one case this resulted in treatment failure. A similar interaction would be expected with ketoconazole.

A

Itraconazole and ketoconazole should be taken at least 2 hours before buffered didanosine. Consider changing to enteric-coated didanosine as it does not appear to affect absorption of these azoles.

Zidovudine ❓

In one study fluconazole increased the AUC of zidovudine by 74% but other studies have found that fluconazole causes only slight changes in zidovudine pharmacokinetics. Increased zidovudine levels, thought to be caused by itraconazole, have been seen in two cases.

Be aware that concurrent use may rarely result in zidovudine toxicity.

Azoles + NSAIDs ⚠

Fluconazole increases the AUC of celecoxib by 130%. The AUC of the active metabolite of parecoxib (valdecoxib) is increased by 62% by fluconazole.

The manufacturers recommend that half the dose of celecoxib should be used in patients taking fluconazole. A dose reduction of parecoxib is recommended in patients taking fluconazole.

Azoles + Opioids

Alfentanil or Fentanyl ⚠

Some patients experience prolonged and increased alfentanil effects if they are also given fluconazole. There is a single case report of opioid toxicity when itraconazole was given to a patient with a fentanyl patch.

Be alert for evidence of prolonged alfentanil or fentanyl effects and respiratory depression. Consider using smaller doses of alfentanil.

Buprenorphine ⚠

Ketoconazole increased the maximum serum levels and AUC of buprenorphine by about 70% and 50%, respectively.

The buprenorphine dose should be halved when starting treatment with ketoconazole.

Methadone ⚠

Fluconazole may increase the levels and AUC of methadone by about 30%; a single case reports opioid toxicity. Ketoconazole and voriconazole appear to interact with methadone to a greater extent (methadone levels raised by 50% or more).

Patients given these azoles with methadone should be monitored for signs of opioid toxicity and a methadone dose alteration should be considered. However, note that the interaction with fluconazole is considered unlikely to be of general clinical significance.

Azoles + **Phenobarbital**

Itraconazole, Posaconazole, or Voriconazole ❌

Phenobarbital (given with carbamazepine or phenytoin) has been shown to decrease itraconazole levels resulting in treatment failure. Phenobarbital is predicted to decrease posaconazole and voriconazole levels. Note that primidone is metabolised to phenobarbital and therefore may interact similarly with these azoles.

> Concurrent use should be avoided unless the benefits are expected to outweigh the risks, although note that the manufacturers contraindicate the use of voriconazole. If concurrent use is necessary it seems likely that the antifungal dose will need to be increased. It would seem prudent to use other alternatives wherever possible or monitor concurrent use very closely.

Ketoconazole ⚠️

Phenobarbital (with phenytoin) has reduced the levels of ketoconazole and its antifungal effects in some patients. Note that primidone is metabolised to phenobarbital and therefore may interact similarly.

> Be alert for any signs of a reduced antifungal response. Consider adjusting the dose of ketoconazole.

Azoles + **Phenytoin**

Fluconazole, or Miconazole ⚠️

Phenytoin toxicity has been seen in some patients given fluconazole or miconazole. Phenytoin may reduce fluconazole levels. Fosphenytoin, a prodrug of phenytoin, may interact similarly.

> Toxicity can develop within 2 to 7 days. Monitor serum phenytoin levels closely and reduce the dosage appropriately. Also be alert for any evidence of reduced antifungal effects and consider increasing the dose. Note that, at high doses, miconazole oral gel has the potential to interact.

Itraconazole or Ketoconazole ❌

Phenytoin reduces itraconazole levels (by about 90%). Ketoconazole may interact similarly with phenytoin, and fosphenytoin, a prodrug of phenytoin, may interact similarly with these azoles.

> Concurrent use of phenytoin and itraconazole (and probably ketoconazole) should be avoided unless the benefits are expected to outweigh the risks. It seems highly likely that these azoles will be ineffective.

Posaconazole or Voriconazole ⚠️

Phenytoin decreases the levels of voriconazole and posaconazole by about 50%. Also, voriconazole increases the maximum serum levels and AUC of phenytoin by 67% and 81%, respectively. Potentially clinically significant increases in phenytoin levels have been reported in some patients taking posaconazole. Fosphenytoin, a prodrug of phenytoin, may interact similarly.

> Concurrent use should be avoided unless the benefits outweigh the risks. If both

A

drugs are used be alert for evidence of phenytoin toxicity (blurred vision, nystagmus, ataxia or drowsiness) and, if necessary, adjust the dose based on phenytoin levels. The dose of oral voriconazole should be increased from 200 to 400 mg twice daily, or from 100 mg to 200 mg twice daily in patients who weigh less than 40 kg, and intravenous voriconazole should be increased from 4 to 5 mg/kg twice daily. Similarly, consideration should be given to increasing the posaconazole dose.

Azoles + **Phosphodiesterase type-5 inhibitors** ⊗

Ketoconazole markedly raises the levels of tadalafil and very markedly raises the levels of vardenafil. There is some evidence that ketoconazole also reduces sildenafil clearance. Itraconazole is predicted to interact similarly. Other azole antifungals that are potent inhibitors of CYP3A4 such as posaconazole and voriconazole would also be expected to interact similarly.

The manufacturers of sildenafil recommend that a starting dose of 25 mg of sildenafil should be used for treating erectile dysfunction. The manufacturers say that the use of sildenafil for pulmonary hypertension is contraindicated (UK) or not recommended (US) with ketoconazole or itraconazole. If itraconazole or ketoconazole is given with tadalafil, decrease the dose of tadalafil if adverse effects become troublesome. The US manufacturer advises that the dose of tadalafil should not exceed 10 mg in a 72-hour period, or 2.5 mg daily for patients taking ketoconazole (and therefore probably itraconazole). The UK manufacturer of vardenafil advises avoiding the concurrent use of ketoconazole in all patients, but specifically contraindicates concurrent use in those over 75-years-old. In contrast, the US manufacturer recommends that the dose of vardenafil should not exceed 5 mg in 24 hours when used with itraconazole or ketoconazole 200 mg daily, or 2.5 mg in 24 hours with itraconazole or ketoconazole 400 mg daily.

Azoles + **Praziquantel** ❓

Ketoconazole almost doubles the AUC of praziquantel, which appears to increase the incidence of mild adverse effects (headache and gastrointestinal adverse effects, including nausea and vomiting).

Information is limited, but all azoles have the potential to interact, to a greater or lesser extent. It may be prudent to be alert for an increase in the adverse effects of praziquantel, although an increase in efficacy is also possible.

Azoles + **Protease inhibitors**

Tipranavir/Ritonavir with Fluconazole ⚠

Fluconazole increases tipranavir bioavailability and levels by about 50%.

The manufacturer of tipranavir states that fluconazole, in doses of greater than 200 mg daily is not recommended. No dosage adjustments are recommended for lower doses of fluconazole.

Protease inhibitors with Itraconazole ⚠

Itraconazole increases the levels of amprenavir, indinavir, lopinavir/ritonavir, and saquinavir, and may theoretically increase the levels of other protease inhibitors. Some protease inhibitors, especially ritonavir and possibly indinavir, may increase itraconazole levels.

The manufacturers of indinavir advise modestly reducing the indinavir dose to 600 mg every 8 hours if it is to be given with itraconazole. Most manufacturers say that doses of itraconazole greater than 200 mg a day are not recommended with protease inhibitors. Be alert for itraconazole adverse effects (e.g. abdominal pain, dyspepsia).

Protease inhibitors with Ketoconazole ❓

Most protease inhibitors increase the levels of ketoconazole (up to about 3.5-fold with ritonavir). Ketoconazole may increase the levels of protease inhibitors, but this is usually not clinically significant. The exception may be indinavir, see below.

Ritonavir alone, ritonavir combined with darunavir, fosamprenavir, lopinavir, saquinavir and theoretically tipranavir may increase the adverse effects of ketoconazole. Most protease inhibitor manufacturers (except amprenavir, see below) say that doses greater than 200 mg a day of ketoconazole are not recommended. Dose changes of the protease inhibitors are generally not needed (but see indinavir, below).

Amprenavir with Ketoconazole ❓

Amprenavir increases the levels of ketoconazole by about 50%. Ketoconazole only modestly increases the AUC of amprenavir..

Dose adjustments of ketoconazole or amprenavir are not usually needed, but monitor high-dose ketoconazole for adverse effects.

Indinavir with Ketoconazole ⚠

Ketoconazole raises the AUC of indinavir by 62%.

The US manufacturer of indinavir recommends that the dose of indinavir be reduced to 600 mg every 8 hours when used with ketoconazole.

Protease inhibitors with Posaconazole ⚠

Any interaction between posaconazole and the protease inhibitors is not established but levels of the protease inhibitors are predicted to be increased on concurrent use.

Monitor for protease inhibitor adverse effects.

Protease inhibitors with Voriconazole ⚠

In vitro studies suggest that the concurrent use of protease inhibitors with voriconazole may inhibit the metabolism of both drugs. See also ritonavir with voriconazole, below.

The manufacturers suggest that patients be carefully monitored for evidence of drug toxicity during concurrent use.

Ritonavir with Voriconazole ✖

Ritonavir decreases the AUC of voriconazole by 82%.

Ritonavir, in doses of 400 mg twice daily or more, is contraindicated with

A

voriconazole. Low doses of ritonavir (pharmacokinetic booster doses) should only be given if essential.

Azoles + Proton pump inhibitors ⚠

The bioavailability of ketoconazole is reduced by omeprazole (AUC reduced by about 80%) and rabeprazole (bioavailability reduced by 30%). Other proton pump inhibitors are expected to behave similarly. Omeprazole also markedly reduces the absorption of itraconazole capsules (AUC decreased by 65%), but not the oral solution. Posaconazole absorption is predicted to be reduced by proton pump inhibitors. Omeprazole levels may be increased by ketoconazole (and therefore possibly itraconazole), and markedly increased by fluconazole and voriconazole. Voriconazole may more than double the levels of esomeprazole.

An increase in the antifungal dose has been suggested to overcome this interaction, as has giving ketoconazole or itraconazole with an acidic drink such as cola, which increases its bioavailability. The manufacturers of posaconazole advise avoiding concurrent use. Fluconazole and oral itraconazole solution appear to be unaffected, and they may therefore be alternatives. However, as fluconazole significantly increases omeprazole levels, a dose adjustment may be required with long-term treatment. Voriconazole does not require a dose adjustment when given with omeprazole. However, the manufacturers of voriconazole recommend halving the dose of omeprazole, but this is probably only necessary with higher doses. The dose of esomeprazole will only need adjusting in those taking voriconazole if the esomeprazole dose is very high (e.g. 240 mg).

Azoles + Quinidine

Itraconazole ⚠

Itraconazole increases the plasma levels of quinidine 1.6-fold.

Monitor concurrent use closely, reducing the dose of quinidine accordingly.

Ketoconazole ✕

Ketoconazole caused a marked increase in quinidine levels in one patient.

The clinical relevance of this interaction is uncertain.

Posaconazole ✕

Posaconazole increases quinidine levels and therefore increases the risks of QT prolongation. Quinidine may also increase posaconazole levels.

Concurrent use is contraindicated.

Voriconazole ✕

Voriconazole is predicted to increase quinidine levels, which may lead to potentially fatal torsade de pointes arrhythmias.

Concurrent use is contraindicated.

Azoles + Reboxetine ❌

Ketoconazole decreases the clearance of reboxetine, without apparently altering its adverse effect profile. Other azoles are predicted to interact similarly.

It has been suggested that caution should be used, and a reduction in reboxetine dosage considered, if it is given with ketoconazole. The manufacturers recommend that azoles should not be given with reboxetine as it has a narrow therapeutic index, but this seems overly cautious.

Azoles + Rifabutin

Fluconazole ⚠

The AUC of rifabutin is increased by about 80% by fluconazole. This carries an increased risk of uveitis.

Concurrent use with fluconazole can be advantageous but because of the increased risk of uveitis, the CSM in the UK says that the dosage of rifabutin should be reduced to 300 mg daily.

Itraconazole or Ketoconazole ⚠

Rifabutin reduces the plasma levels of itraconazole. Uveitis was attributed to the concurrent use of rifabutin and itraconazole in one report. Ketoconazole is predicted to interact similarly.

Information is sparse, but based on what is known monitor for reduced antifungal activity, raising the azole dosage as necessary, and watch for increased rifabutin levels and toxicity (in particular uveitis).

Posaconazole ⚠

Rifabutin reduces posaconazole levels by about 50% and posaconazole increases the AUC of rifabutin. Uveitis has been attributed to the concurrent use of these drugs.

Concurrent use should be avoided unless the benefits are expected to outweigh the risks. If used together, the efficacy of posaconazole and toxicity of rifabutin should both be closely monitored, particularly full blood counts and uveitis.

Voriconazole ⚠

Rifabutin decreases voriconazole levels, while voriconazole dramatically increases rifabutin levels.

Concurrent use should be avoided unless the benefits are expected to outweigh the risks. The dose of voriconazole should be increased from 200 mg twice daily to 350 mg twice daily (and from 100 to 200 mg twice daily in patients under 40 kg). The intravenous dose should also be increased from 4 to 5 mg/kg twice daily. The manufacturers of voriconazole advise careful monitoring for rifabutin adverse effects (e.g. check full blood counts, monitor for uveitis).

A

Azoles + **Rifampicin (Rifampin)**

Fluconazole ⚠

Although rifampicin causes only a modest increase in fluconazole clearance, the reduction in its effects may possibly be clinically important. Fluconazole does not appear to affect rifampicin pharmacokinetics.

Monitor concurrent use and increase the fluconazole dosage if necessary.

Itraconazole, Posaconazole, or Voriconazole ✖

Rifampicin causes a marked reduction in itraconazole and voriconazole serum levels (almost undetectable in some instances). Posaconazole is predicted to interact similarly.

Avoid concurrent use.

Ketoconazole ⚠

Ketoconazole levels can be reduced by 50 to 80% by rifampicin. Rifampicin levels can be halved by ketoconazole, but are possibly unaffected if the drugs are given 12 hours apart.

Wherever possible avoid concurrent use. If the combination must be used, monitor efficacy closely, being aware that a reduced effect is highly likely. Consider increasing the doses of both drugs.

Azoles + **Rimonabant** ⚠

Ketoconazole doubles the AUC of rimonabant. Other azoles that are potent inhibitors of CYP3A4, such as itraconazole, are predicted to interact similarly.

The manufacturers of rimonabant recommend caution. Monitor for signs of increased rimonabant adverse effects.

Azoles + **Sibutramine** ⚠

Ketoconazole (and therefore probably itraconazole) can cause moderate increases in the serum levels of sibutramine and its two metabolites. Small increases in heart rates have also been reported seen although there were no associated ECG changes.

The manufacturers caution concurrent use with both ketoconazole and itraconazole. Note that sibutramine alone can cause an increase in heart rate, and a rate increase of 10 bpm is an indication to stop the drug.

Azoles + **Sirolimus**

Clotrimazole and Posaconazole ⚠

Clotrimazole and posaconazole are predicted to interact in the same way as ketoconazole and voriconazole, see below.

Fluconazole ⚠

In one case fluconazole caused a significant increase in sirolimus levels despite dose reductions from 4 mg to 2 mg.

Close monitoring of sirolimus levels is recommended.

Ketoconazole or Itraconazole ✖

Ketoconazole increases the maximum serum levels of sirolimus by 4.3-fold. Itraconazole increases the levels of sirolimus and dosage reductions of up to 90% have been required.

Concurrent use is not recommended.

Miconazole ⚠

Miconazole oral gel may be swallowed in large enough quantities to have a systemic interaction with sirolimus, which would be expected to result in raised sirolimus levels.

The manufacturers of miconazole oral gel recommend close monitoring and possible dose reduction of sirolimus if both drugs are given. An interaction with intravaginal miconazole would not normally be expected.

Voriconazole ✖

Voriconazole raised the maximum serum levels and AUC of a single 2 mg dose of sirolimus by about 5.5-fold and 10-fold respectively.

These rises are probably too large to be easily accommodated by reducing the dosage of the sirolimus. Concurrent use is contraindicated.

Azoles + **Solifenacin** ⚠

Ketoconazole increases solifenacin levels 2- to 3-fold by inhibiting CYP3A4. The manufacturers predict that other CYP3A4 inhibitors (e.g. itraconazole) will have the same effect.

It is recommended that only 5 mg of solifenacin should be used in patients taking itraconazole or ketoconazole. The concurrent use of solifenacin and these azoles is contraindicated in patients with severe renal impairment or moderate hepatic impairment.

Azoles + **Statins**

Atorvastatin ⚠

The AUC of atorvastatin is raised by 150% by itraconazole. Rhabdomyolysis has been seen when atorvastatin and fluconazole have been given.

Because of the potentially serious reactions that can result, any patient given atorvastatin with an azole should be told to report any unexplained muscle pain, tenderness or weakness. Because large increases in atorvastatin levels can occur (most likely with itraconazole or ketoconazole), consider temporarily withdrawing the statin. The manufacturers of voriconazole recommend a dose reduction of atorvastatin (and lovastatin and simvastatin) during concurrent use. For posaconazole, see Simvastatin or Lovastatin, below.

Fluvastatin ❓

Fluconazole increases the AUC and maximum plasma levels of fluvastatin by 84% and 44%, respectively.

The clinical relevance of the modest changes in fluvastatin levels with fluconazole is unclear. However, because of the potentially serious reactions that can result, any patient given fluvastatin, with fluconazole (or miconazole, including the oral gel) should be told to report any unexplained muscle pain, tenderness or weakness.

Pravastatin, or Rosuvastatin ⚠

CYP3A4 is not the main enzyme involved in the metabolism of pravastatin, or rosuvastatin, and so no interaction would generally be expected. However, rare cases of rhabdomyolysis have been reported in patients given one of these statins with an azole.

Because of the potentially serious reactions that can result, any patient given pravastatin or rosuvastatin with an azole should be told to report any unexplained muscle pain, tenderness or weakness.

Simvastatin or Lovastatin ❌

Statins that are largely metabolised by CYP3A4 have their levels greatly raised by azoles that are potent inhibitors of this isoenzyme. The drug pairs that are affected by this interaction are:

- lovastatin with itraconazole (20-fold rises seen)
- lovastatin with ketoconazole
- simvastatin with itraconazole (17-fold rises seen)
- simvastatin with ketoconazole
- atorvastatin, lovastatin or simvastatin with posaconazole (predicted by the manufacturers)

This interaction has resulted in severe muscle toxicity, including rhabdomyolysis, in a number of cases.

Concurrent use of itraconazole, ketoconazole or posaconazole with simvastatin or lovastatin is contraindicated. The manufacturers of posaconazole also contraindicate atorvastatin. If a short course of an azole is essential, the statin should be temporarily withdrawn. For voriconazole, see atorvastatin, above.

Azoles + Sucralfate ⚠

Sucralfate reduces ketoconazole absorption by about 25%, but no significant changes appear to occur if ketoconazole is given 2 hours after sucralfate.

Separate the administration by 2 to 3 hours to ensure maximal absorption.

Azoles + **Tacrolimus** ⚠

When tacrolimus is given orally, its serum levels are considerably increased (within 3 days) by oral fluconazole. *In vitro* study suggests miconazole may interact similarly. Itraconazole, ketoconazole, posaconazole, voriconazole, and possibly oral clotrimazole or miconazole oral gel, also raise tacrolimus levels. There is some evidence that the levels of *intravenous* tacrolimus are minimally affected by fluconazole and ketoconazole.

> One study specifically examining dose adjustments suggests that fluconazole can be safely used if 60% of the original tacrolimus dose is given. Nearly all patients are expected to need dose reductions if azoles are given: the manufacturers of posaconazole and voriconazole suggest a reduction of two-thirds. Monitor tacrolimus levels closely if any azole is given.

Azoles + **Theophylline** ✅

No clinically significant interaction is expected between theophylline and the azoles, although a fall in theophylline levels has been seen in rare cases with ketoconazole and a rise in theophylline levels has been seen in rare cases with fluconazole.

> Bear these reports in mind in case of an unexpected response to treatment.

Azoles + **Tolterodine** ⚠

The AUC of tolterodine is raised by more than 2-fold by ketoconazole. Itraconazole is predicted to interact similarly.

> The UK manufacturers advise avoiding concurrent use. The US manufacturers suggest reducing the tolterodine dose to 1 mg twice daily, which seems practical. If both drugs are given monitor carefully for tolterodine adverse effects, and further reduce the dose if necessary.

Azoles + **Toremifene** ⚠

Inhibitors of CYP3A4, such as ketoconazole, are predicted to decrease toremifene metabolism, which may lead to toxicity (e.g. hot flushes, uterine bleeding, fatigue, nausea, dizziness).

> These warnings are based on indirect evidence and therefore their clinical importance awaits confirmation.

Azoles + **Trazodone** ⚠

Ketoconazole or itraconazole may inhibit the metabolism of trazodone.

> A lower dose of trazodone should be considered if it is given with these azoles, although in the UK it has been suggested that the combination should be avoided where possible. Monitor for increased trazodone adverse effects such as sedation, if concurrent use is required.

Azoles + Tricyclics ❓

Case reports describe increased amitriptyline or nortriptyline levels in patients also taking fluconazole (tricyclic antidepressant levels at least doubled). There is also a report of a patient who developed a prolonged QT interval and torsades de pointes arrhythmias, which were associated with the concurrent use of amitriptyline and fluconazole. Consider also drugs that prolong the QT interval, page 237.

> The general importance of this interaction is unclear, but bear it in mind in case of an unexpected response to treatment.

Azoles + Triptans

Fluconazole ⚠️

Fluconazole modestly increases the plasma levels of eletriptan by 40%.

> Be aware that the effects of eletriptan may be increased in those taking fluconazole. Other triptans would be expected to have little or no interaction with the azoles and may be suitable alternatives.

Itraconazole or Ketoconazole ✖️

Ketoconazole raises the plasma levels of eletriptan 2.7-fold. Itraconazole is expected to interact similarly.

> The manufacturer states that the concurrent use of ketoconazole and itraconazole with eletriptan should be avoided. The US manufacturers further recommend that eletriptan should not be given within 72 hours of these azoles. Other triptans would be expected to have little or no interaction with the azoles and may be suitable alternatives.

Azoles + Warfarin and other oral anticoagulants ⚠️

Case reports describe raised INRs and bleeding when fluconazole, ketoconazole, or itraconazole were given with warfarin. The anticoagulant effects of acenocoumarol, ethyl biscoumacetate, fluindione, phenindione, phenprocoumon, tioclomarol and warfarin can be markedly increased if miconazole is given orally, and bleeding can occur. The interaction can occur with buccal gel, intravaginal miconazole, and in one case, with miconazole cream. Voriconazole decreases the metabolism of warfarin resulting in a doubling of the prothrombin time. Acenocoumarol appears to interact similarly.

> Monitor the INR if an azole is given with an oral anticoagulant and adjust the dose accordingly. Oral miconazole, fluconazole and voriconazole interfere with the main metabolic pathway of warfarin (and acenocoumarol) and are therefore likely to interact more frequently than the other azoles.

Aztreonam

A

Aztreonam + Warfarin and other oral anticoagulants ❓

Aztreonam occasionally causes a prolongation in prothrombin times, which in theory might possibly be additive with the effects of conventional anticoagulants.

The clinical importance of this interaction is unknown, but bear it in mind in case of an increased response to anticoagulant treatment.

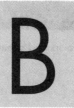

Baclofen

Baclofen + Levodopa ⚠

Unpleasant adverse effects (hallucinations, confusion, headache, nausea) and worsening of the symptoms of parkinsonism have occurred in patients taking levodopa who were also given baclofen.

Information is limited, but what is known suggests that baclofen should be used cautiously in patients taking levodopa.

Baclofen + Lithium ❓

Two patients with Huntington's chorea taking showed an aggravation of their hyperkinetic symptoms within a few days of starting lithium and baclofen. One patient took lithium first, the other baclofen.

The clinical significance of this interaction is unclear. Bear it in mind in case of an unexpected response to treatment.

Baclofen + NSAIDs ❓

An isolated report describes baclofen toxicity (confusion, disorientation, bradycardia, blurred vision, hypotension and hypothermia) in a patient who took ibuprofen. It appeared that the toxicity was caused by ibuprofen-induced acute renal impairment leading to baclofen accumulation.

The general importance of this interaction is likely to be very small. There appears to be no information about baclofen and other NSAIDs, and little reason for avoiding concurrent use.

Balsalazide

Balsalazide + Digoxin ❓

Because digoxin levels can be reduced by up to 50% by *sulfasalazine* the manufacturers cautiously suggest that an interaction may occur with balsalazide. However, no interactions appear to have been reported.

No action needed.

Benzodiazepines

Benzodiazepines + Beta blockers ✅

Only small and clinically unimportant pharmacokinetic interactions occur between most benzodiazepines and beta blockers, but there is some evidence that patients taking diazepam may possibly be more accident prone while taking metoprolol.

The current evidence does not seem to justify any particular caution, but bear this interaction in mind in case of an unexpected response to treatment.

Benzodiazepines + Calcium-channel blockers

Midazolam or Triazolam ⚠

The serum levels and effects of midazolam are markedly increased by diltiazem or verapamil. This also occurs with triazolam and diltiazem, and is predicted to occur with triazolam and verapamil.

Monitor the outcome of concurrent use. Consider using a lower initial dose of midazolam or triazolam.

Other benzodiazepines ❓

There appear to be no significant interactions between diazepam and diltiazem, felodipine or nimodipine; between midazolam and nitrendipine; between temazepam and diltiazem; or between triazolam and isradipine. Lercanidipine absorption is increased by 40% by midazolam, but the clinical significance of this is unclear.

No action needed.

Benzodiazepines + Carbamazepine

Clobazam ✅

Carbamazepine reduces the levels of clobazam and increases the levels of its principal metabolite. A case report describes a small rise in carbamazepine levels resulting in

B

toxicity in a patient also taking clobazam, whereas a small study suggested that clobazam increased the metabolism of carbamazepine.

The clinical significance of these findings is unknown. The changes in clobazam levels are not expected to be clinically significant.

Midazolam ▲

Carbamazepine reduces the AUC and peak serum levels of midazolam by about 90%, when compared with control subjects not taking antiepileptics. The effects of midazolam were also reduced.

Expect to need to use a much larger dose of midazolam in the presence of carbamazepine. An alternative hypno-sedative may be needed.

Other benzodiazepines ✓

The use of benzodiazepines with carbamazepine is common, although some evidence suggests that the effects of the benzodiazepines are sometimes reduced (alprazolam, clonazepam, diazepam, zopiclone).

No action needed, but be aware that sometimes the effects of the benzodiazepines may be reduced.

Benzodiazepines + Digoxin ❓

Digoxin toxicity occurred in two elderly patients, and rises in serum digoxin levels have been seen in others, when they were given alprazolam. This interaction seems to occur particularly in patients over 65 years of age.

Monitor the effects of digoxin (e.g. bradycardia) in any patient if alprazolam is added and reduce the digoxin dosage as necessary.

Benzodiazepines + Disulfiram ❓

An isolated and unconfirmed report describes temazepam toxicity, possibly due to disulfiram. The serum levels of chlordiazepoxide and diazepam are increased by the use of disulfiram and some patients may possibly experience increased drowsiness.

If sedation occurs reduce the dosage of the benzodiazepine if necessary. Other benzodiazepines that are metabolised similarly may possibly interact in the same way (e.g. bromazepam, clobazam, clonazepam, clorazepate, flurazepam, ketazolam, medazepam, nitrazepam, prazepam) but this needs confirmation. Alprazolam, lorazepam and oxazepam appear to be non-interacting alternatives.

Benzodiazepines + Felbamate ▲

A retrospective study found that felbamate increases the levels of the clobazam metabolite, norclobazam.

The clinical significance of this interaction is unknown but it would seem prudent to monitor for increased clobazam effects (e.g. sedation).

Benzodiazepines + H₂-receptor antagonists ✓

The serum levels of adinazolam, alprazolam, chlordiazepoxide, clobazam, clorazepate, diazepam, flurazepam, nitrazepam, triazolam, zaleplon, zolpidem (and probably halazepam and prazepam) are raised by cimetidine, but normally this appears to be of little or no clinical importance, and only the occasional patient may experience an increase in effects (sedation). Clotiazepam, lorazepam, lormetazepam, oxazepam and temazepam are not normally affected by cimetidine. Famotidine, nizatidine and ranitidine do not interact with most benzodiazepines, except possibly triazolam. The picture with midazolam is somewhat confused.

In general no clinically significant interaction occurs, but note that individual patients may rarely experience increased sedation.

Benzodiazepines + Herbal medicines or Dietary supplements

Echinacea ❓

The bioavailability of oral midazolam was increased by 50% by echinacea in one study although another study found no effects. In contrast, the clearance of intravenous midazolam appears to be increased by echinacea.

The clinical importance of this interaction is uncertain. Bear it in mind if intravenous midazolam effects are reduced, or oral midazolam effects are increased.

Kava ❓

A man taking alprazolam became semicomatose a few days after starting to take kava.

The clinical importance of this interaction is uncertain, but bear it in mind in case of an unexpected response to treatment.

St John's wort (Hypericum perforatum) ✓

The bioavailability of oral midazolam is reduced by about 50% by long-term use of St John's wort. St John's wort decreases the metabolism of quazepam, although this did not increase its effects.

No action needed, but bear this interaction in mind if an inadequate response to oral midazolam is seen.

Benzodiazepines + Isoniazid ⚠

Isoniazid reduces the clearance of both diazepam and triazolam. Some increase in their effects would be expected.

The degree of sedation will depend on the individual patient. However, warn all patients of the potential effects, and counsel against driving or undertaking other skilled tasks. Reduce the benzodiazepine dose as necessary. Clotiazepam and oxazepam appear to be non-interacting alternatives.

Benzodiazepines + **Lamotrigine** ❓

Lamotrigine appears to lower clonazepam levels by about 40% in some patients.

The general significance of this interaction is unclear.

Benzodiazepines + **Levodopa** ❓

On rare occasions it seems that the therapeutic effects of levodopa can be reduced by chlordiazepoxide, diazepam or nitrazepam, but this is not an established interaction.

There is no need to avoid concurrent use, but bear these reports in mind in case of an unexpected response to treatment.

Benzodiazepines + **Lithium** ❓

Neurotoxicity and increased serum lithium levels were reported in 5 patients when they took clonazepam with lithium.

It has been recommended that lithium levels should be measured more frequently if clonazepam is added, and the effects of concurrent use should be well monitored.

Benzodiazepines + **Macrolides**

Midazolam, Triazolam or Zopiclone ⚠

The serum levels and effects of midazolam and triazolam are markedly increased and prolonged by erythromycin. Similar effects occur when triazolam is given with clarithromycin, josamycin and possibly telithromycin, and when midazolam is given with clarithromycin and possibly telithromycin. Plasma levels of zopiclone are markedly increased by erythromycin.

The benzodiazepine dose should be reduced in the presence of these macrolides if excessive effects (marked drowsiness, memory loss) are to be avoided. Note that the hypnotic effects may also be prolonged. Other macrolides may also interact, although it seems unlikely that they all will, see macrolides, page 310.

Other benzodiazepines ❓

Roxithromycin has a weak effect on the metabolism of midazolam and triazolam, and erythromycin has a weak effect on the metabolism of diazepam, flunitrazepam, nitrazepam, temazepam and zaleplon. Erythromycin possibly increases the effects of alprazolam.

The general significance of these modest interactions are unclear, but it may be prudent to monitor the outcome of concurrent use, reducing the dose of the benzodiazepine if necessary.

Benzodiazepines + **MAOIs** ❓

Isolated cases of adverse reactions (chorea, severe headache, facial flushing, massive oedema, and prolonged coma) attributed to interactions between phenelzine and chlordiazepoxide, clonazepam or nitrazepam, and between isocarboxazid and chlordiazepoxide have been described.

The case reports of adverse interactions appear to be isolated, and it is by no means certain that all the responses were in fact due to drug interactions.

Benzodiazepines + Mirtazapine ⚠

Additive adverse effects on psychomotor skills and sedation have been reported with diazepam and mirtazapine.

Patients should be warned that the sedative effects of benzodiazepines in general may be potentiated by concurrent use with mirtazapine. Note that the US manufacturer actually recommends that patients taking mirtazapine avoid the use of diazepam and similar drugs, but this is probably overly cautious.

Benzodiazepines + Modafinil ⚠

Modafinil reduced the maximum plasma concentration of triazolam by 42% and reduced its elimination half-life by about one hour. Alprazolam and midazolam may be similarly affected. In contrast, diazepam levels may be increased by modafinil.

Dosage adjustments may be necessary on concurrent use. Monitor to ensure that the benzodiazepine effects are adequate, and, in the case of diazepam, not excessive.

Benzodiazepines + Moxonidine ⚠

Moxonidine increases the cognitive impairment caused by lorazepam. Sedation and dizziness may occur with moxonidine alone, which the manufacturers suggest may be additive with the effects of benzodiazepines.

The degree of impairment will depend on the individual patient. However, warn all patients of the potential effects, and counsel against driving or undertaking other skilled tasks.

Benzodiazepines + NRTIs ❓

Oxazepam causes a modest increase in the bioavailability of zidovudine and can increase the incidence of headaches. *In vitro* studies suggest that lorazepam may interact similarly.

It has been suggested that if headaches occur during concurrent use, the benzodiazepine should be stopped.

Benzodiazepines + Opioids ❓

As would be expected, increased sedative and respiratory depressant effects may occur in patients given opioids with benzodiazepines. Other minor pharmacokinetic interactions may occur, but there is insufficient evidence to suggest that any of these are of general significance.

The degree of impairment will depend on the individual patient. However, warn all patients of the potential effects, and counsel against driving or undertaking other skilled tasks.

Benzodiazepines + Phenobarbital ❓

Clonazepam appears to markedly raise the levels of primidone in children, and toxicity has been seen. The concurrent use of primidone and clorazepate was thought to have caused irritability, aggression and depression in a small number of patients. Note that primidone is metabolized to phenobarbital.

> The clinical importance of this interaction is unknown, but bear it in mind in case of an unexpected response to treatment. Indicators of phenobarbital and primidone toxicity include drowsiness, ataxia, and dysarthria.

Benzodiazepines + Phenytoin

Midazolam ⚠

Phenytoin reduced the AUC of midazolam by about 95%, and the peak serum levels by about 90% when compared with control subjects not taking anticonvulsants. The effects of midazolam were also reduced.

> Expect to need to use a much larger dose of midazolam in the presence of phenytoin. An alternative hypnotic may be needed.

Other benzodiazepines ⚠

Reports are inconsistent: benzodiazepines can cause serum phenytoin levels to rise (chlordiazepoxide, clobazam, clonazepam, diazepam), occasionally resulting in toxicity; or fall (clonazepam, diazepam); or remain unaltered (alprazolam, clonazepam). In addition phenytoin may cause a fall in the serum levels of clobazam, clonazepam, diazepam, midazolam (see above) and oxazepam.

> Warn the patient to monitor for indicators of phenytoin toxicity (blurred vision, nystagmus, ataxia or drowsiness). Take phenytoin levels as necessary. Be aware that the benzodiazepine may be less effective than expected.

Benzodiazepines + Pregabalin ❓

The manufacturer notes that there was no clinically relevant pharmacokinetic interaction between pregabalin and lorazepam, and that concurrent use caused no clinically important effect on respiration. However, they note that pregabalin may potentiate the effects of lorazepam (presumably sedation). All benzodiazepines seem likely to increase sedation when given with pregabalin.

> The degree of impairment will depend on the individual patient. However, warn all patients of the potential effects, and counsel against driving or undertaking other skilled tasks.

Benzodiazepines + Probenecid ⚠

Probenecid reduces the clearance of adinazolam, lorazepam and nitrazepam. Increased therapeutic and adverse effects (sedation) may be expected. There seems to be no direct information about other benzodiazepines, but those that are metabolised like lorazepam and nitrazepam (e.g. oxazepam) may also interact.

Monitor the outcome of concurrent use for increased sedation and decrease the benzodiazepine dose if this becomes troublesome. Limited evidence suggests that temazepam does not interact.

B

Benzodiazepines + **Protease inhibitors**

Midazolam and Triazolam

The protease inhibitors appear to increase the levels and effects of midazolam and triazolam. Increased and prolonged sedation may occur.

The UK manufacturers of the protease inhibitors contraindicate the concurrent use of *oral* midazolam, but advise that *intravenous* midazolam may be used with close monitoring within an intensive care unit or similar setting so that the appropriate management of respiratory depression is available. They also suggest that dosage reductions should be considered. The authors of one study suggest that continuous intravenous midazolam doses should be reduced by 50%, but do not consider dose adjustments to single intravenous doses necessary. Triazolam would be expected to interact in the same way as midazolam, and therefore the UK manufacturers generally contraindicate its use. The US manufacturers however do not differentiate between oral or intravenous midazolam, and in general contraindicate the concurrent use of midazolam and triazolam with protease inhibitors.

Other benzodiazepines ⊗

Ritonavir is predicted to raise the levels of a number of benzodiazepines and related drugs, which would be expected to result in increased and prolonged sedation.

Clorazepate, diazepam, estazolam, and flurazepam are contraindicated by the UK manufacturer of ritonavir, but cautioned by the US manufacturers of ritonavir, amprenavir, and fosamprenavir, and both the UK and US manufacturers of saquinavir: some advise that a reduction in the dose of these benzodiazepines may be necessary. Alprazolam is contraindicated by the UK and US manufacturers of indinavir. The manufacturer of ritonavir notes that zolpidem may be given concurrently with careful monitoring for excessive sedative effects and consideration of reducing the dose of zolpidem.

Benzodiazepines + **Proton pump inhibitors** ⚠

Gait disturbances (attributed to benzodiazepine toxicity) occurred in 2 patients given triazolam, and lorazepam or flurazepam, with omeprazole. Another patient taking diazepam and omeprazole became wobbly and sedated. Lansoprazole, pantoprazole, or rabeprazole appear not to interact with diazepam to a clinically relevant extent. Diazepam serum levels are increased by esomeprazole but the clinical relevance of this is unknown.

Information is sparse. Bear this interaction in mind if excessive benzodiazepine effects occur.

B

Benzodiazepines + **Rifampicin (Rifampin)** ✖

Rifampicin causes a very marked increase in the clearance of diazepam (4-fold), midazolam (AUC reduced by 96%), nitrazepam (83%), triazolam (AUC reduced by 95%), zaleplon (AUC reduced by 80%), zolpidem (AUC reduced by 73%) and zopiclone (AUC reduced by 82%). Benzodiazepines that are metabolised similarly (e.g. chlordiazepoxide, flurazepam) are expected to interact in the same way.

The effects of these benzodiazepines may be almost completely abolished if rifampicin is given. Temazepam appears to be a non-interacting alternative.

Benzodiazepines + **SSRIs** ✖

On the whole, no clinically significant interaction appears to occur between the SSRIs and the benzodiazepines or related drugs, such as cloral hydrate or zaleplon. However, there is some evidence to suggest that the metabolism of some benzodiazepines (such as alprazolam, bromazepam and diazepam, and also possibly midazolam, nitrazepam and triazolam) may be reduced by some SSRIs (such as fluoxetine and fluvoxamine). There is some evidence to support the suggestion that sedation is likely to be increased by the concurrent use of SSRIs and benzodiazepines. Rare cases of hallucinations have been seen with zolpidem and some SSRIs.

No particular action is necessary but remember that the degree of sedation will depend on the individual patient and drug combination. Warn all patients of the potential effects, and counsel caution with driving or undertaking other skilled tasks.

Benzodiazepines + **Theophylline** ❓

Theophylline and aminophylline may antagonise the effects of the benzodiazepines and zopiclone. Alprazolam levels may also be reduced by theophylline (and therefore probably aminophylline).

The extent to which these xanthines actually reduce the anxiolytic effects of the benzodiazepines remains uncertain but be alert for reduced benzodiazepine effects.

Benzodiazepines + **Tricyclics** ⚠

The concurrent use of tricyclic antidepressants and benzodiazepines is not uncommon, and normally appears to be uneventful. However, there have been reports of increased drowsiness and incoordination following the use of the combination.

No particular action is necessary but remember that the degree of sedation will depend on the individual patient and drug combination. Warn all patients of the potential effects, and counsel caution with driving or undertaking other skilled tasks.

Beta blockers

Beta blockers + Calcium-channel blockers

B

Diltiazem ⚠

The cardiac depressant effects of diltiazem and beta blockers are additive, although concurrent use can be beneficial. A number of patients, usually those with pre-existing ventricular failure or conduction abnormalities, have developed serious and potentially life-threatening bradycardia.

Monitor the outcome of concurrent use for additive haemodynamic effects (e.g. bradycardia, hypotension or heart failure).

Nifedipine or Nisoldipine ❓

Isolated cases of severe hypotension and heart failure have been seen in patients taking beta blockers with nifedipine or nisoldipine. Patients with impaired left ventricular function (which is a caution for the use of nifedipine) and/or those taking high-dose beta blockers are most at risk. Note that all cases of an interaction involved short-acting nifedipine (which is now considered unsuitable in angina or hypertension) or when extended-release nifedipine was crushed.

Monitor the outcome of concurrent use for additive haemodynamic effects (e.g. hypotension or heart failure).

Verapamil ⚠

The cardiac depressant effects of verapamil and beta blockers are additive, and although concurrent use can be beneficial, serious cardiodepression (bradycardia, asystole, sinus arrest) sometimes occurs. An adverse interaction can occur even with beta blockers given as eye drops.

Concurrent use should only be undertaken if the patient can initially be closely monitored. The doses should be carefully titrated to effect. It has been suggested that verapamil injections should not be given to patients recently given beta blockers because of the risk of hypotension and asystole.

Other calcium-channel blockers ❓

The use of beta blockers with felodipine, isradipine, lacidipine, nicardipine, and nimodipine normally appears to be useful and safe. Changes in the pharmacokinetics of the beta blockers and calcium-channel blockers may also occur, but these changes do not appear to be clinically important. Note that additive hypotensive effects are likely, see antihypertensives, page 77.

Monitor the outcome of concurrent use for additive haemodynamic effects (e.g. hypotension or heart failure).

Beta blockers + Ciclosporin (Cyclosporine) ❓

There is some evidence that carvedilol can cause a small to moderate rise in ciclosporin levels (requiring a gradual ciclosporin dose reduction of 20%, over about 3 months, to maintain levels within the therapeutic range).

> This interaction is unconfirmed and of uncertain clinical significance. There is insufficient evidence to recommend increased monitoring, but be aware of the potential for an interaction in case of an unexpected response to treatment.

Beta blockers + Clonidine ⚠

The use of clonidine with beta blockers can be therapeutically valuable, but a sharp and serious rise in blood pressure, rebound hypertension', can follow the sudden withdrawal of clonidine, which may be worsened by the presence of a beta blocker. Note that additive hypotensive effects are likely, see antihypertensives, page 77.

> Control this adverse effect by stopping the beta blocker several days before starting a gradual withdrawal of clonidine. A successful alternative is to replace the clonidine and the beta blocker with labetalol. The patient may experience tremor, nausea, apprehension and palpitations, but no serious blood pressure rise or headaches occur. If a hypertensive episode develops, control it with phentolamine. Re-introduction of oral or intravenous clonidine should also stabilise the situation. It is clearly important to emphasise to patients taking clonidine and beta blockers that they must keep taking both drugs.

Beta blockers + Co-artemether ❌

The manufacturer of co-artemether notes that *in vitro* lumefantrine significantly inhibits CYP2D6. They therefore contraindicate any drug that is metabolised by CYP2D6, and they name metoprolol. Additive QT-prolonging effects are likely with sotalol, see drugs that prolong the QT interval, page 237.

> This seems very restrictive as metoprolol is not contraindicated with proven CYP2D6 inhibitors. Until more is known, it would be prudent to at least monitor the effects of concurrent use.

Beta blockers + Contraceptives ✔

The blood levels of metoprolol are increased in women taking hormonal contraceptives, but the clinical importance of this is probably very small. Acebutolol, oxprenolol and propranolol pharmacokinetics are minimally affected by contraceptives.

> No action needed. However, be aware that hormonal contraceptives are cautioned or contraindicated in some of the patient groups who may be treated with beta blockers, and oestrogens can raise blood pressure, which may antagonise the effects of the beta blockers.

Beta blockers + Digoxin ❓

In general digoxin and beta blockers appear not to interact. However there is always the risk of additive bradycardia. Carvedilol appears to increase the bioavailability of digoxin (14% increase in AUC seen in adults, cases suggest a doubling of levels in children).

> Normally uneventful, no immediate action needed. If bradycardia does occur dose

adjustment may be necessary, and this seems more likely to be necessary in children.

B

Beta blockers + **Disopyramide** ✖

Severe bradycardia has been described after the use of disopyramide with beta blockers including practolol (3 cases, 1 fatal) pindolol (1 fatal case) and metoprolol (1 case). Another patient given disopyramide and intravenous sotalol developed asystole (see also drugs that prolong the QT interval, page 237). Oral propranolol and disopyramide have been given to healthy subjects without any increase in negative inotropic effects or pharmacokinetic changes.

The manufacturers of disopyramide suggest that the combination of disopyramide and beta blockers should generally be avoided.

Beta blockers + **Ergot derivatives** ❓

The use of ergot derivatives (e.g. ergotamine) with beta blockers is normally safe and beneficial, but cases of peripheral vasoconstriction have been reported following concurrent use.

This interaction is unlikely to be of general significance, but it may be prudent to be extra alert for any signs of an adverse response, particularly those suggestive of reduced peripheral circulation (coldness, numbness or tingling of the hands and feet).

Beta blockers + **Flecainide** ⚠

The combined use of flecainide and beta blockers may have additive cardiac depressant effects. A study on cardiac function and drug clearance found that when propranolol was given with flecainide the AUCs of both drugs were increased by 20 to 30%, and they had some additive negative inotropic effects. An isolated case of bradycardia and fatal AV block has been reported during the use of flecainide with sotalol, and bradycardia has been reported in a patient taking flecainide and timolol eye drops.

Careful monitoring has been recommended if beta blockers are given with other antiarrhythmics. Monitor for bradycardia.

Beta blockers + **H$_2$-receptor antagonists** ❓

Cimetidine affects the pharmacokinetics of some beta blockers. The AUC of oral labetalol is increased by 66%, metoprolol peak plasma levels are increased by 70%, the AUC of nebivolol is increased by 48%, the AUC of pindolol is increased by about 40%, and the AUC of propranolol is increased by 47%. However, this only rarely appears to result in clinically significant effects.

Monitor the outcome of concurrent use, adjusting the dose of the beta blocker if necessary. Note that other H$_2$-receptor antagonists (e.g. famotidine, nizatidine and ranitidine) do not appear to interact and so may be suitable alternatives.

Beta blockers + **Hydralazine** ❓

Plasma levels of propranolol and other extensively metabolised beta blockers (metoprolol, oxprenolol) are increased by hydralazine, but an increase in adverse effects does not seem to have been reported.

> Concurrent use is usually valuable in the treatment of hypertension. No particular precautions seem to be necessary, but the outcome should be monitored. Note that additive hypotensive effects are likely, see antihypertensives, page 77.

Beta blockers + **Inotropes and Vasopressors** ⚠

The hypertensive effects of adrenaline (epinephrine) can be markedly increased in patients taking non-selective beta blockers such as propranolol. A severe and potentially life-threatening hypertensive reaction and/or marked bradycardia can develop. Cardioselective beta blockers such as atenolol and metoprolol interact minimally. Some evidence suggests anaphylactic shock in patients taking beta blockers may be resistant to treatment with adrenaline (epinephrine).

> Patients taking non-selective beta blockers such as propranolol should only be given adrenaline (epinephrine) in very reduced dosages because of the marked bradycardia and hypertension that can occur. A less marked effect is likely with the cardioselective beta blockers such as atenolol and metoprolol. Local anaesthetics such as those used in dental surgery usually contain very low concentrations of adrenaline (e.g. 5 to 20 micrograms/mL, i.e. 1:200 000 to 1:50 000) and only small volumes are usually given, so that an undesirable interaction is unlikely. Acute hypertensive episodes have been controlled with chlorpromazine or phentolamine. Reflex bradycardia may be managed with atropine and the pre-emptive use of glycopyrrolate has also been suggested.

Beta blockers + **Lidocaine** ⚠

The plasma levels of lidocaine can be increased by the concurrent use of propranolol, which has resulted in toxicity in isolated cases. Nadolol possibly interacts similarly, but there is uncertainty about metoprolol.

> As it is not clear why this interaction occurs, it would seem prudent to monitor the concurrent use of any beta blocker and lidocaine.

Beta blockers + **Moxonidine** ⚠

Beta blockers can exacerbate the rebound hypertension that follows the withdrawal of clonidine, page 138. Moxonidine is reported to have less affinity for central alpha receptors than clonidine, and no such rebound hypertension has actually been seen when moxonidine is withdrawn.

> For safety's sake the manufacturers advise that any beta blocker should be stopped first, followed by the moxonidine a few days later. Note that additive hypotensive effects are likely, see antihypertensives, page 77.

Beta blockers + **NSAIDs** ❓

The antihypertensive effects of beta blockers may be reduced by NSAIDs. In some cases this interaction has resulted in large changes in blood pressure, although the effect varies with different beta blocker/NSAID combinations. The most significant increases (of 8 to 10 mmHg) appear to be caused by indometacin.

> Only some patients are affected. Monitor blood pressure if an NSAID is started or stopped.

B

Beta blockers + **Phenobarbital** ⚠

The plasma levels and the effects of beta blockers that are mainly metabolised in the liver (e.g. alprenolol, metoprolol, timolol) are reduced by the barbiturates. Alprenolol concentrations are halved, but the others are possibly not affected as much.

> Monitor concurrent use to ensure these beta blockers are effective. Beta blockers that are mainly excreted unchanged in the urine (e.g. atenolol, sotalol, nadolol) would not be expected to be affected by the barbiturates.

Beta blockers + **Phosphodiesterase type-5 inhibitors** ✗

Vardenafil modestly prolongs the QT interval (by 5 to 10 milliseconds). The manufacturers therefore advise against concurrent use of class III antiarrhythmics such as sotalol. Consider also drugs that prolong the QT interval, page 237.

> Avoid concurrent use.

Beta blockers + **Propafenone** ⚠

Plasma metoprolol and propranolol levels can be markedly raised (2- to 5-fold) by propafenone. Toxicity may develop.

> Information is limited. Anticipate the need to reduce the dosage of metoprolol and propranolol. Monitor closely. It is possible that other beta blockers that undergo liver metabolism will interact similarly but not those largely excreted unchanged in the urine (e.g. atenolol, nadolol). This needs confirmation.

Beta blockers + **Quinidine** ❓

An isolated report describes a patient taking quinidine who developed marked bradycardia when using timolol eye drops. Other reports describe orthostatic hypotension with quinidine and atenolol or propranolol. Quinidine can raise plasma metoprolol, propranolol, and timolol levels, but the clinical relevance of this is uncertain. Additive QT-prolonging effects likely with sotalol, see drugs that prolong the QT interval, page 237.

> The general relevance of these case reports is unclear.

Beta blockers + **Rifampicin (Rifampin)** ❓

Rifampicin increases the loss of bisoprolol, carvedilol, celiprolol, metoprolol, propranolol, tertatolol and talinolol from the body, and reduces their serum

B

levels. The extent to which this reduces the effects of these beta blockers is uncertain, but it is probably small. However, one patient taking atenolol experienced a reduction in exercise tolerance when given rifampicin.

> The significance of this interaction is unclear, but bear it in mind in case of an unexpected response to treatment.

Beta blockers + SSRIs ❓

In general no significant interaction appears to occur between beta blockers and SSRIs. The concurrent use of citalopram or escitalopram and metoprolol does not significantly affect heart rate and blood pressure. However, the plasma levels of metoprolol are increased by up to 2-fold, which may decrease its cardioselectivity. Paroxetine significantly increases the AUC of metoprolol, which results in more sustained beta-blocking effects and a more pronounced reduction in exercise systolic blood pressure.

> The clinical significance of these potential interactions is unclear, but they seem more likely to be important in those given metoprolol for heart failure. Bear it in mind if the effects of metoprolol seem excessive.

Beta blockers + Terbinafine ⚠

In vitro studies suggest that terbinafine is an inhibitor of CYP2D6. It may therefore be expected to increase the plasma levels of other drugs that are substrates of this enzyme. The manufacturers suggest that the levels of some beta blockers may be raised. Carvedilol, metoprolol, nebivolol, propranolol and timolol are all metabolized, at least in part, by CYP2D6.

> Until more is known it would seem wise to be aware of the possibility of an increase in adverse effects if any of these drugs is given with terbinafine and consider a dose reduction if necessary. The interaction is most likely to be of clinical significance when drugs such as metoprolol are given for heart failure.

Beta blockers + Triptans ⚠

No clinically important interaction occurs between most triptans and propranolol, but the plasma levels of rizatriptan are almost doubled by propranolol.

> If propranolol is also given the manufacturers recommend a dosage reduction to 5 mg of rizatriptan, with a maximum of two or three doses in 24 hours. In the UK it is additionally recommended that dosing should be separated by 2-hours, but the basis for this is unclear, as studies have found that this does not modify the interaction.

Bexarotene

B

Bexarotene + Contraceptives ⚠

The manufacturer suggests that bexarotene may theoretically increase the metabolism of contraceptives, thereby reducing both their serum levels and their efficacy.

The manufacturer advises that additional non-hormonal contraception (such as a barrier method) should be used to avoid the risk of contraceptive failure. They point out that this is particularly important because if contraceptive failure were to occur, the foetus might be exposed to the teratogenic effects of bexarotene.

Bexarotene + Corticosteroids ❓

The manufacturers say that, in theory, dexamethasone may reduce bexarotene levels.

This interaction does not appear to have been studied in patients, so the clinical importance of this prediction is unknown.

Bexarotene + Fibrates ❌

A population analysis of patients with cutaneous T-cell lymphoma found that gemfibrozil substantially increased the plasma levels of bexarotene.

The manufacturers say that concurrent use should be avoided.

Bexarotene + Grapefruit juice ❓

The manufacturers say that, in theory, grapefruit juice may raise bexarotene levels.

This interaction does not appear to have been studied in patients, so the clinical importance of this prediction is unknown.

Bexarotene + Macrolides ❓

The manufacturers say that, in theory, clarithromycin and erythromycin may raise bexarotene levels.

This interaction does not appear to have been studied in patients, so the clinical importance of this prediction is unknown. If this prediction is clinically relevant other macrolides may also interact, although it seems unlikely that they all will, see macrolides, page 310.

Bexarotene + Phenobarbital ❓

The manufacturers say that, in theory, phenobarbital (and therefore probably primidone) may reduce bexarotene levels.

This interaction does not appear to have been studied in patients, so the clinical importance of this prediction is unknown.

Bexarotene + **Phenytoin** ❓

The manufacturers say that, in theory, phenytoin (and therefore probably fosphenytoin) may reduce bexarotene levels.

This interaction does not appear to have been studied in patients, so the clinical importance of this prediction is unknown.

Bexarotene + **Protease inhibitors** ⚠

The manufacturers say that, in theory, protease inhibitors may raise bexarotene levels.

This interaction does not appear to have been studied in patients, so the clinical importance of this prediction is unknown.

Bexarotene + **Rifampicin (Rifampin)** ❓

The manufacturers say that, in theory, rifampicin may reduce bexarotene levels.

This interaction does not appear to have been studied in patients, so the clinical importance of this prediction is unknown.

Bexarotene + **Vitamin A** ❓

Bexarotene is related to vitamin A.

Vitamin A supplements should be limited to 15 000 units or less daily to avoid potentially additive toxic effects.

Bicalutamide

Bicalutamide + **Warfarin and other oral anticoagulants** ❓

The suggestion that bicalutamide might interact with warfarin appears to be based on protein-binding studies, which have now largely been discredited as the sole mechanism of drug interactions.

Until more is known, it would be prudent to keep this potential interaction in mind when giving both drugs.

Bisphosphonates

Bisphosphonates + **Food** ⚠

The absorption of the bisphosphonates is reduced by food.

Recommendations on the timing of administration of bisphosphonates in relation to food and other drugs vary. Alendronate and risedronate should be given at least 30 minutes before the first food of the day. Clodronate should be given at least 1 hour before or after food, ibandronate should be given with water on an empty stomach at least one hour before the first food of the day, and etidronate and tiludronate should be given on an empty stomach at least 2 hours before or after food.

Bisphosphonates + **Iron** ⚠

The oral absorption of bisphosphonates is significantly reduced (90% reduction with clodronate) by aluminium/magnesium hydroxide. Other polyvalent cations, such as iron, are expected to interact similarly.

Bisphosphonates should be prevented from coming into contact with iron. Recommendations on the timing of administration of bisphosphonates in relation to food and other drugs varies. Alendronate and risedronate should be taken at least 30 minutes before taking the first food or drink of the day, clodronate should probably be taken at least 1 hour before or after iron, ibandronate should be taken 1 hour before iron, and etidronate and tiludronate should be taken at least 2 hours apart from iron.

Bisphosphonates + **NSAIDs** ⚠

Indometacin increases tiludronate bioavailability by about 2-fold.

The manufacturer advises that indometacin and tiludronate should be given 2 hours apart.

Bisphosphonates + **Zinc** ⚠

The oral absorption of bisphosphonates is significantly reduced (90% reduction with clodronate) by aluminium/magnesium hydroxide. Other polyvalent cations, such as zinc, are expected to interact similarly.

Bisphosphonates should be prevented from coming into contact with zinc. Recommendations on the timing of administration of bisphosphonates in relation to food and other drugs varies. Alendronate and risedronate should be taken at least 30 minutes before taking the first food or drink of the day, clodronate should probably be taken at least 1 hour before or after zinc, ibandronate should be taken 1 hour before zinc, and etidronate and tiludronate should be taken at least 2 hours apart from zinc.

Bosentan

B

Bosentan + Ciclosporin (Cyclosporine) ❌

Bosentan decreases the AUC of ciclosporin by 50%, and ciclosporin increases bosentan levels by up to 4-fold.

The manufacturer of bosentan contraindicates the combination, because of the possible increased risk of liver toxicity.

Bosentan + Contraceptives ⚠

Bosentan reduces the levels of ethinylestradiol and norethisterone given as a combined oral contraceptive, which may result in contraceptive failure.

The manufacturer recommends that an additional or an alternative reliable method of contraception should be used.

Bosentan + Phosphodiesterase type-5 inhibitors ⚠

Bosentan markedly reduces the AUC of sildenafil (by about 70%) and modestly reduces the AUC of tadalafil (by about 40%). Bosentan levels are modestly reduced by sildenafil and not affected to a clinically relevant extent by tadalafil.

The efficacy of sildenafil and possibly tadalafil may be reduced in patients taking bosentan, whereas the effects of bosentan may be increased in those taking sildenafil (but probably not tadalafil). The outcome of concurrent use should be closely monitored.

Bosentan + Protease inhibitors ⚠

Ritonavir inhibits the metabolism of bosentan and increases its levels 2-fold.

The manufacturer says that dosage adjustments are not necessary. However, they note that in patients with low levels of CYP2C9 greater increases may occur. Monitoring is therefore advisable as it is unlikely that CYP2C9 phenotype will be known.

Bosentan + Statins ⚠

Bosentan modestly reduces the AUC of simvastatin (by 34%) and its active metabolite (by 46%), which could lead to a reduction in simvastatin efficacy.

Monitor the outcome to ensure that simvastatin is effective.

Bosentan + Warfarin and other oral anticoagulants ❓

Bosentan may reduce the anticoagulant effects of warfarin by 23%, and a case report describes a reduction in INR due to this interaction. However, the manufacturer of bosentan notes that clinical use of bosentan with warfarin did not result in clinically relevant changes in the INR or warfarin dose.

It is recommended that the INR should be closely monitored in any patient taking warfarin during the period that bosentan is started or stopped, or if the dose is altered.

Bupropion

Bupropion + Carbamazepine ⚠

Carbamazepine decreases the maximum plasma levels and AUC of bupropion by about 81 to 96%. The AUC of the active metabolite of bupropion is increased by 50%.

Monitor for any evidence of reduced efficacy (which is likely) and/or increased toxicity (due to the raised metabolite). Note that bupropion is contraindicated in patients with epilepsy.

Bupropion + Clopidogrel ⚠

Clopidogrel increases the AUC of bupropion by 60% and decreases the AUC of its active metabolite, hydroxybupropion, by about 50%.

Dose adjustments may be needed. It would seem prudent to monitor for increased bupropion adverse effects (lightheadedness, gastrointestinal effects) and efficacy.

Bupropion + Dextromethorphan ❓

Bupropion may reduce the metabolism of dextromethorphan in some patients.

Dextromethorphan is generally considered to have a wide therapeutic range and its dose is not individually titrated; therefore, the interaction with bupropion is unlikely to be clinically relevant. Nevertheless, it is possible that some patients might become more sensitive to the adverse effects of dextromethorphan while taking bupropion. Note that dextromethorphan is widely found in non-prescription preparations such as cough suppressants.

Bupropion + Flecainide ⚠

The manufacturers warn that bupropion may raise flecainide levels (by inhibiting CYP2D6). This seems a reasonable prediction as other CYP2D6 substrates are affected in this way.

If flecainide is added to treatment with bupropion, doses at the lower end of the range should be used. If bupropion is added to existing treatment, decreased dosages should be considered.

Bupropion + **Herbal medicines or Dietary supplements** ❓

Mania and dystonia have been reported in patients taking St John's wort (*Hypericum perforatum*) and bupropion.

No general conclusions can be drawn from these isolated reports.

Bupropion + **Levodopa** ⚠

The manufacturer says that the concurrent use of bupropion and levodopa should be undertaken with caution because limited clinical data suggests a higher incidence of undesirable effects (nausea, vomiting, excitement, restlessness, postural tremor).

Good monitoring is advisable and patients should be given small initial bupropion doses, which should be increased gradually.

Bupropion + **MAOIs** ✖

The manufacturers of bupropion contraindicate the concurrent use of MAOIs.

At least 14 days should elapse between stopping non-selective MAOIs and starting bupropion.

Bupropion + **Moclobemide** ✖

The manufacturers of bupropion contraindicate the concurrent use of moclobemide.

At least 24 hours should elapse between stopping non-selective MAOIs and starting bupropion.

Bupropion + **Phenobarbital** ⚠

Carbamazepine decreases the maximum plasma levels and AUC of bupropion by about 81 to 96%. The AUC of the active metabolite of bupropion is increased by 50%. The manufacturers predict that phenobarbital (and therefore probably primidone) will interact similarly.

Monitor for any evidence of reduced efficacy (which is likely) and/or increased toxicity (due to the raised metabolite). Note that bupropion is contraindicated in patients with epilepsy.

Bupropion + **Phenytoin** ⚠

Carbamazepine decreases the maximum plasma levels and AUC of bupropion by about 81 to 96%. The AUC of the active metabolite of bupropion is increased by 50%. The manufacturers predict that phenytoin (and therefore possibly fosphenytoin) will interact similarly.

Monitor for any evidence of reduced efficacy (which is likely) and/or increased toxicity (due to the raised metabolite). Note that bupropion is contraindicated in patients with epilepsy.

Bupropion + **Propafenone** ⚠

The manufacturers warn that bupropion may raise propafenone levels (by inhibiting CYP2D6). This seems a reasonable prediction as other CYP2D6 substrates are affected in this way.

> If propafenone is added to treatment with bupropion, doses at the lower end of the range should be used. If bupropion is added to existing treatment, decreased dosages should be considered.

Bupropion + **Protease inhibitors** ⚠

Ritonavir, both at boosted doses and higher doses, *decreases* bupropion levels, and reduced efficacy might be expected. This is the opposite effect to that which was originally predicted.

> The extent of reduction in bupropion levels seen suggests that the dose of bupropion might need to be doubled. It would seem prudent to start bupropion at the recommended starting dose and titrate to effect. Nevertheless, because of the original *in vitro* data, the UK manufacturers of bupropion currently caution that the recommended doses should not be exceeded.

Bupropion + **Rifampicin (Rifampin)** ⚠

Rifampicin markedly increases the clearance of both bupropion and its active metabolite hydroxybupropion. Reduced efficacy might be anticipated on concurrent use.

> Monitor the efficacy of bupropion in any patient requiring rifampicin, and titrate the bupropion dose as necessary.

Bupropion + **SSRIs** ⚠

SSRIs that inhibit CYP2D6 (such as paroxetine and fluoxetine) may raise bupropion levels. Concurrent use has lead to psychosis, mania, seizures, serotonin syndrome and hypersexuality.

> The manufacturers of bupropion recommend caution with SSRIs (fluoxetine, paroxetine and sertraline named). Bupropion should be started at the lower end of the dose range in patients taking an SSRI. Note that, a maximum bupropion dose of 150 mg daily is recommended if it is given with other drugs that reduce the seizure threshold.

Bupropion + **Ticlopidine** ⚠

Ticlopidine increases the AUC of bupropion by about 80% and decreases the AUC of its active metabolite, hydroxybupropion, by about 80%.

> Dose adjustments may be needed. It would seem prudent to monitor for increased bupropion adverse effects (lightheadedness, gastrointestinal effects) and efficacy.

B

Bupropion + Tricyclics ❓

Bupropion may increase the levels of desipramine, imipramine, and nortriptyline. Adverse effects including confusion, lethargy and unsteadiness have been reported with nortriptyline and bupropion. Because there is a small risk of seizures (up to 0.4%) in those given bupropion at doses of up to 450 mg daily, the manufacturers caution other drugs that can lower the convulsive threshold, such as the tricyclic antidepressants. A seizure occurred in a patient given trimipramine and bupropion.

> It has been recommended that tricyclic doses at the lower end of the range should be used in patients taking bupropion. If bupropion is added to existing treatment, decreased dosages should be considered. However, there appear to be no reports of problems with the concurrent use of any of these drugs. The clinical significance of the increased seizure risk is unknown, but it should be considered when prescribing this combination.

Bupropion + Valproate ⚠

A study found that the AUC of the active metabolite of bupropion was almost doubled when bupropion was given with valproate. An increase in valproate levels of almost 30% was seen in one patient.

> Monitor for any evidence of increased toxicity (due to the raised bupropion metabolites or valproate). Note that bupropion is contraindicated in patients with epilepsy.

Buspirone

Buspirone + Calcium-channel blockers ⚠

Diltiazem and verapamil inhibit CYP3A4, and they can therefore raise the peak levels of buspirone by 3- to 4-fold, which increases the likelihood of adverse effects.

> The US manufacturers suggest adjusting the buspirone dose according to response, while the UK manufacturers suggest starting with buspirone 2.5 mg twice daily. Information about other calcium-channel blockers appears to be lacking, but most do not commonly appear to interact by inhibiting CYP3A4.

Buspirone + Grapefruit juice ⚠

Grapefruit juice can significantly increase plasma levels of buspirone (peak level increased by more than 4-fold, but a only minor increase in effects seen).

> Consideration should be given to using a lower dose of buspirone, e.g. 2.5 mg twice daily, or avoidance of large quantities of grapefruit juice.

Buspirone + **Herbal medicines or Dietary supplements** ❓

A patient taking buspirone developed marked CNS adverse effects after starting to take herbal medicines including St John's wort (*Hypericum perforatum*), melatonin and *Ginkgo biloba*. The serotonin syndrome, page 392, has been reported in a patient who took buspirone with St John's wort (*Hypericum perforatum*).

B

> The general significance of these cases is unclear, but they highlight the importance of considering the adverse effects of herbal medicines when they are used with conventional medicines.

Buspirone + **Macrolides** ⚠

In one study the maximum levels and AUC of buspirone were increased 5-fold and 6-fold, respectively, by erythromycin, which resulted in psychomotor impairment and an increase in adverse effects.

> Monitor the outcome of concurrent use carefully, expecting to need to reduce the buspirone dosage. The manufacturers suggest a starting dose of buspirone 2.5 mg twice daily. Other macrolides (such as clarithromycin and telithromycin) may also interact, although it seems unlikely that all macrolides will, see macrolides, page 310.

Buspirone + **MAOIs** ✖

Elevated blood pressure has been reported in 4 patients taking buspirone with either phenelzine or tranylcypromine.

> The manufacturers of buspirone recommend that it should not be used concurrently with any MAOI.

Buspirone + **Protease Inhibitors** ⚠

Ritonavir, and possibly indinavir, are predicted to reduce the metabolism of buspirone. A single case report describes Parkinson-like symptoms attributed to concurrent use of buspirone with ritonavir and also possibly indinavir.

> This appears to be an isolated case. However, the UK manufacturer of buspirone recommends that a lower dose of buspirone, 2.5 mg twice daily, should be used with potent inhibitors of CYP3A4, such as ritonavir.

Buspirone + **Rifampicin (Rifampin)** ⚠

Rifampicin can cause an 87% reduction in the peak levels of buspirone and therefore diminish its effects.

> This interaction would appear to be clinically important. If both drugs are used be alert for the need to use an increased buspirone dosage.

Buspirone + SSRIs ❓

An isolated report describes the development of the serotonin syndrome, page 392, with buspirone and citalopram. The combination of buspirone and fluoxetine can be effective, but seizures and worsening of symptoms have been reported. Fluvoxamine may possibly reduce the effects of buspirone.

> The general importance of, and reasons for, these adverse reactions are not well understood, but there would seem to be little reason for avoiding concurrent use. However, bear these interactions in mind when buspirone is given with an SSRI.

Busulfan

Busulfan + Phenytoin ❓

Phenytoin increases the clearance of busulfan and reduces its AUC by about 20%. Subtherapeutic levels of phenytoin may occur in the presence of busulfan.

> The changes in busulfan clearance are relatively small, but nevertheless it has been suggested that phenytoin should be avoided in patients taking busulfan. Note that the US manufacturer of parenteral busulfan gives a dose assuming that phenytoin will also be given, and notes that if other antiepileptics are used instead, the busulfan plasma levels may be increased and monitoring is recommended. If both drugs are given monitor closely to ensure that busulfan remains effective, and that phenytoin levels remain therapeutic.

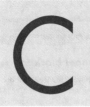

Calcium-channel blockers

Both verapamil and diltiazem are principally metabolised by CYP3A4, and also inhibit this isoenzyme. They are therefore affected by drugs that induce or inhibit CYP3A4, and also themselves affect drugs metabolised by CYP3A4. Many of the dihydropyridine-type calcium-channel blockers are also metabolised by CYP3A4, and are affected by inducers or inhibitors of this isoenzyme. However, they do not generally inhibit CYP3A4 or other isoenzymes to a clinically relevant extent. The exception is perhaps nicardipine, which may cause a clinically relevant inhibition of CYP3A4.

Calcium-channel blockers + Calcium-channel blockers ⚠

Plasma levels of both nifedipine and diltiazem are increased by concurrent use and blood pressure is reduced accordingly. This has been claimed to be an advantageous interaction but caution is advised. There are isolated reports of intestinal occlusion attributed to the concurrent use of nifedipine and diltiazem. If nimodipine is used with another calcium-channel blocker, monitoring, with possible dose reduction or discontinuation of the other calcium-channel blocker, is recommended.

Monitor blood pressure on concurrent use and adjust the dose or stop one calcium-channel blocker as appropriate.

Calcium-channel blockers + Carbamazepine

Diltiazem or Verapamil ⚠

Carbamazepine levels are raised by diltiazem (up to 4-fold), and verapamil has caused carbamazepine toxicity.

Monitor carbamazepine levels and adjust the dose accordingly. Indicators of carbamazepine toxicity include nausea, vomiting, ataxia and drowsiness. Oxcarbazepine appears to be a non-interacting alternative.

Nimodipine ✗

Nimodipine levels are decreased by 85% by carbamazepine.

The manufacturers advise against concurrent use.

Other calcium-channel blockers ⚠

Felodipine, nifedipine and nilvadipine levels are decreased by carbamazepine. All calcium-channel blockers are metabolised by CYP3A4, and carbamazepine would therefore be expected to decrease their levels to some extent.

Monitor the outcome of concurrent use, being aware that the dose of the calcium-channel blocker may need to be raised.

Calcium-channel blockers + Ciclosporin (Cyclosporine)

Lercanidipine ✗

The plasma levels of lercanidipine were raised 3-fold by ciclosporin, and the ciclosporin AUC was raised by 21% by lercanidipine.

The manufacturers contraindicate concurrent use.

Other calcium-channel blockers ⚠

Diltiazem, nicardipine and verapamil markedly raise serum ciclosporin levels but also appear to possess kidney protective effects. Amlodipine has modestly increased ciclosporin levels in some studies, but not in others, and it may also have kidney protective properties. A single case describes elevated ciclosporin levels caused by nisoldipine. Nifedipine normally appears not to interact, but rises and falls in ciclosporin levels have been seen in a few patients.

Ciclosporin levels should be well monitored (especially with diltiazem, nicardipine and verapamil) and dosage reductions made as necessary. With diltiazem and verapamil the ciclosporin dosage can apparently be reduced by about 25 to 50% and even greater reductions may be necessary with nicardipine.

Calcium-channel blockers + Cilostazol

Nifedipine or Verapamil ⚠

The UK manufacturers of cilostazol advise caution when it is given with drugs that are substrates of CYP3A4, especially those with a narrow therapeutic index. They specifically mention nifedipine and verapamil.

Monitor the outcome of concurrent use for an increase in the effects of verapamil or nifedipine (e.g. hypotension or bradycardia).

Diltiazem ⚠

Diltiazem increases the AUC of cilostazol by about 40%.

In the UK the manufacturers contraindicate the combination, whereas in the US the manufacturers suggest halving the cilostazol dose.

Calcium-channel blockers + **Corticosteroids** ⚠

Diltiazem increases the AUC of intravenous and oral methylprednisolone.

> The clinical significance of this interaction is unclear. It has been suggested that patients should be monitored for methylprednisolone adverse effects (e.g. fluid retention, hypertension and hyperglycaemia), and this seems a prudent precaution.

Calcium-channel blockers + **Darifenacin** ⚠

Erythromycin almost doubles the AUC of darifenacin by inhibiting its metabolism by CYP3A4. Other moderate inhibitors of CYP3A4, such as diltiazem and verapamil are expected to interact similarly.

> The US manufacturers suggests that no dosage adjustments are necessary with these calcium-channel blockers, whereas the UK manufacturer suggests increasing the darifenacin dose with caution. Bear in mind the possibility of an interaction if antimuscarinic effects (dry mouth, constipation, drowsiness) are increased.

Calcium-channel blockers + **Digoxin**

Diltiazem ⚠

Serum digoxin levels were found to be unchanged by diltiazem in a number of studies but other studies describe increases ranging from 20 to 85%.

> All patients taking digoxin with diltiazem should be well monitored for signs of over-digitalisation (e.g. bradycardia) and dosage reductions should be made if necessary.

Verapamil ⚠

Serum digoxin levels are increased by about 40% by verapamil 160 mg daily, and by about 70% by verapamil 240 mg daily. Digoxin toxicity may develop if the dosage is not reduced. Deaths have occurred as a result of this interaction.

> An initial 33 to 50% dosage reduction has been recommended for digoxin. The interaction develops within 2 to 7 days, reaching a maximum within 14 days or so. Monitor digoxin levels during this period.

Other calcium-channel blockers ✓

Felodipine, gallopamil, lacidipine, lercanidipine, nicardipine and nisoldipine cause small increases in digoxin levels (maximum rise seen was about 30%, which was not considered clinically significant). The situation with nitrendipine is uncertain but it possibly causes only a small rise in digoxin levels. Serum digoxin levels are normally unchanged or increased only to a small extent by the concurrent use of nifedipine. However, one isolated study indicated that a 45% rise could occur.

> Bear this interaction in mind if patients are treated with both drugs concurrently. The possibility of a serious interaction seems small, but if undesirable bradycardia or other symptoms of over-digitalisation occur consider taking digoxin levels.

Calcium-channel blockers + **Disopyramide** ⚠

Profound hypotension and collapse has occurred in a small number of patients taking verapamil with disopyramide.

> The manufacturers warn about combining disopyramide and verapamil (because of additive negative inotropic effects), but they do point out that in some specific circumstances the combination may be beneficial. Monitor concurrent use carefully.

Calcium-channel blockers + **Diuretics** ⚠

Mild to moderate inhibitors of CYP3A4 (such as diltiazem and verapamil) cause a 2-fold increase in eplerenone levels, which increases the risks of hyperkalaemia. Additive hypotensive effects likely when calcium-channel blockers are given with any diuretic, see antihypertensives, page 77.

> It is generally recommended that the dose of eplerenone should not exceed 25 mg daily in patients taking diltiazem or verapamil.

Calcium-channel blockers + **Dutasteride** ❓

In one study diltiazem and verapamil were found to decrease the clearance of dutasteride by 44% and 37%, respectively. However, this was not thought to be clinically significant due to the wide therapeutic range of dutasteride.

> No action needed, although bear this interaction in mind if dutasteride adverse effects are troublesome.

Calcium-channel blockers + **Flecainide** ⚠

Although flecainide and verapamil have been used together successfully, serious and potentially life-threatening cardiogenic shock and asystole have been seen in a few patients. This is probably because the cardiac depressant effects of the two drugs can be additive.

> The additive cardiac depressant effects are probably of little importance in many patients, but may represent the last straw' in a few who have seriously compromised cardiac function. Monitor concurrent use carefully.

Calcium-channel blockers + **Food** ❓

The bioavailability of manidipine may be increased by food and the plasma levels of other lipophilic calcium-channel blockers (lercanidipine, nisoldipine) may also be affected.

> It has been recommended that manidipine should be given with food. Because of the potential increase in peak plasma concentrations, the manufacturers of lercanidipine and nisoldipine advise giving them before meals (at least 15 minutes before has been recommended).

Calcium-channel blockers + **Grapefruit juice** ✖

Grapefruit juice very markedly increases the bioavailability of felodipine and nisoldipine, and alters their haemodynamic effects. The bioavailability of nicardipine, nifedipine, nimodipine or nitrendipine is increased without significantly altering haemodynamic effects, whereas the bioavailability of amlodipine, diltiazem and verapamil is only minimally affected. However, with verapamil some ECG changes were seen.

The manufacturers of felodipine say that it should not be taken with grapefruit juice. It has been suggested that whole grapefruit or products made from grapefruit peel such as marmalade should also be avoided in patients taking felodipine. The manufacturers of lercanidipine, nifedipine, nimodipine, nisoldipine and verapamil also contraindicate grapefruit juice, although this interaction is normally of little relevance with most calcium-channel blockers in the majority of patients.

C

Calcium-channel blockers + **H₂-receptor antagonists** ✔

The plasma levels of diltiazem, isradipine and nifedipine are increased by cimetidine and it may be necessary to reduce their dosages. High doses of cimetidine may increase the bioavailability of lercanidipine. Although studies suggest no important interactions occur between nicardipine or nisoldipine and cimetidine, the manufacturers advise caution. Plasma felodipine, lacidipine, nimodipine, and nitrendipine levels are also increased but this does not seem to be clinically significant.

Monitor concurrent use. If adverse effects (such as hypotension, dizziness, flushing and palpitations) become troublesome decrease the calcium-channel blocker dose.

Calcium-channel blockers + **Herbal medicines or Dietary supplements** ⚠

St John's wort *(Hypericum perforatum)* reduces the bioavailability of verapamil by over 70%.

It would seem prudent to avoid concurrent use, or at least closely monitor to ensure that verapamil remains effective.

Calcium-channel blockers + **Lithium** ⚠

The concurrent use of lithium and verapamil can be uneventful, but neurotoxicity, bradycardia, choreoathetosis, and decreases in serum lithium levels have been seen in a few patients. An acute parkinsonian syndrome and marked psychosis has been seen in at least one patient taking lithium with diltiazem.

The adverse reactions cited above contrast with other reports describing uneventful concurrent use. This unpredictability emphasises the need to monitor the effects closely where it is thought appropriate to give lithium with these calcium-channel blockers.

Calcium-channel blockers + **Macrolides**

Lercanidipine ⊗

Because potent inhibitors of CYP3A4 have raised lercanidipine levels by 15-fold the manufacturers predict that erythromycin will raise lercanidipine levels.

> Concurrent use is contraindicated. Other macrolides may also interact, although it seems unlikely that they all will, see macrolides, page 310.

Other calcium-channel blockers ⚠

Erythromycin markedly increases the bioavailability of felodipine. Isolated reports describe increased felodipine, nifedipine or verapamil effects and toxicity in patients when given erythromycin, clarithromycin or telithromycin. Note that the calcium-channel blockers are all metabolised by CYP3A4, so all have the potential to interact.

> Monitor concurrent use. If adverse effects become troublesome (such as hypotension, dizziness, flushing and palpitations) adjust the calcium-channel blocker dose.

Calcium-channel blockers + **Magnesium**

Two pregnant women developed muscular weakness and then paralysis when they were given nifedipine and intravenous magnesium sulfate.

> If concurrent use is essential monitor patients very carefully. If problems occur, note that in the two cases of paralysis the interaction resolved rapidly when magnesium was stopped.

Calcium-channel blockers + **NSAIDs** ?

A meta-analysis of 50 studies in patients or healthy subjects found that NSAIDs elevated mean supine blood pressure by 5 mmHg. Ibuprofen, indometacin and piroxicam produced the greatest increases. Aspirin and sulindac produced the smallest increases in blood pressure and the effects of diclofenac, flurbiprofen, naproxen and tiaprofenic acid were intermediate. However, there seems to be little evidence that a clinically significant interaction occurs in most patients taking calcium-channel blockers.

> Although the risks of NSAIDs with calcium-channel blockers may be less than those with other antihypertensive drugs, until more information is available, caution has been recommended. It has been suggested that the use of NSAIDs should be kept to a minimum in patients with hypertension. The effects may be greater in the elderly and in those with blood pressures that are relatively high, as well as in those with high salt intake.

Calcium-channel blockers + **Phenobarbital**

Nimodipine ⊗

Nimodipine levels are decreased by 85% by phenobarbital. Note that primidone is metabolised to phenobarbital and therefore may interact similarly.

> The manufacturers advise against concurrent use.

Other calcium-channel blockers ❌

Phenobarbital decreases the levels of felodipine (bioavailability reduced by more than 90%), nifedipine (AUC reduced by 60%) and verapamil (bioavailability reduced 5-fold). Other calcium-channel blockers are expected to interact similarly with phenobarbital. Note that primidone is metabolised to phenobarbital and therefore may also interact.

> Monitor the outcome of concurrent use, being aware that the dose of calcium-channel blocker may need to be raised. Given the size of the reductions seen it may be prudent to consider alternatives.

C

Calcium-channel blockers + **Phenytoin**

Diltiazem or Nifedipine ❓

Case reports describe phenytoin toxicity in patients given diltiazem or nifedipine.

> The general importance of this interaction is unknown, but bear it in mind in case of an unexpected response to treatment. Indicators of phenytoin toxicity include blurred vision, nystagmus, ataxia or drowsiness.

Nimodipine or Nisoldipine ❌

Phenytoin (with carbamazepine) reduces nimodipine levels by 85% and phenytoin reduces the AUC of nisoldipine 10-fold. Fosphenytoin, a prodrug of phenytoin, may interact similarly.

> The manufacturers contraindicate concurrent use.

Other calcium-channel blockers ⚠

Phenytoin reduces the levels of verapamil and felodipine (bioavailability reduced by more than 90%). Fosphenytoin, a prodrug of phenytoin, may interact similarly.

> Monitor the outcome of concurrent use, being aware that the dose of calcium-channel blocker may need to be raised. Given the size of the reductions seen it may be prudent to consider alternatives.

Calcium-channel blockers + **Protease inhibitors** ⚠

Nelfinavir, ritonavir, and saquinavir are predicted to increase the levels of calcium-channel blockers that are substrates of CYP3A4 (see calcium-channel blockers, page 153). The manufacturers of amprenavir similarly predict that it will increase the levels of diltiazem, nicardipine, nifedipine and nisoldipine. Atazanavir has been seen to raise diltiazem levels (2- to 3-fold) and is therefore predicted to raise verapamil levels.

> Undertake concurrent use with caution. Monitor for toxicity, such as hypotension, dizziness, flushing and palpitations.

Calcium-channel blockers + **Quinidine**

Verapamil 🔺

Verapamil reduces the clearance of quinidine and in one patient the serum quinidine levels doubled and quinidine toxicity developed. Acute hypotension has also been seen in 3 patients taking quinidine with intravenous verapamil.

A reduction in the dosage of quinidine (of up to 50%) may be needed to avoid toxicity.

Other calcium-channel blockers 🔺

The quinidine levels of a number of patients have increased when nifedipine was stopped, but no interaction has occurred in others. One study even suggests that quinidine serum levels may be slightly raised by nifedipine. One study with diltiazem found that it did not interact with quinidine, whereas another found that diltiazem increased the quinidine AUC by 51%, with resulting significant increases in QTc and PR intervals, and a significant decrease in heart rate and diastolic blood pressure.

Monitor the outcome of concurrent use, being aware that the quinidine dose may need to be reduced.

Calcium-channel blockers + **Rifampicin (Rifampin)** 🔺

The plasma levels of diltiazem, nifedipine, nilvadipine, verapamil and possibly those of barnidipine, isradipine, lercanidipine, manidipine, nicardipine, nimodipine, and nisoldipine are markedly reduced by rifampicin. They may become therapeutically ineffective unless their dosages are raised.

Increase the frequency of blood pressure monitoring and adjust the antihypertensive dose, or use an alternative drug, as necessary. Note that the manufacturers of nifedipine and nisoldipine contraindicate their use with rifampicin, and the manufacturer of nimodipine advises against the combination.

Calcium-channel blockers + **Sirolimus** 🔺

The maximum serum levels of sirolimus are raised by diltiazem (43%) and verapamil (over 2-fold). Dosage adjustments may be necessary. Nicardipine is predicted to interact similarly.

The manufacturers recommend monitoring and possible sirolimus dosage adjustment if these calcium-channel blockers are used concurrently.

Calcium-channel blockers + **Statins** 🔺

Marked rises in statin plasma levels have been seen when lovastatin was given with diltiazem, and when simvastatin was given with diltiazem or verapamil. Isolated cases of rhabdomyolysis have been seen when atorvastatin or simvastatin were given with diltiazem or verapamil. However, it seems that problems with combinations of statins and calcium-channel blockers are rare.

It has been suggested that treatment with a statin in those taking diltiazem (and probably verapamil) should be started with the lowest possible dose and titrated upwards, or considerably reduced if either of these calcium-channel blockers is started. The manufacturers recommend a maximum simvastatin dose of 20 mg in patients taking verapamil and 40 mg in patients taking diltiazem. Patients should be told to be alert for any signs of possible rhabdomyolysis (i.e. otherwise unexplained muscle tenderness, pain or weakness or dark coloured urine).

Calcium-channel blockers + Tacrolimus ⚠

Nifedipine causes a moderate rise in serum tacrolimus levels and also appears to be kidney protective. Diltiazem and felodipine also appear to elevate tacrolimus levels. Nicardipine, nilvadipine and verapamil are predicted to interact similarly.

Tacrolimus levels and/or effects (e.g. on renal function) should be monitored as a matter of routine, but consider increasing monitoring if one of these calcium-channel blockers is started or stopped.

Calcium-channel blockers + Theophylline ✅

Giving calcium-channel blockers to patients taking theophylline normally has no adverse effect on the control of asthma, despite the small or modest alterations that occur in theophylline levels with diltiazem, felodipine, nifedipine and verapamil. However, there are isolated case reports of unexplained theophylline toxicity in 2 patients given nifedipine and 2 patients given verapamil.

The clinical significance of the cases is unclear, but generally no adverse interaction would be expected.

Calcium-channel blockers + Tricyclics ❓

Diltiazem and verapamil can increase plasma imipramine levels, possibly accompanied by undesirable ECG changes. Two isolated reports describe increased nortriptyline and trimipramine levels in 2 patients given diltiazem.

The general importance of this interaction is unclear, but bear it in mind in case of an unexpected response to treatment.

Calcium-channel blockers + Valproate ⚠

In a group of patients taking sodium valproate, the AUC of nimodipine was found to be about 50% higher than in a control group not taking sodium valproate.

Monitor concurrent use carefully, bearing in mind it may be necessary to adjust the dose of nimodipine.

Capecitabine

Capecitabine + **Folates** ⚠

A patient died after treatment with capecitabine possibly because the concurrent use of folic acid enhanced capecitabine toxicity. The maximum tolerated dose of capecitabine is decreased by folinic acid.

> The UK manufacturers say that the maximum tolerated capecitabine dose when used alone in the intermittent regimen is 3000 mg/m^2, but it is reduced to 2000 mg/m^2 if folinic acid 30 mg twice daily is also given. Consider the use of folate supplements as a contributory factor in the case of troublesome capecitabine adverse effects.

Capecitabine + **Phenytoin** ⚠

Phenytoin toxicity occurred in a patient given capecitabine. Fosphenytoin, a prodrug of phenytoin, may interact similarly.

> As this interaction is in line with the way fluorouracil interacts, it would seem prudent to warn the patient to monitor for signs of phenytoin toxicity (blurred vision, nystagmus, ataxia or drowsiness). Take phenytoin levels and adjust the dose as necessary.

Capecitabine + **Warfarin and other oral anticoagulants** ⚠

Capecitabine has been reported to markedly increase the anticoagulant effects of phenprocoumon and warfarin in some patients. The interaction may occur within several days or even after months of concurrent use.

> The INR should be regularly monitored in patients taking capecitabine with these and other coumarins.

Carbamazepine

Carbamazepine is extensively metabolised by CYP3A4 to the active 10,11-epoxide metabolite, which is then further metabolised. Concurrent use of CYP3A4 inhibitors or inducers may therefore lead to toxicity or reduced efficacy. However, importantly, carbamazepine also induces CYP3A4 and so induces its own metabolism (auto-induction). Because of this, it is important that drug interaction studies are multiple-dose and carried out at steady state. Auto-induction also means that moderate inducers of CYP3A4 may have less effect on steady-state carbamazepine levels than expected. Carbamazepine can also act as an inhibitor of CYP2C19.

Carbamazepine + Caspofungin ▲

Population pharmacokinetic data suggests that carbamazepine may reduce caspofungin levels.

> The manufacturers say that consideration should be given to increasing the dose of caspofungin from 50 to 70 mg daily.

Carbamazepine + Ciclosporin (Cyclosporine) ▲

Carbamazepine has caused reductions of 50% or more in ciclosporin levels. This has occurred within 3 days of concurrent use.

> Ciclosporin levels and/or effects (e.g. on renal function) should be monitored as a matter of routine, but it may be prudent to increase monitoring and adjust the ciclosporin dose as needed if carbamazepine is stopped, started, or the dose altered.

Carbamazepine + Contraceptives ▲

Combined hormonal contraceptives, progestogen-only pills and emergency hormonal contraceptives are less reliable during treatment with carbamazepine. Breakthrough bleeding and spotting can take place and unintended pregnancies have occurred. Controlled studies have shown that carbamazepine can reduce contraceptive steroid levels.

> Because of the consequences of an unwanted pregnancy, especially with drugs that may cause foetal abnormalities, adjustments should be made. For general advice on the use of enzyme inducers, such as carbamazepine, and contraceptives, see contraceptives, page 199.

Carbamazepine + Corticosteroids ▲

The clearance of methylprednisolone and prednisolone is increased in patients taking carbamazepine. Dexamethasone clearance is also increased, and therefore the results of the dexamethasone adrenal suppression test may be invalid in those taking carbamazepine. More study is needed but it is likely that other corticosteroids such as hydrocortisone and prednisone may be affected.

> Patients taking carbamazepine are likely to need increased doses of dexamethasone, methylprednisolone or prednisolone. Prednisolone is less affected than methylprednisolone and is probably preferred.

Carbamazepine + Danazol ▲

Serum carbamazepine levels can be doubled by danazol and carbamazepine toxicity may occur.

> Consider monitoring carbamazepine levels and adjust the dose if necessary. Carbamazepine toxicity may present as nausea, vomiting, ataxia or drowsiness.

Carbamazepine + **Diuretics** ❌

Because St John's wort (*Hypericum perforatum*) decreases the AUC of eplerenone by 30% the manufacturers say that more potent enzyme inducers (such as carbamazepine) may have a greater effect on eplerenone.

Concurrent use is not recommended by the manufacturers.

Carbamazepine + **Ethosuximide** ⚠

Some, but not all studies suggest that carbamazepine reduces ethosuximide levels by about 20% and reduces its half-life.

The concurrent use of antiepileptics is common and often advantageous. Information on this interaction is sparse, and its clinical importance is uncertain, although probably small.

Carbamazepine + **Gestrinone** ❓

The manufacturers warn that carbamazepine may increase the metabolism of gestrinone and thereby reduce its effects.

The clinical significance of this warning is unclear. There appear to be no reports of an interaction in practice.

Carbamazepine + **Grapefruit juice** ⚠

Grapefruit juice increases carbamazepine levels by about 40%. A case of possible carbamazepine toxicity has been seen in a man taking carbamazepine after he started to eat grapefruit.

The manufacturers advise monitoring levels and adjusting the dose of carbamazepine as necessary. If monitoring is not practical, or regular intake of grapefruit is not desired, it would seem prudent to avoid grapefruit or grapefruit juice.

Carbamazepine + **H$_2$-receptor antagonists** ❓

Epileptic patients and subjects taking carbamazepine long-term show a transient increase in serum levels, possibly accompanied by an increase in adverse effects, for the first few days after starting to take cimetidine, but these adverse effects rapidly disappear.

An increase in carbamazepine adverse effects may be seen, and patients should be warned. However, because the serum levels are only transiently increased the adverse effects normally disappear by the end of a week. Ranitidine appears to be a non-interacting alternative to cimetidine, and oxcarbazepine appears to be a non-interacting alternative to carbamazepine.

Carbamazepine + **Herbal medicines or Dietary supplements** ✓

St John's wort (*Hypericum perforatum*) modestly increased the clearance of single-dose carbamazepine, but had no effect on multiple-dose carbamazepine in one study.

Before the publication of these studies the CSM in the UK had advised that patients taking carbamazepine should not take St John's wort. This advice was based on predicted pharmacokinetic interactions. In the light of the above studies, this advice may no longer apply.

C

Carbamazepine + **HRT** ❓

Enzyme-inducing drugs (such as carbamazepine), which increase the metabolism of contraceptive steroids, may reduce the efficacy of HRT.

This effect is most noticeable where HRT is prescribed for menopausal vasomotor symptoms, but might be difficult to detect where the indication is osteoporosis. Any interaction may be less likely with transdermal HRT. However, as yet the clinical significance of any interaction is unclear.

Carbamazepine + **Imatinib** ⚠

Rifampicin decreases the AUC of imatinib by 74%. No specific studies have been carried out with imatinib and other CYP3A4 inducers, but the manufacturers suggest that carbamazepine will interact similarly.

The manufacturers suggest that concurrent use should be avoided. However, if this is not possible it would be prudent to monitor the outcome of concurrent use, and increase the imatinib dose as necessary.

Carbamazepine + **Isoniazid** ⚠

Carbamazepine serum levels are markedly and very rapidly increased by isoniazid, and toxicity can occur. Rifampicin (rifampin) has been reported both to augment and negate this interaction. Limited evidence suggests that carbamazepine may potentiate isoniazid hepatotoxicity.

Carbamazepine toxicity can develop quickly (within 1 to 5 days) and also seems to disappear quickly if the isoniazid is withdrawn. Concurrent use should not be undertaken unless the effects can be closely monitored and suitable downward dosage adjustments made (a carbamazepine dose reduction to between one-half or one-third was effective in some patients). Carbamazepine toxicity may present as nausea, vomiting, ataxia or drowsiness.

Carbamazepine + **Lamotrigine** ⚠

Most studies have found that lamotrigine has no effect on the pharmacokinetics of carbamazepine or its active epoxide metabolite. However, some studies have found that lamotrigine raises the serum levels of carbamazepine-epoxide. Carbamazepine reduces lamotrigine levels. Toxicity has been seen irrespective of changes in levels.

> Overall lamotrigine does not appear to significantly alter carbamazepine levels. However, toxicity has occurred, therefore patients should be well monitored if lamotrigine is added, and the carbamazepine dose reduced if CNS adverse effects occur. Carbamazepine induces the metabolism of lamotrigine, and the recommended starting dose and long-term maintenance dose of lamotrigine in patients already taking carbamazepine is twice that of patients receiving lamotrigine monotherapy. However, if they are also taking valproate in addition to carbamazepine, the lamotrigine dose should be reduced.

Carbamazepine + Levothyroxine ❓

Clinical hypothyroidism can occur in patients stabilised taking levothyroxine when they start carbamazepine.

> The general importance of this interaction seems small, but be alert for any evidence of changes in thyroid status if carbamazepine is added or withdrawn from patients taking levothyroxine.

Carbamazepine + Lithium ⚠️

Although the combined use of lithium and carbamazepine is beneficial in many patients, mild to severe neurotoxicity is reported to have developed in some, and possibly sinus node dysfunction in others.

> Monitor the outcome of concurrent use carefully, but note that signs of toxicity have developed even with lithium levels within the normal range. Risk factors appear to be a history of neurotoxicity with lithium therapies and compromised medical or neurological functioning.

Carbamazepine + Macrolides

Erythromycin ❌

Erythromycin raises carbamazepine levels by as much as 5-fold, which has resulted in toxicity in several cases.

> Avoid concurrent use unless carbamazepine levels can be closely monitored and suitable dosage reductions made. Symptoms commonly begin within 24 to 72 hours of starting erythromycin. In most cases toxicity resolves within 5 days of stopping the erythromycin. Carbamazepine toxicity may present as nausea, vomiting, ataxia or drowsiness.

Telithromycin ❌

The manufacturer predicts that carbamazepine will reduce the levels of telithromycin, and that telithromycin may raise carbamazepine levels.

> The manufacturers say to avoid telithromycin use during and for up to 2 weeks after carbamazepine treatment. If concurrent use is essential, monitor carbamazepine levels and telithromycin efficacy. Carbamazepine toxicity may present as nausea, vomiting, ataxia or drowsiness.

Other macrolides ⚠

Clarithromycin raises carbamazepine levels by 20 to 50%, despite dosage reductions of up to 40%. Several cases of toxicity have been seen.

Monitor carbamazepine levels and adjust the dose accordingly. It has been recommended that carbamazepine doses are reduced by 30 to 50% and patients monitored within 3 to 5 days of starting clarithromycin. Carbamazepine toxicity may present as nausea, vomiting, ataxia or drowsiness. Azithromycin appears not to interact and may therefore be a suitable alternative.

Carbamazepine + MAOIs ✗

Although there is no evidence that the MAOIs interact with carbamazepine the manufacturers advise avoidance as carbamazepine is structurally related to the tricyclics, page 323. However, note that there have been several reports of successful use of MAOIs with carbamazepine.

The manufacturers advise avoiding concurrent use. Note that, rarely, the MAOIs have been seen to cause convulsions.

Carbamazepine + Mebendazole ⚠

Carbamazepine appears to lower the plasma levels of mebendazole.

When treating systemic worm infections it may be necessary to increase the mebendazole dosage in patients taking carbamazepine. Monitor the outcome of concurrent use. This interaction is of no importance when mebendazole is used for intestinal worm infections where its action is a local effect on the worms in the gut.

Carbamazepine + Methylphenidate ❓

Limited evidence suggests that carbamazepine may decrease methylphenidate levels.

It would seem wise to monitor the response to methylphenidate treatment carefully in patients taking carbamazepine. Note that the manufacturer says methylphenidate should be used with caution in patients with epilepsy, as it can, rarely, cause an increase in seizure frequency. If seizure frequency increases, methylphenidate should be discontinued.

Carbamazepine + Mianserin ⚠

Plasma levels of mianserin can be markedly reduced by the concurrent use of carbamazepine.

Monitor the response to mianserin and increase the dose as necessary.

Carbamazepine + Mirtazapine ⚠

Carbamazepine decreases the AUC and maximum plasma levels of mirtazapine, by

63% and 44%, respectively. Mirtazapine does not appear to affect the pharmacokinetics of carbamazepine.

The mirtazapine dose may need to be increased. Monitor concurrent use to assess mirtazapine efficacy, and adjust the dose accordingly.

Carbamazepine + **NNRTIs** ⚠

The concurrent use of carbamazepine and efavirenz leads to a modest reduction in the plasma levels of both drugs. The use of nevirapine and carbamazepine may also result in decreased levels of both drugs.

The manufacturers of efavirenz note that an alternative to carbamazepine should be considered (especially with doses of greater than 400 mg daily). If both drugs are given it would seem prudent to their monitor plasma levels (where possible), and efficacy.

Carbamazepine + **Opioids**

Dextropropoxyphene (Propoxyphene) ⚠

Dextropropoxyphene has caused rises in trough serum carbamazepine levels of around 60 to 600%. Several cases of toxicity have been seen.

Monitor carbamazepine levels and adjust the dose if necessary. Carbamazepine toxicity may present as nausea, vomiting, ataxia or drowsiness.

Other opioids ⚠

Carbamazepine appears to reduce the serum levels of fentanyl (48 to 144% dose increase needed), methadone (opiate withdrawal seen), and tramadol.

Be alert for the need to increase opioid doses. Note that tramadol should be avoided in patients with a history of epilepsy.

Carbamazepine + **Phenobarbital** ❓

Carbamazepine serum levels are reduced to some extent by the concurrent use of phenobarbital, but the levels of its active metabolite are unchanged; seizure control remains unaffected. Primidone seems to interact similarly. In children, phenobarbital clearance is decreased by carbamazepine.

This interaction seems to be of little clinical importance as seizure control is not affected. However, it would be prudent to monitor phenobarbital levels in children also given carbamazepine as changes in clearance may affect dose requirements.

Carbamazepine + **Phenytoin** ⚠

Some reports describe rises in serum phenytoin levels, with toxicity, whereas others describe falls in phenytoin levels. Genetic differences in the metabolism of these drugs may be an explanation for the differences. Falls in carbamazepine serum levels, sometimes with rises in carbamazepine-epoxide levels, have been described.

Monitor antiepileptic levels during concurrent use (where possible including carbamazepine-epoxide, the active metabolite of carbamazepine) so that steps can be taken to avoid the development of toxicity or lack of efficacy. Not all patients appear to have an adverse interaction, and, at present, it does not seem possible to identify those potentially at risk.

C

Carbamazepine + Phosphodiesterase type-5 inhibitors ⚠

Carbamazepine is predicted to reduce the levels of phosphodiesterase type-5 inhibitors, because other inducers of CYP3A4 have been shown to do so. For example, sildenafil levels are reduced by 70% by *bosentan* and tadalafil levels are reduced by 88% by *rifampicin*. Vardenafil is also metabolised by CYP3A4, and therefore its levels may possibly be lowered by carbamazepine.

If these phosphodiesterase type-5 inhibitors are not effective in patients taking carbamazepine, it would seem sensible to try a higher dose with close monitoring.

Carbamazepine + Praziquantel ⚠

Carbamazepine markedly reduces the serum levels of praziquantel by 90%, but whether this results in neurocysticercosis treatment failures is unclear; one study found that concurrent use was still effective for neurocysticercosis.

When treating systemic worm infections such as neurocysticercosis some authors advise increasing the praziquantel dosage from 25 to 50 mg/kg if carbamazepine is being taken, but in one study this dose was not effective. Note that the manufacturers current recommended dose of praziquantel for neurocysticercosis is 50 mg/kg daily in 3 divided doses. The interaction with carbamazepine is of no importance when praziquantel is used for intestinal worm infections (where its action is a local effect on the worms in the gut).

Carbamazepine + Protease inhibitors ⚠

Case reports suggest that ritonavir, lopinavir/ritonavir and nelfinavir markedly increases carbamazepine levels resulting in toxicity. Carbamazepine reduces indinavir and tipranavir levels and efficacy, and would also be expected to decrease the levels of other protease inhibitors.

Although the evidence is limited, these interactions seem to be established. It would therefore appear that the combination of carbamazepine and protease inhibitors should be avoided where possible (mainly because of the risk of antiviral treatment failure). If both must be used then extremely close monitoring of both protease inhibitor levels/efficacy and carbamazepine levels/toxicity is warranted. Indicators of carbamazepine toxicity include nausea, vomiting, ataxia and drowsiness. The authors of one report suggest that amitriptyline or gabapentin would be possible alternatives for carbamazepine when used for pain, or valproic acid or lamotrigine for carbamazepine when used for seizures.

Carbamazepine + Rimonabant ❓

The manufacturers predict that potent inducers of CYP3A4 such as carbamazepine may lower the serum levels of rimonabant. This is based on the fact that potent *inhibitors* of CYP3A4 *increase* rimonabant levels (see under azoles, page 122).

Caution is recommended with concurrent use of carbamazepine and rimonabant and patients should be monitored to ensure rimonabant remains effective.

Carbamazepine + Sirolimus ⚠

The manufacturers predict that carbamazepine may lower the serum levels of sirolimus, probably because rifampicin (rifampin), another CYP3A4 inducer, has been shown to do so.

The extent of any change in sirolimus levels is uncertain, but it would seem prudent to increase the frequency of monitoring of sirolimus levels during concurrent use.

Carbamazepine + Solifenacin ⚠

Ketoconazole increases solifenacin levels 2- to 3-fold by *inhibiting* CYP3A4. The manufacturers predict that potent CYP3A4 *inducers* (e.g. carbamazepine) will decrease solifenacin levels.

Be alert for a reduction in the efficacy of solifenacin in patients taking carbamazepine.

Carbamazepine + SSRIs ⚠

Case reports indicate that carbamazepine levels can be increased by fluoxetine and fluvoxamine. Toxicity may develop. Citalopram, paroxetine and sertraline do not normally affect carbamazepine levels, but carbamazepine may reduce their levels. Isolated cases of a Parkinsonian and serotonin syndrome have occurred when fluoxetine was given with carbamazepine, and an isolated case of pancytopenia has been reported when sertraline was given with carbamazepine. Consideration should be given to the fact that SSRIs have been known to cause seizures.

Reports of an adverse interaction seem rare, but bear these reactions in mind during concurrent use. Carbamazepine toxicity may present as nausea, vomiting, ataxia or drowsiness. Consider monitoring carbamazepine levels if fluoxetine or fluvoxamine is started.

Carbamazepine + Statins ⚠

Carbamazepine reduces the levels of simvastatin and its active metabolite by around 80%.

A simvastatin dose increase seems likely to be necessary. Monitor concurrent use to check that simvastatin is effective.

Carbamazepine + Tacrolimus ⚠

Phenytoin decreased tacrolimus levels in one case, and has been used to reduce tacrolimus levels after an overdose. Other CYP3A4 inducers such as carbamazepine are predicted to interact similarly.

No interaction is established, but based on the known metabolism of these drugs it would be prudent to monitor tacrolimus levels in a patient given carbamazepine.

Carbamazepine + Tetracyclines ⚠

The serum levels of doxycycline are reduced and may fall below the accepted therapeutic minimum in patients taking carbamazepine long-term.

It has been suggested that the doxycycline dosage could be doubled to counteract this interaction. Tetracycline, oxytetracycline and chlortetracycline appear not to interact and may therefore be suitable alternatives.

Carbamazepine + Theophylline ⚠

Two case reports describe a marked fall in theophylline levels when carbamazepine was given. Another single case report and a pharmacokinetic study describe a fall in serum carbamazepine levels when theophylline was given.

The general importance of these reports is uncertain. Concurrent use need not be avoided, but it would be prudent to check that the serum concentrations of each drug (and their effects) do not become subtherapeutic.

Carbamazepine + Tiagabine ⚠

The plasma concentrations of tiagabine may be reduced 1.5- to 3-fold by carbamazepine.

The manufacturers recommend that tiagabine 30 to 45 mg (in divided doses) should be given to patients taking enzyme-inducing antiepileptics such as carbamazepine. A lower maintenance dose of 15 to 30 mg should be given to patients who are not taking enzyme-inducing drugs.

Carbamazepine + Tibolone ❓

The manufacturers warn that carbamazepine may increase the metabolism of tibolone and thereby reduce its effects.

The clinical significance of this warning is unclear. There appear to be no reports of an interaction in practice.

Carbamazepine + Topiramate ⚠

Topiramate serum levels may be reduced by about 40% by carbamazepine. Carbamazepine levels are not affected by topiramate. However, one report suggests that the toxicity seen when topiramate was added to the maximum tolerated doses of carbamazepine may respond to a reduction in the carbamazepine dose.

Monitor the outcome of concurrent use, increasing the topiramate dose if it seems less effective than desired.

Carbamazepine + Toremifene ⚠

Carbamazepine can reduce the serum levels of toremifene.

The manufacturers of toremifene suggest that its dosage may need to be doubled in the presence of carbamazepine.

Carbamazepine + Trazodone ❓

A single case report describes a moderate rise in serum carbamazepine levels in a patient given trazodone. Carbamazepine may moderately decrease trazodone levels.

Monitor trazodone efficacy and increase the dose as needed. The clinical significance of the rise in carbamazepine levels is likely to be small. Indicators of carbamazepine toxicity include nausea, vomiting, ataxia, drowsiness.

Carbamazepine + Tricyclics ❓

The serum levels of amitriptyline, desipramine, doxepin, imipramine and nortriptyline, but possibly not clomipramine, can be reduced (halved or more) by the concurrent use of carbamazepine but there is evidence to suggest that this is not necessarily clinically important.

It seems unlikely that any action is needed, but bear this interaction in mind in case of a reduced response to a tricyclic. Note that the tricyclics can lower the convulsive threshold and should therefore be used with caution in patients with epilepsy.

Carbamazepine + Vaccines ✔

Carbamazepine levels rose modestly 14 days after influenza vaccination in one study. A case report describes carbamazepine toxicity and markedly increased carbamazepine levels in a teenager 13 days after influenza vaccination.

The moderate increase in serum carbamazepine levels seen in the study is unlikely to have much clinical relevance. However, the case report of markedly increased carbamazepine levels introduces a note of caution. Carbamazepine toxicity may present as nausea, vomiting, ataxia or drowsiness.

Carbamazepine + Valproate ⚠

The serum levels of carbamazepine are usually only slightly affected by sodium valproate, valproic acid or valpromide although a moderate to marked rise in the levels of its active epoxide metabolite may occur. Carbamazepine may reduce the serum levels of sodium valproate by 60% or more. Concurrent use may possibly increase the incidence of sodium valproate-induced hepatotoxicity.

Monitor valproate levels, and adjust the dose if necessary. Also monitor for carbamazepine toxicity (due to raised carbamazepine-epoxide levels), which may present as nausea, vomiting, ataxia or drowsiness.

Carbamazepine + **Warfarin and other oral anticoagulants** ⚠

The anticoagulant effects of warfarin can be markedly reduced (by around 50% in many reports) by carbamazepine. Acenocoumarol is expected to interact similarly, and cases of this interaction have been seen with phenprocoumon.

Monitor the INR if carbamazepine is added to warfarin therapy. Continue monitoring until the carbamazepine dose is stabilised. Also monitor the INR if the carbamazepine is withdrawn as the effects of warfarin may become excessive within a week.

Carbamazepine + **Zonisamide** ❓

Carbamazepine can cause a small to moderate reduction in the serum levels of zonisamide, and zonisamide has been reported to cause increases, decreases or no changes to carbamazepine serum levels.

The clinical importance of this interaction is unknown, but be aware of the possibility of changes in the levels of both drugs if they are given together.

Carbimazole

Carbimazole + **Digoxin** ❓

Carbimazole slightly lowers digoxin levels in euthyroid subjects. However, the drug-disease interaction that also occurs is probably of more importance. Hyperthyroid subjects are relatively resistant to the effects of digoxin and so need higher doses. As treatment with carbimazole progresses and they become euthyroid, the dosage of digoxin will need to be decreased.

Monitor the outcome of resolving hyperthyroidism, checking for digoxin overdosage, by symptoms of bradycardia etc. Monitor digoxin levels as necessary.

Carbimazole + **Theophylline** ⚠

Thyroid status may affect the rate at which theophylline is metabolised. In hyperthyroidism it is increased, and so patients require higher theophylline dosages. As thyroid function is corrected (e.g. with carbimazole) theophylline metabolism decreases and so smaller doses are needed. Two case reports describe theophylline toxicity in patients being treated for hyperthyroidism.

Monitor the outcome of resolving hyperthyroidism, checking for theophylline adverse effects (headache, nausea, palpitations). Monitor theophylline levels and adjust the dose as necessary.

Carbimazole + Warfarin and other oral anticoagulants ⚠

Thyroid status affects the response to warfarin: correction of hyperthyroidism will increase the amount of warfarin needed.

Weekly monitoring of the INR is advisable for any patient taking an oral anticoagulant until they become euthyroid.

Caspofungin

Caspofungin + Ciclosporin (Cyclosporine) ⚠

Ciclosporin increases the AUC of caspofungin by 35% and causes increases in AST and ALT of up to 3-fold. Retrospective studies found no serious hepatic adverse events with the combination, but 2 of 40 patients had discontinued therapy because of abnormalities in hepatic enzymes. However, other studies suggest adverse hepatic events are increased by the combination.

The manufacturer advises that ciclosporin and caspofungin should only be used if the benefits outweigh the risks of treatment, and if they are used, close monitoring of liver enzymes is recommended.

Caspofungin + NNRTIs ⚠

Population data suggests that efavirenz and nevirapine may reduce caspofungin levels. This is in line with the known enzyme-inducing properties of these NNRTIs.

The manufacturers say that consideration should be given to increasing the dose of caspofungin from 50 to 70 mg daily.

Caspofungin + Phenytoin ⚠

Population data suggests that phenytoin may reduce caspofungin levels. This is in line with the known enzyme-inducing properties of phenytoin.

The manufacturers say that consideration should be given to increasing the dose of caspofungin from 50 to 70 mg daily.

Caspofungin + **Rifampicin (Rifampin)** ⚠

Rifampicin initially increases the trough levels of caspofungin by 170%, but after 2 weeks the trough levels of caspofungin decrease, and are about 30% lower than in patients not receiving rifampicin. Antifungal treatment failure has been seen in a patient taking rifampicin with caspofungin 70 mg daily.

The manufacturers say that consideration should be given to increasing the dose of caspofungin from 50 to 70 mg daily in patients taking enzyme-inducing drugs. However, close monitoring is still required because of the isolated report of treatment failure even at the higher dose.

Caspofungin + **Tacrolimus** ⚠

Caspofungin decreases trough tacrolimus levels by 26%. Tacrolimus does not affect the pharmacokinetics of caspofungin.

Tacrolimus levels and/or effects (e.g. on renal function) should be monitored as a matter of routine, but it is advisable to increase monitoring if caspofungin is started or stopped, and adjust the dose of tacrolimus if required.

Cephalosporins

Cephalosporins + **Ciclosporin (Cyclosporine)** ❓

Isolated reports suggest that ceftazidime, ceftriaxone, and latamoxef may increase ciclosporin levels, whereas one report suggested ceftazidime, ceftriaxone, and cefuroxime did not, although ceftazidime caused deterioration in some measures of renal function.

Information about these cephalosporins is very limited. The general relevance of these reports is uncertain, but bear them in mind in the event of an unexpected response to treatment.

Cephalosporins + **Contraceptives** ⚠

A few anecdotal cases of combined oral contraceptive failure have been reported with the cephalosporins. The interaction (if such it is) appears to be very rare indeed.

For guidance on the use of antibacterials with contraceptives, see contraceptives, page 199.

Cephalosporins + **H_2-receptor antagonists** ⚠

Ranitidine and famotidine reduce the bioavailability of cefpodoxime proxetil. Ranitidine (with sodium bicarbonate) reduces the bioavailability of cefuroxime axetil.

In most cases the interactions between the cephalosporins and H_2-receptor antagonists are not clinically significant. The clinical importance of the interaction with cefpodoxime has not been studied, but the manufacturer recommends that it should be given at least 2 hours before H_2-receptor antagonists. As it is thought that a change in gastric pH is responsible for this interaction it would seem likely that all H_2-receptor antagonists will interact similarly. As long as cefuroxime is taken with food (as is recommended), any interaction is minimal.

Cephalosporins + **Probenecid** ✓

Overall, probenecid reduces the clearance, raises the serum levels and sometimes prolongs the half-lives of the cephalosporins.

No special precautions are normally needed. However, be aware that elevated serum levels of some cephalosporins might possibly increase the risk of toxicity.

Cephalosporins + **Proton pump inhibitors** ⚠

Ranitidine and *famotidine* reduce the bioavailability of cefpodoxime proxetil. *Ranitidine* (with sodium bicarbonate) reduces the bioavailability of cefuroxime axetil.

As it is thought that a change in gastric pH is responsible for this interaction it would seem likely that the proton pump inhibitors will interact in the same way as the H_2-receptor antagonists. However, as long as cefuroxime is taken with food (as is recommended), any interaction is minimal.

Cephalosporins + **Warfarin and other oral anticoagulants** ⚠

Cephalosporins with an *N*-methylthiotetrazole side-chain can cause bleeding alone or more severely in the presence of an anticoagulant. The cephalosporins implicated are cefaclor, cefaloridine, cefalotin, cefamandole, cefazaflur, cefazolin, cefixime, cefmenoxime, cefmetazole, cefminox, cefonicid, cefoperazone, ceforanide, cefotetan, cefotiam, cefoxitin, cefpiramide, ceftriaxone, and latamoxef.

Severe bleeding events have been seen with some cephalosporins. As this usually occurs after about 3 days it would seem prudent to monitor the INR at this point and adjust the anticoagulant dose accordingly. If dose alterations are needed further INR monitoring will be required when the cephalosporin is stopped.

Chloramphenicol

Chloramphenicol + **Ciclosporin (Cyclosporine)** ⚠

Four patients have shown marked rises in serum ciclosporin levels when treated with chloramphenicol. A small study supports these findings.

Ciclosporin levels and/or effects (e.g. on renal function) should be monitored as a matter of routine, but it may be prudent to increase monitoring if chloramphenicol is started or stopped. Adjust the dose of ciclosporin as necessary. It seems doubtful that there will be enough chloramphenicol absorbed from eye drops to interact with ciclosporin, but this needs confirmation.

Chloramphenicol + **Contraceptives** ⚠

One or two cases of combined oral contraceptive failure have been reported with chloramphenicol. These isolated cases are anecdotal and unconfirmed, and the interaction (if such it is) appears to be very rare indeed.

For guidance on the use of antibacterials with contraceptives, see contraceptives, page 199.

Chloramphenicol + **Iron** ❌

In addition to the serious and potentially fatal bone marrow depression that can occur with chloramphenicol, it may also cause a milder, reversible bone marrow depression, which can oppose the treatment of anaemia with iron.

It has been suggested that chloramphenicol dosages of 25 to 30 mg/kg are usually adequate for treating infections without running the risk of elevating serum levels to 25 micrograms/mL or more, which is when this type of marrow depression can occur. Monitor the effects of using iron concurrently. Where possible it would be preferable to use a different antibacterial.

Chloramphenicol + **Paracetamol (Acetaminophen)** ✓

Although there is limited evidence to suggest that paracetamol may affect chloramphenicol pharmacokinetics its validity has been criticised. Evidence of a clinically relevant interaction appears lacking.

No action needed.

Chloramphenicol + **Phenobarbital** ⚠

Studies in children show that phenobarbital can markedly reduce chloramphenicol levels. An isolated case describes markedly increased phenobarbital levels in an adult caused by the use of chloramphenicol. Note that primidone is metabolised to phenobarbital and therefore may interact similarly.

Concurrent use should be well monitored to ensure that chloramphenicol serum levels are adequate. Make appropriate dosage adjustments as necessary. The case of raised phenobarbital levels is of uncertain importance.

Chloramphenicol + **Phenytoin** ⚠

Serum phenytoin levels can be raised by the concurrent use of chloramphenicol. Also, evidence from children suggests that phenytoin may reduce or raise serum chloramphenicol levels. Fosphenytoin, a prodrug of phenytoin, may interact similarly.

> Concurrent use should be avoided unless the effects can be closely monitored and appropriate phenytoin dosage reductions made as necessary. The use of a single prophylactic dose of phenytoin or fosphenytoin may be an exception to this. If both drugs are given, monitor for phenytoin toxicity (indicators include blurred vision, nystagmus, ataxia or drowsiness). Take phenytoin levels as necessary and adjust the dose accordingly. Also monitor for chloramphenicol efficacy and toxicity.

Chloramphenicol + Rifampicin (Rifampin) ⚠

Four case reports describe seriously reduced chloramphenicol levels in children also given rifampicin.

> It has been suggested that rifampicin prophylaxis should be delayed in patients with invasive Haemophilus influenzae infections until the end of chloramphenicol treatment.

Chloramphenicol + Tacrolimus ⚠

A marked rise in serum tacrolimus levels has been reported in several patients also given systemic chloramphenicol. This is expected to be an interaction of general importance.

> Tacrolimus levels and/or effects (e.g. on renal function) should be monitored as a matter of routine, but it may be prudent to increase monitoring if chloramphenicol is started or stopped.

Chloramphenicol + Vitamin B$_{12}$ ✖

In addition to the serious and potentially fatal bone marrow depression that can occur with chloramphenicol, it may also cause a milder, reversible bone marrow depression, which can oppose the treatment of anaemia with iron or vitamin B$_{12}$.

> It has been suggested that chloramphenicol dosages of 25 to 30 mg/kg are usually adequate for treating infections without running the risk of elevating serum levels to 25 micrograms/mL or more, which is when this type of marrow depression can occur. Monitor the effects of using iron or vitamin B$_{12}$ concurrently. Where possible it would be preferable to use a different antibacterial.

Chloramphenicol + Warfarin and other oral anticoagulants ❓

Some limited, and poor quality evidence suggests that the anticoagulant effects of acenocoumarol and dicoumarol can be increased by oral chloramphenicol. An isolated report attributes a marked INR rise in a patient taking warfarin to the use of chloramphenicol eye drops.

> This interaction is by no means adequately established. There would therefore appear to be little reason for avoiding concurrent use, but be aware that increases

in INR are possible. The interaction with chloramphenicol eye drops seems unlikely to be generally relevant.

Chloroquine

Chloroquine + **Ciclosporin (Cyclosporine)** ⚠

Three patients had rapid rises in serum ciclosporin levels, with evidence of nephrotoxicity in two of them, when they were given chloroquine. Some loss of renal function has been seen even when low doses of ciclosporin are used with chloroquine for rheumatoid arthritis. Note that hydroxychloroquine may interact similarly.

Ciclosporin levels and/or effects (e.g. on renal function) should be monitored as a matter of routine, but it may be prudent to increase monitoring if chloroquine is started or stopped. Adjust the dose of ciclosporin as necessary.

Chloroquine + **Digoxin** ⚠

The blood levels of digoxin were found to be markedly increased by 70% in two elderly patients when they took hydroxychloroquine. A similar increase has been seen with chloroquine in *dogs*.

The clinical significance of this interaction is uncertain, but it would seem sensible to be aware of this potential interaction if both drugs are used.

Chloroquine + **H₂-receptor antagonists** ⚠

Cimetidine reduces the metabolism and halves the clearance of chloroquine.

The clinical importance of this interaction is uncertain, but it would seem prudent to be alert for any signs of chloroquine toxicity during concurrent use. Hydroxychloroquine is expected to be similarly affected. Ranitidine may be a suitable alternative as it does not appear to interact.

Chloroquine + **Kaolin** ⚠

Kaolin can reduce the absorption of chloroquine by about 30%. Hydroxychloroquine is predicted to interact similarly.

Separate the dosages of chloroquine and kaolin as much as possible (at least 2 to 3 hours) to minimise the interaction. Be alert for any signs of reduced chloroquine efficacy.

Chloroquine + **Leflunomide** ✗

The manufacturers say that the concurrent use of leflunomide and chloroquine or hydroxychloroquine has not yet been studied, but it would be expected to increase the risk of serious adverse reactions (haematological toxicity or hepatotoxicity).

The manufacturers advise avoiding concurrent use. As the active metabolite of leflunomide has a long half life of 1 to 4 weeks a washout with colestyramine or activated charcoal should be given if patients are to be switched to other DMARDs.

Chloroquine + Mefloquine ❌

In theory there is an increased risk of convulsions if mefloquine is given with chloroquine. The manufacturers suggest that concurrent use increases the risks of ECG abnormalities. Note that hydroxychloroquine may interact similarly.

The manufacturers suggest that concurrent use should be avoided.

Chloroquine + Penicillamine ❌

The concurrent use of chloroquine and penicillamine may result in increased toxicity, possibly as a result of increased penicillamine levels.

If problems occur consider this drug interaction as a possible cause. Note that chloroquine, hydroxychloroquine and penicillamine are associated with serious haematological adverse effects, and therefore the US manufacturers suggest that the use of penicillamine with either of these drugs should be avoided.

Chloroquine + Praziquantel ⚠

Chloroquine reduces the bioavailability of praziquantel, which would be expected to reduce its efficacy in systemic worm infections such as schistosomiasis. Note that hydroxychloroquine may interact similarly.

It has been suggested that an increased dosage of praziquantel should be considered in the presence of chloroquine, particularly in anyone who does not respond to initial treatment with praziquantel. This interaction is not of importance when praziquantel is used for intestinal worm infections (where its action is a local effect on the worms in the gut).

Ciclosporin (Cyclosporine)

Ciclosporin (Cyclosporine) + Colchicine ⚠

A handful of cases of ciclosporin toxicity and serious muscle disorders (myopathy, rhabdomyolysis) have been seen when colchicine was given with ciclosporin.

Concurrent use should be carefully monitored and treatment stopped at the earliest signs of myopathy.

Ciclosporin (Cyclosporine) + **Contraceptives** ❓

Hepatotoxicity has been described in 2 patients taking ciclosporin with oral contraceptives containing ethinylestradiol or desogestrel plus levonorgestrel. The use of norethisterone 10 or 15 mg daily has caused raised ciclosporin levels.

The interactions between ciclosporin and hormonal contraceptives or norethisterone are unconfirmed and of uncertain clinical significance. There is insufficient evidence to recommend increased monitoring, but be aware of the potential for an interaction in case of an unexpected response to treatment.

C

Ciclosporin (Cyclosporine) + **Corticosteroids** ❓

The concurrent use of ciclosporin and corticosteroids is very common, but some evidence suggests that ciclosporin serum levels are raised by corticosteroids (2-fold by methylprednisolone, and by up to 20% with prednisolone or prednisone). Ciclosporin can moderately increase corticosteroid levels, which may lead to symptoms of overdosage (cushingoid symptoms such as steroid-induced diabetes, osteonecrosis of the hip joints). Convulsions have also been described during concurrent use.

The combination is commonly used, and the case reports and studies document effects well known to be adverse effects of both drugs. The clinical importance of this interaction is probably limited, but if abnormal results occur, remember that this drug combination could perhaps be a cause.

Ciclosporin (Cyclosporine) + **Co-trimoxazole** ❓

Although co-trimoxazole can increase the serum creatinine levels in kidney transplant patients taking ciclosporin, concurrent use normally appears to be safe and effective.

This interactions is not firmly established. Serious interactions with co-trimoxazole seem rare, and so no additional monitoring would seem to be necessary, at least for low-dose prophylactic co-trimoxazole.

Ciclosporin (Cyclosporine) + **Danazol** ⚠

Marked increases in ciclosporin levels (3-fold in one case) have been seen in patients taking danazol.

Ciclosporin levels and/or effects (e.g. on renal function) should be monitored as a matter of routine, but it may be prudent to increase monitoring if danazol is started or stopped.

Ciclosporin (Cyclosporine) + **Digoxin** ⚠

Ciclosporin causes 3- to 4-fold rises in serum digoxin levels in some patients.

The effects of concurrent use should be monitored very closely, and the digoxin dosage should be adjusted according to levels.

Ciclosporin (Cyclosporine) + **Diuretics** ❓

Isolated cases of nephrotoxicity have been described in patients taking ciclosporin with either amiloride/hydrochlorothiazide or metolazone. The concurrent use of ciclosporin with thiazides may increase serum magnesium levels, and the concurrent use of ciclosporin with potassium-sparing diuretics may cause hyperkalaemia. The concurrent use of ciclosporin and eplerenone may increase potassium levels and lead to renal impairment.

> The general importance of these adverse interactions is not clear, but some caution is clearly prudent. Consider monitoring potassium levels if a potassium-sparing diuretic is given. The manufacturers of eplerenone advise avoiding concurrent use wherever possible. If concurrent use is necessary, monitor ciclosporin levels, potassium and renal function frequently until stable.

Ciclosporin (Cyclosporine) + **Etoposide** ⚠

High-dose ciclosporin markedly raises etoposide serum levels and increases the suppression of white blood cell production. Severe toxicity has been reported in one patient.

> Some have suggested reducing the dose of etoposide by 40 or 50%. The use of high-dose ciclosporin for multidrug resistant tumour modulation remains experimental and should only be used in clinical studies. Concurrent use should be very well monitored.

Ciclosporin (Cyclosporine) + **Ezetimibe** ⚠

Ciclosporin may elevate ezetimibe levels by as much as 3.4-fold.

> The manufacturers advise that ciclosporin levels and ezetimibe adverse effects should be closely monitored. Be aware of the risks of increased ezetimibe toxicity (abdominal pain, headache, nausea and rarely myopathy). Patients should be advised to report any muscle pain, tenderness or weakness.

Ciclosporin (Cyclosporine) + **Fibrates** ⚠

Bezafibrate significantly increased serum creatinine and tended to reduce ciclosporin levels in one study. Deterioration in renal function has also been reported in 5 patients, 4 of whom had no change in ciclosporin levels, and one of whom had increased serum ciclosporin levels. The use of fenofibrate has also been associated with reduced renal function and possibly reduced serum ciclosporin levels. Two studies found no pharmacokinetic interaction between ciclosporin and gemfibrozil while a third found gemfibrozil caused a significant reduction in ciclosporin levels.

> Ciclosporin levels and effects (e.g. on renal function) should be monitored as a matter of routine, but it may be prudent to increase monitoring if a fibrate is started or stopped. Adjust the dose of ciclosporin as necessary.

Ciclosporin (Cyclosporine) + Grapefruit juice ❌

A considerable number of single and multiple dose studies have shown that if oral ciclosporin is taken with 150 to 250 mL of grapefruit juice, the trough and peak serum levels and the bioavailability of ciclosporin may be increased. Increases in trough serum levels range from 23 to 85%. Intravenous ciclosporin does not appear to be affected.

The increases appear to be variable and this interaction is difficult, if not impossible, to control. This is because batches of grapefruit juice vary so much, and also because considerable patient variation occurs with this interaction. The US manufacturers suggest that patients on ciclosporin should avoid whole grapefruit, as well as the juice.

Ciclosporin (Cyclosporine) + Griseofulvin ❓

The ciclosporin levels of a man were roughly halved when he took griseofulvin 500 mg daily, despite an approximately 70% increase in the ciclosporin dosage.

This interaction is unconfirmed and of uncertain clinical significance. There is insufficient evidence to recommend increased monitoring, but be aware of the potential for an interaction in the case of an unexpected response to treatment.

Ciclosporin (Cyclosporine) + H₂-receptor antagonists ❓

Although some reports suggest that cimetidine (and possibly famotidine) can rarely increase ciclosporin levels, the majority of the information suggests no interaction occurs. Note that raised creatinine levels have been seen following the combination, but this does not appear to be related to renal toxicity or reduced renal function.

There is little to suggest that concurrent use should be avoided, but good initial monitoring is advisable.

Ciclosporin (Cyclosporine) + Herbal medicines or Dietary supplements

Alfalfa and/or Black cohosh ❌

An isolated report describes acute rejection and vasculitis when a renal transplant patient taking ciclosporin also took black cohosh and/or alfalfa.

The evidence of for this interaction is limited, but as the effects were so severe in this case it would seem prudent to avoid concurrent use.

Berberine ❓

Berberine appears to increase the bioavailability and trough blood levels of ciclosporin.

Although the increase seen was not sufficient to suggest that concurrent use should be avoided, it may make ciclosporin levels less stable. If concurrent use is undertaken it should be well monitored.

Geum chiloense ❓

A single report describes a marked (more than 5-fold), rapid increase in the ciclosporin levels of a man who drank an infusion of *Geum chiloense*.

There is insufficient evidence to make any strong recommendations, but be aware of the potential for an interaction.

Red yeast rice (Monascus purpureus) ⚠

Red yeast rice has been reported to cause rhabdomyolysis in a kidney transplant patient taking ciclosporin.

Ciclosporin is well known to interact with the statins, and this interaction appeared to be mediated by a statin-like component in the red yeast rice. Patients should report any unexplained muscle pain, tenderness or weakness.

St John's wort (Hypericum perforatum) ✖

Marked falls in ciclosporin levels (resulting in transplant rejection in some cases) can occur with a few weeks of starting St John's wort.

It is possible to accommodate this interaction by increasing the ciclosporin dosage. However, the advice of the CSM in the UK is that patients taking ciclosporin should avoid or stop taking St John's wort. In the latter situation, the serum ciclosporin levels should be well monitored. Some evidence suggests that monitoring should continue for up to 2 weeks after stopping the St John's wort.

Ciclosporin (Cyclosporine) + Lanreotide ⚠

Octreotide causes a marked fall in the serum levels of ciclosporin, and inadequate immunosuppression may result. Lanreotide is predicted to interact similarly.

Ciclosporin levels and effects (e.g. on renal function) should be monitored as a matter of routine, but it may be prudent to increase monitoring if lanreotide is started or stopped.

Ciclosporin (Cyclosporine) + Macrolides ⚠

Ciclosporin levels can be markedly raised by clarithromycin (commonly 2- to 3-fold), erythromycin (4- to 5-fold or more, intravenous use seems to have less effect than oral), josamycin (commonly 2- to 3-fold), midecamycin (2-fold) and pristinamycin (65% in one study). Rokitamycin, telithromycin and troleandomycin are predicted to interact similarly. Although major studies have found no interaction with azithromycin, there have been several case reports.

Ciclosporin levels and effects (e.g. on renal function) should be monitored as a matter of routine, but it may be prudent to increase monitoring if macrolides are started or stopped. With erythromycin, also consider increased monitoring if the route of administration is changed. Other macrolides may also interact, although it seems unlikely that they all will, see macrolides, page 310. There is some evidence to suggest that roxithromycin and spiramycin interact minimally or not at all.

Ciclosporin (Cyclosporine) + Methotrexate ⚠

Previous or concurrent treatment with methotrexate may possibly increase the risk of liver and other toxicity, but effective and valuable concurrent use has also been reported. Ciclosporin causes a moderate rise in serum methotrexate levels.

Monitor the outcome of concurrent use carefully. The dose of either drug may need to be reduced and drug toxicity (renal and hepatic) may be more common.

Ciclosporin (Cyclosporine) + Metoclopramide ⚠

Metoclopramide increases the absorption of ciclosporin and raises its peak serum levels by 46%.

Ciclosporin levels and effects (e.g. on renal function) should be monitored as a matter of routine, but it may be prudent to increase monitoring if metoclopramide is started or stopped.

Ciclosporin (Cyclosporine) + Modafinil ❓

Ciclosporin serum levels were reported to be reduced by modafinil in one patient.

This is seems to be the only reported case of an interaction between ciclosporin and modafinil, and its general importance is unknown.

Ciclosporin (Cyclosporine) + NNRTIs ❓

The ciclosporin levels of one patient dramatically decreased following the addition of efavirenz.

Although this is an isolated case it is in line with the way both drugs are known to interact. It would seem prudent to closely monitor ciclosporin levels in any patient given efavirenz.

Ciclosporin (Cyclosporine) + NSAIDs ⚠

Some NSAIDs (diclofenac, indometacin, ketoprofen, mefenamic acid, naproxen, piroxicam and sulindac) sometimes reduce renal function in individual patients, which is reflected in serum creatinine level rises and possibly in changes in ciclosporin levels, but concurrent use can also be uneventful. Diclofenac serum levels can be doubled by ciclosporin.

Concurrent use in rheumatoid arthritis need not be avoided but renal function should be closely monitored. The manufacturers of ciclosporin also specifically recommend that patients with rheumatoid arthritis taking ciclosporin and an NSAID should also have their liver function measured, because hepatotoxicity is a potential adverse effect of both drugs. It is difficult to generalise about what will or will not happen if any particular NSAID is given, but in the case of diclofenac, it has been recommended that doses at the lower end of the range should be used initially, because its serum levels can be doubled by ciclosporin.

Ciclosporin (Cyclosporine) + Octreotide ⚠

Octreotide causes a marked fall in the serum levels of ciclosporin, and inadequate immunosuppression may result.

> Ciclosporin levels and effects (e.g. on renal function) should be monitored as a matter of routine, but it may be prudent to increase monitoring if octreotide is started or stopped.

Ciclosporin (Cyclosporine) + Orlistat ⚠

The absorption of ciclosporin is significantly reduced by orlistat (by more than 50% in some cases). In one case, orlistat appeared to have less effect on the microemulsion formulation (*Neoral*) of ciclosporin than the older formulation (*Sandimmun*). Nevertheless, a non-significant episode of acute graft rejection has been reported with the microemulsion formulation.

> Ciclosporin levels and effects (e.g. on renal function) should be monitored as a matter of routine, but it would be prudent to increase monitoring if orlistat is started or stopped. Adjust the dose of ciclosporin as necessary.

Ciclosporin (Cyclosporine) + Phenobarbital ⚠

Several cases describe large reductions in ciclosporin levels in patients given phenobarbital. In one case the ciclosporin dose had to be increased 3-fold to keep the levels within the therapeutic range. As primidone is metabolised to phenobarbital it seems likely that it will interact similarly.

> Ciclosporin levels and effects (e.g. on renal function) should be monitored as a matter of routine, but it may be prudent to increase monitoring if these drugs are stopped, started, or the dose altered.

Ciclosporin (Cyclosporine) + Phenytoin ⚠

A study and several case reports describe a reduction in ciclosporin levels (37% reduction in the study) following the addition of phenytoin. Other reports describe the need to make 2- to 4-fold increases in the ciclosporin dose in patients also taking phenytoin.

> Ciclosporin levels and effects (e.g. on renal function) should be monitored as a matter of routine, but it may be prudent to increase monitoring if phenytoin is stopped, started, or the dose altered.

Ciclosporin (Cyclosporine) + Protease inhibitors ⚠

Increased ciclosporin levels have been seen in patients taking fosamprenavir, lopinavir, ritonavir and saquinavir. Other protease inhibitors would be expected to interact similarly.

Ciclosporin levels should be carefully monitored and the dose adjusted accordingly if a protease inhibitors are also given, bearing in mind that large dose reductions may be required in some patients.

Ciclosporin (Cyclosporine) + Proton pump inhibitors ❓

Studies suggest that omeprazole 20 mg daily does not affect ciclosporin levels, but isolated reports describe doubled serum ciclosporin levels in one patient, and more than halved serum ciclosporin levels in another. Both patients were taking omeprazole 40 mg daily.

This interaction is unlikely to be of general importance, but bear it in mind in case of an unexpected response to treatment, particularly with doses of omeprazole 40 mg daily or above.

Ciclosporin (Cyclosporine) + Quinolones ⚠

Ciclosporin serum levels are normally unchanged by the use of ciprofloxacin, but increased serum levels and nephrotoxicity may occur in a small number of patients. One study, and two case reports describe rises in ciclosporin levels in patients given norfloxacin, but another study found no change. Similar results have been found with levofloxacin.

Increased monitoring of ciclosporin levels and effects would seem prudent in patients given ciprofloxacin, levofloxacin or norfloxacin, although note that evidence for an adverse interaction is limited. There seem to be no reports of problems with enoxacin, ofloxacin, pefloxacin or trovafloxacin.

Ciclosporin (Cyclosporine) + Rifabutin ⚠

Rifabutin appears to increase the clearance of ciclosporin by about 20%.

Information is limited so it would still be prudent to consider increasing the monitoring of ciclosporin levels and effects (e.g. on renal function) if rifabutin is started or stopped.

Ciclosporin (Cyclosporine) + Rifampicin (Rifampin) ⚠

Ciclosporin serum levels are markedly reduced (in some cases within one day) by the concurrent use of rifampicin. Transplant rejection can rapidly develop if the ciclosporin dosage is not increased.

Ciclosporin levels and effects (e.g. on renal function) should be monitored as a matter of routine, but it is essential to increase monitoring if rifampicin is started or stopped. The ciclosporin dose will need to be increased substantially when rifampicin is added (3- to 5-fold increases have been needed in some cases). It has been suggested that other antituberculars should be used in patients taking ciclosporin.

C

Ciclosporin (Cyclosporine) + Sevelamer ⚠

One study suggests sevelamer does not appear to alter ciclosporin levels, but a report describes markedly reduced ciclosporin levels in a patient who took sevelamer.

The manufacturers advise that ciclosporin should be taken at least 1 hour before or 3 hours after sevelamer.

Ciclosporin (Cyclosporine) + Statins

Rosuvastatin ⊗

The AUC of rosuvastatin is increased 7-fold by ciclosporin.

The manufacturers of rosuvastatin contraindicate its use with ciclosporin.

Other statins ⚠

Ciclosporin can cause marked rises in the plasma levels of atorvastatin, fluvastatin, lovastatin, pravastatin and simvastatin, and for some of the statins this had led to the development of serious myopathy (rhabdomyolysis) accompanied by kidney failure. The plasma levels of ciclosporin appear not to be affected by fluvastatin, lovastatin or pravastatin, but some moderate changes have been seen when atorvastatin or simvastatin were used.

Concurrent use should be very well monitored, a precautionary recommendation being to start (or reduce) the statin at the lowest daily dose, appropriate to the patient's condition. It has been suggested by some manufacturers that the dose of simvastatin should not exceed 10 mg daily, and the dose of lovastatin should not exceed 20 mg daily, in patients taking ciclosporin. Patients should be told to report any signs of myopathy and possible rhabdomyolysis (i.e. otherwise unexplained muscle pain, tenderness or weakness or dark coloured urine). If myopathy does occur, withdrawing the statin has been shown to resolve the symptoms. Only simvastatin and atorvastatin appear to affect ciclosporin levels, and it may be prudent to monitor ciclosporin levels more closely with these two drugs.

Ciclosporin (Cyclosporine) + Sulfinpyrazone ⚠

Sulfinpyrazone can reduce ciclosporin levels (by about 40% in one study), and this is said to have led to transplant rejection, which developed over a period of several months.

If there is a trend towards decreased ciclosporin levels in patients taking sulfinpyrazone it would be prudent to consider this interaction as a cause and adjust treatment accordingly.

Ciclosporin (Cyclosporine) + **Sulfonamides** ❓

In isolated cases sulfadiazine given orally or sulfadimidine with trimethoprim given intravenously have caused a fall in serum ciclosporin levels. Sulfametoxydiazine possibly caused a minor fall in one case.

> These interactions are not firmly established. Until more information is available it would be prudent to check ciclosporin levels if any sulphonamide is added to established treatment with ciclosporin.

Ciclosporin (Cyclosporine) + **Terbinafine** ❓

Terbinafine causes a small, usually clinically unimportant fall in ciclosporin serum levels (maximum levels reduced by 14%).

> This interaction is not usually clinically significant. However, patients whose ciclosporin levels are at the lower end of the therapeutic range should be closely monitored if they are given terbinafine.

Ciclosporin (Cyclosporine) + **Ursodeoxycholic acid (Ursodiol)** ⚠

Ursodeoxycholic acid unpredictably increases the absorption and raises the serum levels of ciclosporin in some patients.

> Ciclosporin levels and effects (e.g. on renal function) should be monitored as a matter of routine, but it may be prudent to increase monitoring if ursodeoxycholic acid is started or stopped. Adjust the dose of ciclosporin as necessary.

Ciclosporin (Cyclosporine) + **Vaccines** ✕

The body's immune response is suppressed by ciclosporin. The antibody response to vaccines may be reduced, and the use of live attenuated vaccines may result in generalised infection.

> For many inactivated vaccines even the reduced response seen is considered clinically useful, and in the case of renal transplant patients influenza vaccination is actively recommended. If a vaccine is given, it may be prudent to monitor the response, so that alternative prophylactic measures can be considered where the response is inadequate. Note that even where effective antibody titres are produced, these may not persist as long as in healthy subjects, and more frequent booster doses may be required. The use of live vaccines is generally considered to be contraindicated.

Ciclosporin (Cyclosporine) + **Warfarin and other oral anticoagulants** ⚠

Case reports describe decreased warfarin or acenocoumarol effects, which were attributed to an interaction with ciclosporin. Warfarin and acenocoumarol have decreased ciclosporin levels in isolated cases, and a further report describes a rise in serum ciclosporin levels when an unnamed anticoagulant was given.

Information is limited. In patients taking an anticoagulant with ciclosporin, it may be prudent to consider an increase in the frequency of the standard monitoring of both drugs.

Cilostazol

Cilostazol + Food ⚠

Food increases the bioavailability of cilostazol and increases the maximum plasma levels by 95%, which may increase adverse effects.

The manufacturer recommends that cilostazol should be taken 30 minutes before or 2 hours after food.

Cilostazol + H₂-receptor antagonists ⚠

Erythromycin increases the maximum plasma level and AUC of cilostazol by 47% and 73%, respectively. Other drugs that inhibit CYP3A4 (such as cimetidine) are predicted to interact similarly.

In view of these effects the US manufacturers suggest halving the dose of cilostazol in the presence of CYP3A4 inhibitors. However, the UK manufacturers contraindicate CYP3A4 inhibitors, and they specifically name cimetidine. This seems a very cautious approach.

Cilostazol + Herbal medicines or Dietary supplements ❓

A study found no significant increase in the antiplatelet effects of single doses of cilostazol when a single dose of *Ginkgo biloba* was added. However, the bleeding time was significantly, although none of the subjects developed any significant adverse effects.

Concurrent use need not be avoided, but, as with any combination of antiplatelet drugs, caution should be exercised if *Ginkgo biloba* is used with drugs that affect platelet aggregation.

Cilostazol + Macrolides ⚠

Erythromycin increases the maximum plasma level and AUC of cilostazol by 47% and 73%, respectively. Other macrolides may also interact, although it seems unlikely that they all will, see macrolides, page 310.

In view of these effects the US manufacturers suggest halving the dose of cilostazol in the presence of CYP3A4 inhibitors such as erythromycin. However, the UK manufacturers contraindicate CYP3A4 inhibitors, and they specifically name erythromycin.

Cilostazol + Protease inhibitors ⚠

Erythromycin increases the maximum plasma level and AUC of cilostazol by 47% and 73%, respectively. Other drugs that inhibit CYP3A4 (e.g. the protease inhibitors) would be expected to have a similar effect.

In view of these effects the US manufacturers suggest halving the dose of cilostazol in the presence of CYP3A4 inhibitors such as erythromycin. However, the UK manufacturers contraindicate CYP3A4 inhibitors, and they specifically name the protease inhibitors.

Cilostazol + Proton pump inhibitors ⚠

Omeprazole increases the AUC of 3,4-dehydro-cilostazol (a metabolite with 4 to 7 times the activity of cilostazol) by about 70%. Lansoprazole may interact similarly.

The US manufacturers suggest that the dose of cilostazol should be halved when given with omeprazole, while the UK manufacturers suggest that concurrent use should be avoided.

Cilostazol + Warfarin and other oral anticoagulants ⚠

No pharmacokinetic interaction appears to occur between cilostazol and warfarin.

As additive pharmacodynamic effects may occur the manufacturers advise that concurrent use should be monitored because of the increased risk of bleeding.

Cinacalcet

Cinacalcet + Food ⚠

Cinacalcet absorption is increased by food (AUC increased by 68%).

Cinacalcet should be taken with food or shortly after a meal to maximise absorption.

Cinacalcet + Macrolides ⚠

Ketoconazole raises cinacalcet levels 2-fold and increased the incidence of cinacalcet adverse effects, probably by inhibiting the metabolism of cinacalcet by CYP3A4. Other potent CYP3A4 inhibitors, such as the macrolides, are predicted to interact similarly, although they differ in their ability to inhibit CYP3A4, see macrolides, page 310.

> It may be prudent to monitor parathyroid hormone and serum calcium more frequently if a macrolide that potently inhibits CYP3A4 is started or stopped.

Cinacalcet + **Protease inhibitors** ⚠

Ketoconazole raises cinacalcet levels 2-fold and increased the incidence of cinacalcet adverse effects, probably by inhibiting the metabolism of cinacalcet by CYP3A4. Potent CYP3A4 inhibitors, such as the protease inhibitors, are predicted to interact similarly.

> It may be prudent to monitor parathyroid hormone and serum calcium more frequently in any patient receiving a protease inhibitor.

Cinacalcet + **Quinolones** ⚠

Ciprofloxacin may decrease the clearance (and therefore increase the levels) of cinacalcet, by inhibiting its metabolism by CYP1A2.

> It may be prudent to monitor parathyroid hormone and serum calcium more frequently if ciprofloxacin is started or stopped. Note that other quinolones may also inhibit CYP1A2, see quinolones, page 382, and may therefore also interact.

Cinacalcet + **Rifampicin (Rifampin)** ⚠

Rifampicin is predicted to decrease cinacalcet levels by inducing its metabolism by CYP3A4. This seems a reasonable prediction as potent CYP3A4 inhibitors raise cinacalcet levels.

> It may be prudent to monitor parathyroid hormone and serum calcium more frequently if rifampicin is started or stopped.

Cinacalcet + **SSRIs** ⚠

Fluvoxamine may decrease the clearance (and therefore increase the levels) of cinacalcet, by inhibiting its metabolism by CYP1A2.

> It may be prudent to monitor parathyroid hormone and serum calcium more frequently if fluvoxamine is started or stopped. Note that other SSRIs do not inhibit CYP1A2 and are therefore unlikely to interact by this mechanism.

Clindamycin

Clindamycin + **Contraceptives** ⚠

One or two cases of combined oral contraceptive failure have been reported with clindamycin. These isolated cases are anecdotal and unconfirmed, and the interaction (if such it is) appears to be very rare indeed.

For guidance on the use of antibacterials with contraceptives, see contraceptives, page 199.

Clonidine

C

Clonidine + Inotropes and Vasopressors ✓

Despite predictions to the contrary, studies suggest that pretreatment with clonidine does not appear to affect the blood pressure responses to noradrenaline (norepinephrine).

No action needed.

Clonidine + Levodopa ❓

Limited evidence suggests that the control of Parkinson's disease with levodopa may be impaired by clonidine.

Be alert for a reduction in the control of the Parkinson's disease during concurrent use. The effects of this interaction appear to be reduced if antimuscarinic drugs are also being used. Be aware that, as with all antihypertensives, additive hypotensive effects may occur with levodopa, see antihypertensives, page 77.

Clonidine + Methylphenidate ✓

There have been fears about serious adverse events when methylphenidate is taken with clonidine due to reports of 3 deaths in children taking both drugs, and because of the theoretical potential for adverse effects such as significant hypertension and/or tachycardia or hypotension and/or bradycardia. Although, studies have failed to establish any link between the use of methylphenidate with clonidine and the reported deaths, adverse effects have been described. Nevertheless, studies have suggested that the combination is both safe and effective for the treatment of attention deficit hyperactivity disorder.

No action needed, although be aware that, rarely, adverse cardiac events may occur.

Clonidine + Tricyclics ⚠

The tricyclic antidepressants, clomipramine, desipramine and imipramine reduce or abolish the antihypertensive effects of clonidine. Other tricyclics are expected to behave similarly. A hypertensive crisis developed when a woman taking clonidine was given imipramine.

This interaction is not seen in all patients. Avoid concurrent use unless the effects on blood pressure can be monitored. Increasing the dosage of clonidine seems to be an effective way of managing this interaction.

Clopidogrel

Clopidogrel + Heparin ⚠

A study showed that the dosage of heparin did not need modification when given with clopidogrel, and the inhibitory effects of clopidogrel on platelet aggregation were unchanged.

Although no pharmacokinetic interaction occurs the manufacturers still advise caution because of the possible risk of increased bleeding.

Clopidogrel + Herbal medicines or Dietary supplements ⚠

Ginkgo biloba has been associated with bleeding, platelet and clotting disorders, and there are isolated reports of serious adverse reactions after its concurrent use with clopidogrel. However, a single-dose study found no increase in adverse effects when *Ginkgo biloba* was given with clopidogrel.

Concurrent use need not be avoided, but, as with any combination of antiplatelet drugs, caution should be exercised if *Ginkgo biloba* is used with drugs that affect platelet aggregation.

Clopidogrel + Low-molecular-weight heparins ⚠

The manufacturers of clopidogrel note that in various large clinical studies in patients with acute coronary syndrome or myocardial infarction, most patients received LMWHs without an obvious difference in the rate of bleeding or the incidence of major bleeding. However, case reports describe occasional serious bleeding events in those given clopidogrel with a LMWH.

Although concurrent use can be beneficial the manufacturers advise caution because of the possible risk of increased bleeding.

Clopidogrel + NSAIDs ❓

The risk of faecal blood loss, gastrointestinal haemorrhage and other bleeding is increased by concurrent use of clopidogrel with naproxen and celecoxib.

The manufacturers advise caution if NSAIDs and clopidogrel are given together. Consider giving additional gastrointestinal prophylaxis such as a proton pump inhibitor in patients at risk of gastrointestinal ulceration and bleeding.

Clopidogrel + SSRIs ❓

The SSRIs may increase the risk of upper gastrointestinal bleeding and the risk appears to be further increased by concurrent clopidogrel.

The manufacturers of the SSRIs warn that patients should be cautioned about the concurrent use of antiplatelet drugs. Consideration should be given to the prescribing of gastroprotective drugs (such as proton pump inhibitors) in those at high risk of gastrointestinal bleeding, such as elderly patients or those with a history of gastrointestinal bleeding.

Clopidogrel + Statins ❓

Some evidence suggests that atorvastatin, and possibly other CYP3A4-metabolised statins (e.g. simvastatin) may interfere with the antiplatelet actions of clopidogrel, but data from some large clinical studies suggests no clinically relevant interaction occurs.

Although an interaction has been demonstrated, the anticipated negative effect on clinical outcomes has not been consistently shown. The beneficial properties of statins may offset any attenuating effects on the antiplatelet action of clopidogrel. Some have suggested that pravastatin and rosuvastatin may be preferred; however others consider there is insufficient data to warrant changing clinical practice, and given the established clinical benefits of the combination, this seems the most appropriate course of action.

Clopidogrel + Warfarin and other oral anticoagulants ⚠

A small study suggests that warfarin and clopidogrel do not interact adversely. However the manufacturers say that the concurrent use of warfarin and clopidogrel is not recommended because it may increase the intensity of bleeding.

If concurrent use is necessary it would seem prudent to monitor the outcome of concurrent use. Monitor for signs of bleeding and check bleeding times as necessary.

Co-artemether

Co-artemether is a combination product containing artemether and lumefantrine, the interaction are discussed under the combined preparation.

Co-artemether + Flecainide ❌

The manufacturer of co-artemether notes that *in vitro* data indicate that lumefantrine significantly inhibits CYP2D6. As a consequence, they contraindicate the use of co-artemether in patients taking any drug that is metabolised by CYP2D6, and specifically name flecainide.

These contraindications seem unnecessarily restrictive, especially as flecainide is not contraindicated with other established inhibitors of CYP2D6. Until more is known, it would be prudent to closely monitor the effects of any CYP2D6 substrate in patients for whom co-artemether is considered the antimalarial drug of choice.

Co-artemether + **Food** ❓

Food, especially high-fat food (including soya milk), markedly increases the absorption of both lumefantrine and artemether.

> As soon as patients can tolerate food, co-artemether should be taken with food to increase absorption. Patients who remain averse to food during treatment should be closely monitored since they may be at greater risk of recrudescence (reappearance of the disease after a period of inactivity).

Co-artemether + **Grapefruit juice** ✅

Grapefruit juice doubles the AUC of artemether.

> Based on the evidence with ketoconazole, page 109, this increase is not expected to be clinically significant.

Co-artemether + **Tricyclics** ❌

The manufacturer of co-artemether notes that *in vitro* data indicate that lumefantrine significantly inhibits CYP2D6. As a consequence, they contraindicate the use of co-artemether in patients taking any drug that is metabolised by CYP2D6 (they include imipramine, amitriptyline, and clomipramine as examples).

> These contraindications seem unnecessarily restrictive, especially since the tricyclics are not contraindicated with other established inhibitors of CYP2D6. Until more is known, it would be prudent to closely monitor the effects of any CYP2D6 substrate in patients for whom co-artemether is considered the antimalarial drug of choice. However, more seriously, note that additive QT-prolonging effects are possible, see drugs that prolong the QT interval, page 237.

Colchicine

Colchicine + **Fibrates** ❓

Case reports suggest that the current use of fibrates and colchicine can result in rhabdomyolysis or neuromyopathy.

> Information is limited, although rhabdomyolysis is associated with both colchicine and the fibrates. Suspect this interaction in any patient presenting with muscle pain or a raised creatinine kinase level taking these drugs.

Colchicine + **Macrolides** ❓

Several case reports describe acute life-threatening colchicine toxicity caused by the concurrent use of erythromycin or clarithromycin. A retrospective study and individual case reports have identified fatalities associated with the combination of clarithromycin and colchicine.

Information on this interaction is limited, but it appears that erythromycin and clarithromycin can provoke acute colchicine toxicity, at the very least in pre-disposed individuals. Other macrolides may also interact, although it seems unlikely that they all will, see macrolides, page 310. If any patient is given colchicine and a potentially interacting macrolide be aware of the potential for toxicity, especially in patients with pre-existing renal impairment.

Colchicine + Statins ❓

Three case reports describe myopathy or rhabdomyolysis in patients given colchicine and fluvastatin, pravastatin or simvastatin. It seems possible that this reaction could occur with colchicine and any statin.

Although this interaction is rare it is serious. Given the evidence available it seems likely to occur with all statins, although this has not been clearly demonstrated. All patients taking statins should be warned about the symptoms of myopathy and told to report muscle pain or weakness. It would be prudent to reinforce this advice if they are given colchicine.

Colchicine + Verapamil ❓

Verapamil may markedly increase colchicine levels, which led to neuromyopathy in one man.

Although this is an isolated case, it is in line with the way both drugs interact with other substances. Therefore it would seem prudent to suspect an interaction in the case of otherwise unexplained colchicine toxicity.

Colestyramine and related drugs

Note that it is usually recommended that other drugs are given one hour before or 4 hours after colestipol and one hour before or 4 to 6 hours after colestyramine. Interactions have therefore only been included where information suggests that different actions may be appropriate.

Colestyramine and related drugs + Diuretics

Loop diuretics ⚠

The 4-hour diuretic response to furosemide can be reduced by 58% and 77% by colestipol and colestyramine, respectively.

Furosemide should be given 2 to 3 hours before taking colestyramine or colestipol to minimise this interaction.

Thiazides ⚠

The absorption of hydrochlorothiazide and chlorothiazide can be reduced by more than one-third if colestipol is given concurrently. Colestyramine also reduces the absorption of hydrochlorothiazide by more than two-thirds.

Separating the dosages of hydrochlorothiazide and colestyramine by 4 hours can reduce, but not totally overcome the effects of this interaction. It may therefore be prudent to ensure a 6-hour separation.

Colestyramine and related drugs + Leflunomide ⊗

Studies have shown that colestyramine reduces the serum levels of the active metabolite of leflunomide by up to 65%.

Patients taking leflunomide should not be given colestyramine unless it is needed to washout' the leflunomide, such as in overdosage or when switching to another DMARD.

Colestyramine and related drugs + NSAIDs

Colestipol ⚠

Simultaneous colestipol modestly reduces the oral absorption of diclofenac, but has no effect on ibuprofen absorption.

The reduction in diclofenac absorption with colestipol may be clinically relevant, so if the combination is required monitor well. Note that it is usually recommended that other drugs are given one hour before or 4 hours after colestipol.

Colestyramine ⚠

Colestyramine, given at the same time as an NSAID, markedly reduced the oral absorption of diclofenac and sulindac, modestly reduced the absorption of ibuprofen, but only delayed and did not reduce the extent of absorption of naproxen. Administration of colestyramine three or more hours after oral sulindac, piroxicam, or tenoxicam still markedly reduced their plasma levels. Colestyramine, given after the NSAID, markedly reduces the levels of *intravenous* meloxicam or tenoxicam.

It is usually recommended that other drugs are given one hour before or 4 to 6 hours after colestyramine. However, meloxicam, piroxicam, sulindac, and tenoxicam undergo enterohepatic recirculation and so the interaction cannot be avoided by separating the doses, and it may be best to avoid using these drug combinations. The effect on ibuprofen and naproxen is probably not clinically important, although the delayed absorption may be relevant in the management of acute pain. Information on many other NSAIDs appears to be lacking.

Colestyramine and related drugs + Raloxifene ⊗

The manufacturers report that the concurrent use of colestyramine reduced the absorption of raloxifene by about 60%, due to an interruption in enterohepatic cycling.

Separating administration is unlikely to be effective as the interaction is via enterohepatic circulation. It is recommended that these two drugs should not be used concurrently. Other drugs, such as colestipol, are expected to interact similarly.

Colestyramine and related drugs + Valproate ⚠

Colestyramine causes a small 20% reduction in the absorption of valproate.

No interaction occurs if administration of the drugs is separated by 3 hours. Note that it is usually recommended that other drugs are given one hour before or 4 to 6 hours after colestyramine. Colesevelam does not appear to interact, and may therefore be a suitable alternative in some patients.

Colestyramine and related drugs + Vancomycin ⚠

Colestyramine binds to vancomycin in the gut, possibly reducing its efficacy.

Administration of oral vancomycin and colestyramine should be separated (it is usually suggested that other drugs should be given 1 hour before or 4 to 6 hours after colestyramine). Note that this combination is no longer recommended in antibiotic-associated colitis.

Colestyramine and related drugs + Warfarin and other oral anticoagulants ⚠

The anticoagulant effects of phenprocoumon and warfarin can be reduced by colestyramine. An isolated and unexplained report describes a paradoxical increase in the effects of warfarin.

Colestyramine given 3 to 6 hours after warfarin has been shown to minimise this interaction. Colestipol does not appear to interact with either warfarin or phenprocoumon and so may be a suitable alternative. However, note that it is usually recommended that other drugs are given one hour before or 4 hours after colestipol and one hour before or 4 to 6 hours after colestyramine.

Contraceptives

As HRT contains many of the same hormones as the contraceptives, studies with contraceptives may be applicable to HRT and *vice versa*, although the relative doses should be borne in mind.

General advice for use with antibacterials

The interaction between the combined oral contraceptives and non-enzyme inducing antibacterials is inadequately established and controversial. Almost all of the evidence is anecdotal with no controls. The total number of failures is extremely small when viewed against the number of women worldwide using combined oral contraceptives (estimated at 70 million in 1996 by WHO). However, because of the personal and

C

ethical consequences of an unwanted pregnancy, where uncertainty remains, it has been recommended that for maximal protection an additional form of contraception (e.g. a barrier method) should be used routinely while taking a short course of antibacterials (less than 3 weeks), and for at least 7 days afterwards. In addition, if fewer than 7 active pills are left in the pack after the antibacterials have stopped, the next packet should be started straight away, without a break, and any inactive pills should be omitted. Progestogen-only contraceptives (including emergency hormonal contraceptives) do not appear to interact. Combined oral contraceptive users who start long-term courses of antibacterials need only use additional contraceptive protection for the first 3 weeks, as after that the gut flora becomes resistant to the antibacterial. Patients who are taking long-term antibacterials for more than 3 weeks who then start a combined oral contraceptive do not need any additional contraceptive protection, unless the antibacterial is changed.

General advice for use with enzyme-inducing drugs

Recommendations when taking enzyme-inducing drugs with hormonal contraceptives (including the patch) include:

- Women taking combined hormonal contraceptives should use an ethinylestradiol dose of at least 50 micrograms daily. The dose may be increased further above 50 micrograms if breakthrough bleeding occurs. Note that, for those using the patch, the use of more than one patch is not recommended. Omitting or reducing the pill-free interval has not been shown to reduce the risk of ovulation with liver enzyme inducers. Additional non-hormonal methods of contraception, such as condoms, should also be used by patients using combined hormonal contraceptives, both when taking the liver enzyme inducers and for at least 4 weeks after stopping the drug. Alternatives to all forms of combined hormonal contraceptives should be considered with long-term use of liver enzyme inducers.
- The progestogen-only implant may be continued with *short* courses of enzyme inducers. Additional non-hormonal methods of contraception, such as condoms, should also be used by patients using the progestogen-only implant, both when taking the liver enzyme inducers and for at least 4 weeks after stopping the drug. Alternatives to the progestogen-only implant should be considered with long-term use of liver enzyme inducers.
- The progestogen-only pill is not recommended for use with liver enzyme inducers and alternative methods of contraception are advised.
- The effectiveness of the progestogen-only *emergency* hormonal contraceptive will be reduced in women taking liver enzyme inducers.

An increased dose of levonorgestrel 1.5 mg immediately followed by another 1.5-mg dose 12 hours later may be used, although this is unlicensed. A copper IUD may be used as an alternative option.

- Copper or levonorgestrel-releasing intrauterine devices (IUD) and depot progestogen-only injections may be used as alternative contraceptive methods, particularly for women requiring hormonal contraception who are likely to be taking the enzyme inducer in the long-term, as these are unaffected by liver enzyme inducers.

Contraceptives + Co-trimoxazole ⚠

Co-trimoxazole modestly *increases* ethinylestradiol levels. However, there are about 15 anecdotal cases on record of contraceptive failure attributed to co-trimoxazole. There are also isolated cases of contraceptive failure attributed to various sulphonamides, and trimethoprim.

Not established. The pharmacokinetic and pharmacodynamic evidence indicates that co-trimoxazole is not likely to reduce the effectiveness of combined hormonal contraceptives. Although there are a number of reports of contraceptive failure attributed to co-trimoxazole, these are anecdotal and unconfirmed. It is possible that these cases are coincidental, and fit within the normal failure rate of combined hormonal contraceptives. It has been said that it is almost certain that co-trimoxazole does not interact with combined hormonal contraceptives.

C

Contraceptives + Danazol ✗

There is a theoretical risk that the effects of both danazol and hormonal contraceptives might be altered or reduced on concurrent use.

The manufacturers say that women of childbearing age taking danazol should use an effective non-hormonal method of contraception.

Contraceptives + Dapsone ⚠

One or two cases of combined oral contraceptive failure have been reported with dapsone. These isolated cases are anecdotal and unconfirmed, and the interaction (if such it is) appears to be very rare.

For guidance on the use of antibacterials with contraceptives, see contraceptives, page 199.

Contraceptives + Felbamate ❓

Felbamate increased the clearance of gestodene from a combined oral contraceptive in one study, but ovulation remained suppressed.

What this change means in terms of the reliability of the hormonal contraceptive is not known, but some reduction in its efficacy might be expected. If both drugs are used tell patients to report any changes in bleeding.

Contraceptives + Fusidic acid ⚠

One or two cases of combined oral contraceptive failure have been reported with fusidic acid. These isolated cases are anecdotal and unconfirmed, and the interaction (if such it is) appears to be very rare.

For guidance on the use of antibacterials with contraceptives, see contraceptives, page 199.

Contraceptives + Gestrinone ✗

There is a theoretical risk that the effects of both gestrinone and hormonal contraceptives might be altered or reduced on concurrent use.

> The manufacturers say that women of childbearing age taking gestrinone should use an effective non-hormonal method of contraception.

Contraceptives + Griseofulvin ❌

The effects of the oral contraceptives may possibly be disturbed (either inter-menstrual bleeding or amenorrhoea) if griseofulvin is taken concurrently. There are reports of 4 women taking oral contraceptives who became pregnant while taking griseofulvin. Similarly, progestogen-only emergency hormonal contraceptives are considered to be less effective in those taking griseofulvin. The situation with progestogen-only oral contraceptives is not clear, but it has been suggested that they are not the contraceptive of choice in those taking griseofulvin because of increased menstrual irregularities.

> As griseofulvin is potentially teratogenic it has been recommended that a barrier method is used during and for 1 month after taking griseofulvin. For general advice on the use of enzyme inducers, such as griseofulvin, and contraceptives, see contraceptives, page 199.

Contraceptives + Herbal medicines or Dietary supplements ❌

Both breakthrough bleeding and contraceptive failure have been seen in women taking St John's wort (*Hypericum perforatum*). In two cases the failure of emergency hormonal contraception has been attributed to the use of St John's wort.

> Since it is not known who is particularly likely to be at risk, women taking hormonal contraceptives should either avoid St John's wort (the recommendation of the CSM in the UK) or they should use an additional form of contraception. For general advice on the use of enzyme inducers, such as St John's wort, and contraceptives, see contraceptives, page 199.

Contraceptives + Isoniazid ⚠️

One or two cases of combined oral contraceptive failure have been reported with isoniazid. However, there is evidence that isoniazid does not cause contraceptive failure when used in combination with other antimycobacterials (without rifampicin (rifampin)). These isolated cases are anecdotal and unconfirmed, and the interaction (if such it is) appears to be very rare.

> For guidance on the use of antibacterials with contraceptives, see contraceptives, page 199.

Contraceptives + Isotretinoin ❓

There seems to be no evidence that the reliability of combined hormonal contraceptives is affected by isotretinoin, and they are the contraceptive method of choice with these teratogenic drugs. Progestogen-only oral contraceptives are not generally considered reliable enough for use with teratogenic drugs. The adverse effects of isotretinoin on lipids may be additive with those of oral contraceptives, but the importance of this is not known.

Contraceptives should be started one month before isotretinoin and continued for one month after stopping isotretinoin. In the USA, it is standard practice to recommend that a second form of contraception, such as a barrier method, should also be used. This is because, even though hormonal methods of contraception are highly effective, they do, on rare occasions, fail.

C

Contraceptives + Lamotrigine ⚠

One study suggests that lamotrigine does not alter the contraceptive efficacy or plasma levels of combined oral contraceptives. Another study found a slight reduction in levonorgestrel levels but no evidence of ovulation. Hormonal contraceptives may reduce the levels of lamotrigine, which can lead to a decrease in seizure control.

The manufacturers suggest that reduced contraceptive efficacy cannot be ruled out, and recommend the use of non-hormonal contraceptives. However, the FFPRHC has found no evidence of reduced contraceptive efficacy and so they suggest that there is no good evidence that non-hormonal methods of contraception are preferable. Lamotrigine can be started as normal in patients already taking hormonal contraceptives. For women already taking lamotrigine and carbamazepine or phenytoin no lamotrigine dosage adjustment is necessary when hormonal contraceptives are started, but in the absence of these other antiepileptics the maintenance dose of lamotrigine may need to be increased by as much as twofold, according to clinical response. Patients should also be advised that an increase in seizure frequency may occur when the combined oral contraceptive is started.

Contraceptives + Macrolides ⚠

The macrolides clarithromycin, dirithromycin, roxithromycin and telithromycin appear unlikely to cause combined hormonal contraceptive failure. Isolated cases of contraceptive failure have been attributed to erythromycin or spiramycin. Conversely, in two studies of contraceptive failures in dermatology patients, no pregnancies were identified in a total of 74 women taking erythromycin with oral contraceptives.

For guidance on the use of antibacterials with contraceptives, see contraceptives, page 199.

Contraceptives + MAO-B inhibitors ⚠

In a small study, the bioavailability of selegiline was markedly higher (mean of about 20-fold) in women taking combined oral contraceptives than in those not taking contraceptives.

One UK manufacturer of selegiline advises caution on the concurrent use of contraceptives, and the other suggests that concurrent use should be avoided.

Contraceptives + Metronidazole ⚠

Isolated cases of oral contraceptive failure have been reported with metronidazole. The interaction (if such it is) appears to be very rare. In a controlled trial, metronidazole did not affect contraceptive steroid levels.

> For guidance on the use of antibacterials with contraceptives, see contraceptives, page 199.

Contraceptives + Modafinil ⚠

Modafinil slightly reduced the levels of ethinylestradiol taken as part of a combined hormonal contraceptive. Emergency hormonal contraceptives and progestogen-only implants may also be less effective if taken with modafinil.

> These small changes may be sufficient to cause the failure of combined hormonal contraceptives in rare cases. For additional advice on the use of enzyme inducers, such as modafinil, and contraceptives, see contraceptives, page 199. It is also recommended that additional or alternative methods should be continued for up to 2 cycles after stopping modafinil.

Contraceptives + Nitrofurantoin ⚠

One or two cases of combined oral contraceptive failure have been reported with nitrofurantoin. These isolated cases are anecdotal and unconfirmed, and the interaction (if such it is) appears to be very rare.

> For guidance on the use of antibacterials with contraceptives, see contraceptives, page 199.

Contraceptives + NNRTIs

Efavirenz ⚠

Efavirenz increases the plasma levels of ethinylestradiol.

> Despite this increase, the manufacturers recommend using a reliable method of barrier contraception as they cannot rule out the potential for contraceptive failure. Note that this is also advisable to reduce the risk of HIV transmission.

Nevirapine ⚠

Nevirapine modestly reduces the plasma concentrations of ethinylestradiol and norethisterone, which could reduce the efficacy of contraception. The efficacy of emergency hormonal contraceptives and progestogen-only implants or injections may also be reduced by nevirapine.

> For general advice on the use of enzyme inducers, such as nevirapine, and contraceptives, see contraceptives, page 199. However, note that the manufacturers of nevirapine recommend that combined hormonal contraceptives should not be used as the sole method of contraception in women taking nevirapine. They suggest that a barrier method (e.g. condoms) should also be used, and note that this is also advisable to reduce the risk of HIV transmission. They also suggest that if combined hormonal contraceptives are used for reasons other than contraception (e.g. endometriosis), that the therapeutic effect should be monitored and the dose increased if necessary.

Contraceptives + **NSAIDs** ❓

A study in women taking ethinylestradiol and norethisterone-containing oral contraceptives found that the addition of etoricoxib increased the steady-state levels of ethinylestradiol by 50 to 60%, but the rise in norethisterone levels was not clinically relevant.

There would appear to be no reason for avoiding concurrent use but the manufacturers suggest that this increase in ethinylestradiol levels should be considered when choosing a hormonal contraceptive. It may be appropriate to use a contraceptive with a lower dose of ethinylestradiol.

C

Contraceptives + **Orlistat** ⚠

Orlistat does not appear to interact with combined oral contraceptives. However, pregnancies have occurred in those taking the combination.

The manufacturers recommend additional contraceptive measures (presumably barrier methods) if severe diarrhoea occurs.

Contraceptives + **Oxcarbazepine** ⚠

Combined hormonal contraceptives and possibly progestogen-only oral contraceptives are less reliable during treatment with oxcarbazepine. Breakthrough bleeding and spotting can take place. Controlled studies have shown that oxcarbazepine can reduce contraceptive steroid levels.

The increase in failure rate appears small, but because of the consequences of an unwanted pregnancy, especially with drugs that may cause foetal abnormalities, adjustments should be made. If possible, change to another suitable, non-interacting antiepileptic. For additional advice on the use of enzyme inducers, such as oxcarbazepine, and contraceptives, see contraceptives, page 199.

Contraceptives + **Penicillins** ⚠

Failure of combined oral contraceptives has been attributed to the concurrent use of penicillins, but the interaction (if such it is) appears to be very rare.

For guidance on the use of antibacterials with contraceptives, see contraceptives, page 199.

Contraceptives + **Phenobarbital** ⚠

Combined hormonal contraceptives and possibly progestogen-only oral contraceptives are less reliable during treatment with phenobarbital. Inter-menstrual breakthrough bleeding and spotting can take place, and pregnancies have occurred. Controlled studies have shown that phenobarbital can reduce contraceptive steroid levels. Similarly, emergency hormonal contraceptives are considered to be less effective in those taking phenobarbital. Note that primidone is metabolised to phenobarbital and therefore may interact similarly.

The increase in failure rate appears small, but because of the consequences of an unwanted pregnancy, especially with drugs that may cause foetal abnormalities, adjustments should be made. If possible, change to another suitable, non-inter-acting antiepileptic. For additional advice on the use of enzyme inducers, such as phenobarbital, and contraceptives, see contraceptives, page 199. Reliable contra-ception in most patients is said to be achievable with 80 to 100 micrograms of ethinylestradiol daily. Additional barrier methods are considered the most appropriate option for the short-term use of enzyme-inducing antiepileptics.

Contraceptives + Phenytoin ⚠

Combined hormonal contraceptives and possibly progestogen-only oral contracep-tives are less reliable during treatment with phenytoin. Inter-menstrual breakthrough bleeding and spotting can take place, and pregnancies have occurred. Controlled studies have shown that phenytoin can reduce contraceptive steroid levels. Similarly, emergency hormonal contraceptives are considered to be less effective in those taking phenytoin. Fosphenytoin, a prodrug of phenytoin, may interact similarly.

The increase in failure rate appears small, but because of the consequences of an unwanted pregnancy, especially with drugs that may cause foetal abnormalities, adjustments should be made. If possible, change to another suitable, non-interacting antiepileptic. For general advice on the use of enzyme inducers, such as phenytoin, and contraceptives, see contraceptives, page 199. Reliable contraception in most patients is said to be achievable with 80 to 100 micrograms of ethinylestradiol daily. Additional barrier methods are considered the most appropriate option for the short-term use of enzyme-inducing antiepileptics.

Contraceptives + Protease inhibitors ⊗

Ethinylestradiol levels are reduced by fosamprenavir with ritonavir, lopinavir/ritonavir, nelfinavir and ritonavir alone, and norethisterone levels are slightly reduced by fosamprenavir with ritonavir, lopinavir/ritonavir, nelfinavir and tipranavir in patients taking combined oral contraceptives. Concurrent use of hormonal contra-ceptives with amprenavir is not recommended, as amprenavir levels are reduced. There is no direct information about progestogen-only pills but since lopinavir/ritonavir and nelfinavir cause small reductions in the levels of norethisterone (given as part of a combined oral contraceptive) it is possible that these protease inhibitors could reduce the contraceptive efficacy of progestogen-only oral contraceptives containing norethisterone. The efficacy of emergency hormonal contraceptives may also be decreased.

There have been unconfirmed reports of contraceptive failure in patients taking indinavir, nelfinavir, ritonavir and saquinavir. To avoid this potential risk, and the risk of breakthrough bleeding, it has been suggested that a contraceptive preparation with a higher dose of ethinylestradiol or an alternative or additional non-hormonal form of contraception should be used during and for one cycle after ritonavir is stopped. Similar advice applies to other protease inhibitors given with ritonavir. Note that the progestogen-only oral contraceptives have a higher failure rate than the combined oral contraceptives. Despite the lack of evidence it would seem prudent to use additional contraceptive measures in this situation as well. For additional advice on the use of enzyme inducers, such as protease inhibitors, and contraceptives, see contraceptives, page 199. Note that whatever other methods of contraception are being used, barrier methods are also advisable to reduce the risk of HIV transmission.

Contraceptives + Quinolones ⚠

Ciprofloxacin, moxifloxacin and ofloxacin have been shown not to affect the pharmacokinetics of the combined oral contraceptives in controlled studies. Contraceptive failure does not appear to have been reported, and ovarian suppression is not affected.

> It is possible that the anecdotal cases of contraceptive failure with antibacterials are indistinguishable from the normal accepted failure rate and no special precautions are required. However, some specialists recommend that additional contraceptives, such as condoms, should be used for short courses of antibacterials. For guidance on the use of antibacterials with contraceptives, see contraceptives, page 199.

C

Contraceptives + Rifabutin ⚠

Combined hormonal contraceptives and progestogen-only oral contraceptives are considered to be less reliable during treatment with rifabutin. Similarly, emergency hormonal contraceptives are considered to be less effective in those taking rifabutin. The etonogestrel implant is also expected to be less effective.

> For advice on the use of enzyme inducers, such as rifabutin, and contraceptives, see contraceptives, page 199. It has been recommended that an alternative or additional form of contraception should also be used for 4 to 8 weeks after stopping rifabutin.

Contraceptives + Rifampicin (Rifampin) ⚠

Combined hormonal contraceptives are less reliable during treatment with rifampicin. Breakthrough bleeding and spotting are common, and pregnancies have occurred. Similarly, progestogen-only oral contraceptives and emergency hormonal contraceptives are considered to be less effective in those taking rifampicin.

> For advice on the use of enzyme inducers, such as rifampicin, and contraceptives, see contraceptives, page 199. It has been recommended that an alternative or additional form of contraception should also be used for 4 to 8 weeks after stopping rifampicin.

Contraceptives + Sulfonamides ⚠

Isolated cases of contraceptive failure have been attributed to various sulfonamides.

> It is possible that the anecdotal cases of contraceptive failure with antibacterials are indistinguishable from the normal accepted failure rate and no special precautions are required. However, some specialists recommend that additional contraceptives, such as condoms, should be used for short courses of antibacterials. For guidance on the use of antibacterials with contraceptives, see contraceptives, page 199.

Contraceptives + **Tacrolimus** ⚠

The manufacturers of tacrolimus say that during clinical use ethinylestradiol has been shown to increase tacrolimus levels, and *in vitro* data suggests that gestodene and norethisterone may do the same. Tacrolimus has the potential to interfere with the metabolism of hormonal contraceptives.

The manufacturers suggest that other (presumably non-hormonal) contraceptive measures should be used.

Contraceptives + **Tetracyclines** ⚠

Contraceptive failure has been attributed to a tetracycline in about 40 reported cases, 7 of which specified long-term antibacterial use. The interaction (if such it is) appears to be very rare. Controlled studies have not found that tetracyclines affect contraceptive steroid levels.

For guidance on the use of antibacterials with contraceptives, see contraceptives, page 199.

Contraceptives + **Tizanidine** ⚠

Hormonal contraceptives increase the levels of tizanidine by up to 4-fold: the blood pressure-lowering effect of tizanidine was increased by 12/8 mmHg.

A clinical response or adverse effect with tizanidine might occur at lower doses of tizanidine in patients taking hormonal contraceptives, therefore during dose titration individual doses should be reduced initially.

Contraceptives + **Topiramate** ⚠

The serum levels of ethinylestradiol are moderately reduced by topiramate, which increases the risk of breakthrough bleeding and possible contraceptive failure in women taking combined hormonal contraceptives. Similarly, emergency hormonal contraceptives are considered to be less effective in those taking topiramate.

Topiramate is a weak enzyme inducer. However, the potential for contraceptive failure still exists. The manufacturers advise that patients should be told to report any changes in their bleeding patterns. For advice on the use of enzyme inducers, such as topiramate, and contraceptives, see contraceptives, page 199.

Contraceptives + **Trimethoprim** ⚠

Isolated cases of contraceptive failure have been attributed to trimethoprim.

It is possible that the anecdotal cases of contraceptive failure with antibacterials are indistinguishable from the normal accepted failure rate and no special precautions are required. However, some specialists recommend that additional contraceptives, such as condoms, should be used for short courses of antibacterials. For guidance on the use of antibacterials with contraceptives, see contraceptives, page 199.

Contraceptives + **Warfarin and other oral anticoagulants** ❓

The anticoagulant effects of dicoumarol and phenprocoumon can be decreased, and those of acenocoumarol increased, by hormonal contraceptives. An isolated report describes a marked INR increase in a woman taking warfarin when she was given levonorgestrel emergency contraception. A report describes a woman who needed more acenocoumarol when her HRT treatment with oral conjugated oestrogens was changed to transdermal estradiol.

> Direct information is limited. Combined hormonal contraceptives are usually contraindicated in patients with thromboembolic disorders. However, if they are used be aware that the anticoagulant response may be affected.

C

Corticosteroids

Corticosteroids + **Digoxin** ⚠

Corticosteroids can cause potassium loss, which increases the risk of digoxin toxicity.

> Monitor concurrent use for digoxin toxicity (e.g. bradycardia). Consider monitoring potassium levels.

Corticosteroids + **Diuretics** ⚠

Loop diuretics such as furosemide, and thiazide diuretics, such as bendroflumethiazide, can cause hypokalaemia. This can be increased by other potassium-depleting drugs such as the corticosteroids. In severe cases the risk of serious cardiac arrhythmias could be increased. The synthetic corticosteroids (glucocorticoids) have a less marked potassium-depleting effect and are therefore less likely to cause problems. These include betamethasone, dexamethasone, prednisolone, prednisone and triamcinolone.

> Consider monitoring potassium levels, based on the severity of the patient's condition, the number of potassium-depleting drugs used, and any predisposing disease states.

Corticosteroids + **Herbal medicines or Dietary supplements** ❓

Glycyrrhizin (liquorice) can increase the AUC of prednisolone by about 50%.

> The clinical significance of this interaction is unclear, but bear it in mind in case of an unexpected response to treatment.

Corticosteroids + **Macrolides** ⚠

Clarithromycin and erythromycin can reduce the clearance of methylprednisolone, thereby increasing both its therapeutic and adverse effects. Other macrolides may also interact, although it seems unlikely that they all will, see macrolides, page 310.

Appropriate dosage reductions (based on symptoms) may need to be made to avoid the development of corticosteroid adverse effects. Prednisolone seems to be a non-interacting alternative, except possibly in those also taking enzyme inducers (e.g. phenobarbital, page 210).

Corticosteroids + **Methotrexate** ⚠

Dexamethasone may increase the acute hepatotoxicity of high-dose methotrexate.

Monitor the outcome of concurrent use: full blood count and liver function tests are likely to already be monitored.

Corticosteroids + **Mifepristone** ⚠

The UK manufacturer of mifepristone says that the efficacy of corticosteroids (including inhaled corticosteroids) is expected to be reduced in the 3 to 4 days following the use of mifepristone.

Patients taking corticosteroids should be monitored in the 3 to 4 days following the use of mifepristone, and consideration given to increasing the corticosteroid dose. The US manufacturer contraindicates the use of mifepristone in those receiving long-term corticosteroid therapy.

Corticosteroids + **Nasal decongestants** ⚠

Ephedrine increased the clearance of dexamethasone by 40% in one study, but the clinical effect of this is unknown.

Monitor the outcome of concurrent use to ensure dexamethasone efficacy. Adjust the dose as necessary.

Corticosteroids + **NSAIDs** ❓

Corticosteroids may increase the incidence and/or severity of ulceration associated with NSAIDs, and increase the possibility of gastrointestinal bleeding.

Concurrent use need not be avoided, but be aware that the risks are increased. Consider the use of mucosal protectants such as H_2-receptor antagonists or proton pump inhibitors.

Corticosteroids + **Phenobarbital** ⚠

The therapeutic effects of systemic dexamethasone, methylprednisolone, predniso-lone and prednisone are decreased by phenobarbital. Other barbiturates (including primidone) probably interact similarly, although direct evidence is lacking. The dexamethasone adrenal suppression test may be expected to be unreliable in those taking phenobarbital.

Prednisone and prednisolone appear to be less affected and therefore may be preferred. Monitor concurrent use to ensure corticosteroid efficacy.

Corticosteroids + **Phenytoin** ⚠

The therapeutic effects of dexamethasone, methylprednisolone, prednisolone, prednisone (and probably other glucocorticoids) can be markedly reduced by phenytoin. Fludrocortisone may similarly be affected. One study suggested that dexamethasone may increase serum phenytoin levels, but another study and two case reports suggest that an important decrease can occur. The results of the dexamethasone adrenal suppression test may prove to be unreliable in those taking phenytoin. Fosphenytoin, a prodrug of phenytoin, may interact similarly with these corticosteroids.

The significance of the falls in corticosteroid levels will depend on the disease the corticosteroid is prescribed for. Monitor the outcome of concurrent use closely, especially in transplant patients, and increase the dose accordingly. Consider monitoring phenytoin levels if dexamethasone is given.

Corticosteroids + **Protease inhibitors** ⚠

Several cases of Cushing's syndrome have been seen in patients taking inhaled or intranasal fluticasone with ritonavir. Ritonavir may reduce the clearance of prednisone, and ritonavir or nelfinavir may increase levels of the active metabolite of ciclesonide. The manufacturers of betamethasone and budesonide predict a similar interaction with ritonavir or nelfinavir. Dexamethasone may reduce the levels of indinavir and saquinavir.

Monitor concurrent use for signs of corticosteroid overdose such as fluid retention, hypertension and hyperglycaemia. The problem may take months to manifest itself with inhaled corticosteroids. Monitor antiviral efficacy if dexamethasone is given with indinavir or saquinavir.

Corticosteroids + **Rifabutin** ⚠

The effects of cortisone, dexamethasone, fludrocortisone, hydrocortisone, methylprednisolone, prednisolone and prednisone can be markedly reduced by rifampicin. The UK manufacturers and the CSM in the UK suggest that rifabutin may interact similarly, although this is likely to be to a lesser extent.

The significance of the falls in corticosteroid levels will depend on the disease the corticosteroid is prescribed for. Monitor the outcome of concurrent use closely, especially in transplant patients, and increase the dose accordingly. Topical preparations are not likely to be affected.

Corticosteroids + **Rifampicin (Rifampin)** ⚠

The effects of cortisone, dexamethasone, fludrocortisone, hydrocortisone, methyl-prednisolone, prednisolone and prednisone can be markedly reduced by rifampicin.

The significance of the falls in corticosteroid levels will depend on the disease the corticosteroid is prescribed for. Monitor the outcome of concurrent use closely, especially in transplant patients, and increase the dose accordingly. Topical preparations are not likely to be affected.

C

Corticosteroids + **Salbutamol (Albuterol) and related bronchodilators** ❓

Beta$_2$ agonists, such as salbutamol, can cause hypokalaemia. This can be increased by other potassium-depleting drugs such as the corticosteroids. In severe cases the risk of serious cardiac arrhythmias could be increased.

The CSM in the UK advises monitoring potassium in severe asthma, because of the probability of multiple potassium-depleting drugs being used, and because some conditions predispose these patients to hypokalaemia (e.g. hypoxia). Consider monitoring based on the severity of the patient's condition, and the number of potassium-depleting drugs used.

Corticosteroids + **Tacrolimus** ⚠

Tacrolimus levels are said to have been increased, decreased and unaltered by methylprednisolone.

The combination of tacrolimus and corticosteroids is commonly used. The clinical importance of this interaction is therefore probably limited, but if abnormal results occur, remember that this drug combination could perhaps be a cause.

Corticosteroids + **Theophylline** ❓

Theophylline and corticosteroids have established roles in the management of asthma and their concurrent use is common. There are isolated reports of increases in serum theophylline levels (sometimes associated with toxicity) when oral or parenteral corticosteroids are given, but other studies have found no changes. The general clinical importance of these findings is uncertain. Both theophylline and corticosteroids can cause hypokalaemia, which may be additive.

The CSM in the UK advises monitoring potassium in severe asthma, because of the probability of multiple potassium-depleting drugs being used, and because some conditions predispose these patients to hypokalaemia (e.g. hypoxia). Consider monitoring based on the severity of the patient's condition, and the number of potassium-depleting drugs used.

Corticosteroids + **Vaccines** ⚠

Patients who are immunised with live vaccines while receiving immunosuppressive doses of corticosteroids may develop generalised, possibly life-threatening, infections.

It has been recommended that live vaccination should be postponed for at least 3 months after high-dose corticosteroids are stopped. Adult patients taking the equivalent of 40 mg of prednisolone daily for more than one week would generally be considered to be immunosuppressed.

Corticosteroids + Warfarin and other oral anticoagulants ❓

Only small increases or decreases in anticoagulation normally occur when low to moderate doses of corticosteroids are given with oral anticoagulants. However, some patients have shown very marked prothrombin time increases when given high-dose corticosteroids.

Monitor the anticoagulant effect if high-dose corticosteroids are started or stopped in patients taking oral anticoagulants.

Co-trimoxazole

Co-trimoxazole is a combination product containing sulfamethoxazole and trimethoprim.

Co-trimoxazole + Dapsone ⚠

The serum levels of both dapsone and trimethoprim are possibly raised by concurrent use. Both increased efficacy and dapsone toxicity have been seen. Note that co-trimoxazole contains trimethoprim.

Be alert for evidence of apparently rare cases of increased dapsone toxicity (methaemoglobinaemia).

Co-trimoxazole + Digoxin ⚠

Serum digoxin levels can be increased by about 22% by trimethoprim, but some individuals may show a much greater rise.

Monitor the effects of digoxin if trimethoprim is given, and consider measuring digoxin levels, particularly in the elderly. Adjust the dose as necessary. Trimethoprim is a constituent of co-trimoxazole but it is not known whether prophylactic doses of co-trimoxazole (160 mg of trimethoprim a day from a 960-mg dose of co-trimoxazole) will interact to a clinically significant degree. An interaction would seem likely with high-dose co-trimoxazole, and care is needed in the elderly with any co-trimoxazole dose.

Co-trimoxazole + **Methotrexate** ⚠

The concurrent use of low-dose methotrexate and co-trimoxazole or has resulted in several cases of severe bone marrow depression, some of which were fatal.

Full blood count should be monitored when methotrexate is used. If any abnormalities arise, consider this interaction as a possible cause.

Co-trimoxazole + **Phenytoin** ⚠

Phenytoin serum levels can be raised by co-trimoxazole. Phenytoin toxicity may develop in some cases.

The risk of toxicity is small and is most likely in those with serum phenytoin levels at the top end of the range. Monitor phenytoin levels and adjust the dose accordingly. Indicators of phenytoin toxicity include blurred vision, nystagmus, ataxia or drowsiness.

Co-trimoxazole + **Procainamide** ⚠

Trimethoprim causes a marked increase in the plasma levels of procainamide and its active metabolite, N-acetylprocainamide. Note that co-trimoxazole contains trimethoprim.

The need to reduce the procainamide dosage should be anticipated if trimethoprim is given to patients already controlled on procainamide.

Co-trimoxazole + **Pyrimethamine** ⚠

Serious pancytopenia and megaloblastic anaemia have been described in patients given pyrimethamine and co-trimoxazole.

Caution should be used in prescribing the combination, especially in the presence of other drugs (e.g. methotrexate, phenytoin) or disease states that may predispose to folate deficiency. Note that the manufacturer of sulfadoxine/pyrimethamine recommends that the concurrent use of sulfonamides (including co-trimoxazole) should be avoided.

Co-trimoxazole + **Rifampicin (Rifampin)** ⚠

Rifampicin reduces the AUCs of trimethoprim and sulfamethoxazole by 56% and 28%, respectively, in HIV-positive subjects, but apparently has no effect on trimethoprim in healthy subjects. Co-trimoxazole can increase rifampicin serum levels in patients with tuberculosis by almost a third.

The efficacy of co-trimoxazole prophylaxis may be reduced in HIV-positive patients taking rifampicin. Bear this in mind when using the combination. The risk of hepatotoxicity may be increased due to raised rifampicin levels. Liver function tests should already be closely monitored so no additional precautions seem necessary.

Co-trimoxazole + **Warfarin and other oral anticoagulants** ⚠

The anticoagulant effects of warfarin, acenocoumarol, and phenprocoumon are increased by co-trimoxazole (sulfamethoxazole with trimethoprim). Bleeding may occur if the anticoagulant dosage is not reduced appropriately.

> The incidence of the interaction with co-trimoxazole appears to be high. If bleeding is to be avoided the INR should be well monitored and the warfarin, acenocoumarol, or phenprocoumon dosage should be reduced. Phenindione is said not to interact.

Cyclophosphamide

Cyclophosphamide + **Digoxin** ⚠

Treatment with cyclophosphamide (as part of antineoplastic regimens) appears to damage the lining of the intestine so that digoxin is much less readily absorbed when given in tablet form.

> In one of the studies this interaction was overcome by giving the digoxin in liquid or liquid-in-capsule form. Monitor carefully, adjusting dose, drug or preparation as appropriate.

Cyclophosphamide + **Vaccines** ⚠

The immune response of the body is suppressed by cytotoxic antineoplastics. The effectiveness of vaccines may be poor and generalised infection may occur in patients immunised with live vaccines. In one study the antibody response to pneumococcal vaccination was reduced by 60% in patients receiving antineoplastics including cyclophosphamide, and suboptimal responses to influenza and measles vaccines have been reported.

> Extreme care should be taken when considering vaccinating immunosuppressed patients, especially with live vaccines, which should generally be avoided. Monitor the immune response to other types of vaccine. Consider whether vaccination can be carried out before or after cyclophosphamide use.

Danazol

Danazol + Sirolimus ⚠

The manufacturers predict that the serum levels of sirolimus will be increased by danazol. Note that similar predictions have proven to be true with ciclosporin (cyclosporine) and tacrolimus.

> Sirolimus levels and/or effects (e.g. on renal function) should be monitored as a matter of routine, but it may be prudent to increase monitoring if danazol is started or stopped.

Danazol + Statins ⚠

Severe rhabdomyolysis and myoglobinuria developed in a man taking lovastatin about 2 months after danazol was added. Another report describes a similar interaction with simvastatin.

> The US manufacturers of lovastatin suggest that the dose should not exceed 20 mg daily in the presence of danazol. Similarly the manufacturers of simvastatin suggest that the dose should not exceed 10 mg daily in the presence of danazol. It would seem prudent to remind patients of the symptoms of myopathy if danazol is given to a patient taking lovastatin or simvastatin, and tell them to report any unexplained muscle pain, tenderness or weakness.

Danazol + Tacrolimus ⚠

An isolated report describes an increase in tacrolimus levels in a patient also given danazol.

> Tacrolimus levels and/or effects (e.g. on renal function) should be monitored as a matter of routine, but it may be prudent to increase monitoring if danazol is started or stopped. Adjust the dose of tacrolimus as necessary.

Danazol + Warfarin and other oral anticoagulants ⚠

Increased anticoagulant effects and bleeding, often developing within 2 to 3 days, have been seen when danazol was given to patients taking warfarin.

If concurrent use cannot be avoided, the dosage of the anticoagulant should be appropriately reduced. One recommendation is that the initial dosage of anticoagulant should be halved. After withdrawal of the interacting drug the anticoagulant dosage will need to be increased.

Dapsone

D

Dapsone + Probenecid ❓

The serum levels of dapsone can be raised by about 50% by probenecid.

The extent of the rise and evidence that the haematological toxicity of dapsone may be dose-related suggests that this interaction may be clinically important. Monitor concurrent use for dapsone adverse effects.

Dapsone + Rifabutin ⚠

Rifabutin increases the clearance of dapsone, but may also increase its toxicity (methaemoglobinaemia).

Concurrent use should be well monitored to confirm that treatment is effective. It may be necessary to raise the dosage of dapsone. Also be alert for any evidence of methaemoglobinaemia.

Dapsone + Rifampicin (Rifampin) ⚠

Rifampicin increases the excretion of dapsone, lowers its serum levels and increases the risk of toxicity (methaemoglobinaemia).

Concurrent use should be well monitored to confirm that treatment is effective. It may be necessary to raise the dosage of dapsone. It has been pointed out that there is a risk of treatment failure for pneumocystis pneumonia as well as for leprosy. Also be alert for any evidence of dapsone toxicity (methaemoglobinaemia).

Dapsone + Trimethoprim ⚠

The serum levels of both dapsone and trimethoprim are possibly raised by concurrent use. Both increased efficacy and dapsone toxicity have been seen.

Concurrent use appears to be an effective form of treatment, but be alert for evidence of apparently rare cases of increased dapsone toxicity (methaemoglobinaemia).

Darifenacin

Darifenacin + Flecainide ⚠

Darifenacin increases the levels of CYP2D6 substrates such as the tricyclics (imipramine AUC increased by 70%). The manufacturers therefore advise caution with other CYP2D6 substrates, and specifically name flecainide.

The clinical importance of this potential interaction does not appear to have been assessed, but be alert for the need to reduce the flecainide dosage if darifenacin is added.

Darifenacin + Macrolides ⚠

Erythromycin almost doubles the AUC of darifenacin by inhibiting its metabolism by CYP3A4. Other macrolides that inhibit CYP3A4 may interact similarly, see macrolides, page 310.

The US manufacturers suggests that no dosage adjustments are necessary with erythromycin, whereas the UK manufacturer suggests increasing the darifenacin dose with caution. Bear in mind the possibility of an interaction if antimuscarinic effects (dry mouth, constipation, drowsiness) are increased.

Darifenacin + Quinidine ⚠

Paroxetine increases the AUC of darifenacin by a modest 33%. Quinidine is predicted to interact similarly (both paroxetine and quinidine are CYP2D6 inhibitors). However, these changes seem unlikely to be clinically relevant.

No dosage adjustments are recommended by the US manufacturer. The UK manufacturer recommends that the dose of darifenacin should be started at 7.5 mg daily and, if well tolerated, titrated to 15 mg. This seems a cautious approach. Bear in mind the possibility of an interaction if antimuscarinic effects (dry mouth, constipation, drowsiness) are increased.

Darifenacin + SSRIs ⚠

Paroxetine increases the AUC of darifenacin by a modest 33%, which is unlikely to be clinically relevant.

No dosage adjustments are recommended by the US manufacturer. The UK manufacturer recommends that the dose of darifenacin should be started at 7.5 mg daily and, if well tolerated, titrated to 15 mg. This seems a cautious approach. Bear in mind the possibility of an interaction if antimuscarinic effects (dry mouth, constipation, drowsiness) are increased.

Darifenacin + Terbinafine ⚠

Paroxetine increases the AUC of darifenacin by a modest 33%. Terbinafine is predicted to interact similarly (both paroxetine and terbinafine are CYP2D6 inhibitors). However, these changes seem unlikely to be clinically relevant.

No dosage adjustments are recommended by the US manufacturer. The UK manufacturer recommends that the dose of darifenacin should be started at 7.5 mg daily and, if well tolerated, titrated to 15 mg. This seems a cautious approach. Bear in mind the possibility of an interaction if antimuscarinic effects (dry mouth, constipation, drowsiness) are increased.

Darifenacin + Tricyclics ⚠

Darifenacin increases the AUC of imipramine by about 70% and increases the AUC of its active metabolite 2.6-fold. Other tricyclics are similarly metabolised and therefore they may all be affected.

Monitor for signs of tricyclic adverse effects (dry mouth, constipation, blurred vision).

D

Dextromethorphan

Dextromethorphan + Linezolid ⚠

Linezolid does not appear to affect the pharmacokinetics of dextromethorphan, but in one case concurrent use resulted in serotonin syndrome.

It would be prudent to monitor for symptoms of serotonin syndrome, page 392, if concurrent use is necessary.

Dextromethorphan + MAO-B inhibitors ✖

Cases of serotonin syndrome, page 392, have been seen when dextromethorphan has been used with non-selective MAOIs. The likelihood of an interaction with MAO-B inhibitors would appear to be very small, but because of the potential severity, some caution would appear to be prudent.

The manufacturer of *rasagiline* contraindicates its use with dextromethorphan. Some consider that patients taking selegiline should also try to avoid dextromethorphan.

Dextromethorphan + MAOIs ✖

Two fatal cases of hyperpyrexia and coma (symptoms similar to serotonin syndrome, page 392) have occurred in patients taking phenelzine with dextromethorphan (in overdosage in one case). Three other serious but non-fatal reactions occurred in patients taking dextromethorphan with isocarboxazid or phenelzine.

MAOIs are contraindicated with dextromethorphan.

Dextromethorphan + **Moclobemide** ✕

Moclobemide inhibits the metabolism of dextromethorphan, and isolated cases of severe CNS reactions have occurred in patients given the combination.

Moclobemide is contraindicated with dextromethorphan.

Dextromethorphan + **NSAIDs** ❓

The manufacturers say that valdecoxib (the pro-drug of parecoxib) caused a 3-fold increase in the serum levels of dextromethorphan.

If the combination is thought necessary, a low dose of dextromethorphan is advisable. Concurrent use should be well-monitored for evidence of toxicity.

Dextromethorphan + **Quinidine** ⚠

Quinidine markedly increased the plasma levels of dextromethorphan in one study. Some of the patients (given dextromethorphan 60 mg) experienced dextromethorphan toxicity (nervousness, tremors, restlessness, dizziness, shortness of breath, confusion etc.).

It seems likely that at normal therapeutic doses of dextromethorphan will cause a problem in most patients taking quinidine, but be aware that some may become more sensitive to its effects.

Dextromethorphan + **Sibutramine** ✕

There are no reports of adverse reactions between sibutramine and dextromethorphan but the manufacturers predict that concurrent use may lead to the potentially fatal serotonin syndrome, page 392.

The manufacturers suggest that concurrent use should be avoided. The extent of the risk with these serotonergic drugs is not known, but because of the potential severity of the reaction this warning would seem to be a prudent precaution.

Dextromethorphan + **SSRIs** ❓

A serotonin-like syndrome has developed in several patients taking SSRIs with dextromethorphan, although in many of these cases the use of other drugs with serotonergic actions may have contributed. Hallucinations have been reported in one patient taking fluoxetine with dextromethorphan. Paroxetine and fluoxetine markedly inhibit the metabolism of dextromethorphan.

It would seem prudent for patients taking any SSRI to be cautious if using dextromethorphan-containing products because serotonin syndrome, page 392, can be serious. The pharmacokinetic interaction between dextromethorphan paroxetine and fluoxetine may increase the risks of this effect.

Digoxin

There is a relatively narrow gap between therapeutic and toxic serum levels of digoxin. Normal therapeutic levels are about one-third of those that are fatal, and serious toxic arrhythmias begin at about two-thirds of the fatal levels. The normal range for digoxin levels is 0.8 to 2 nanograms/mL (or 1.02 to 2.56 nanomol/L). To convert nanograms/mL to nanomol/L multiply by 1.28, or to convert nanomol/L to nanograms/mL multiply by 0.781. Note that micrograms/L is the same as nanograms/mL. If a patient is over-digitalised, signs and symptoms of toxicity will occur, which may include loss of appetite, nausea and vomiting, and bradycardia. These effects are often used as clinical indicators of toxicity, and a pulse rate of less than 60 bpm is usually considered to be an indication of over-treatment. Other symptoms include visual disturbances, headache, drowsiness and occasionally diarrhoea. Death may result from cardiac arrhythmias. Patients treated for cardiac arrhythmias can therefore demonstrate arrhythmias when they are both under- as well as over-digitalised.

Digoxin + Diuretics

Eplerenone ❓

The AUC of digoxin is increased by 16% by eplerenone.

> The manufacturers warn that caution may be warranted in patients with digoxin levels near the upper end of the therapeutic range.

Loop or Thiazide diuretics ❓

Hypokalaemia, which can be caused by potassium-depleting diuretics such as the loop or thiazide diuretics, increases the toxicity of digoxin.

> Potassium levels should be routinely monitored during diuretic therapy. However, if symptoms of digoxin toxicity occur (see above) it may be prudent to re-check potassium levels.

Spironolactone ⚠

Limited evidence suggests that digoxin levels may be increased by about 20% by spironolactone, but because spironolactone or its metabolite, canrenone, can interfere with some digoxin assay methods, the evaluation of this interaction is difficult. In one report, radioimmunoassay (RIA) and affinity-column-mediated immunoassay (ACMIA) were particularly affected by spironolactone and its metabolites. Conversely, falsely low digoxin readings with the AxSym microparticle enzyme immunoassay (MEIA) assay method led to digoxin overdose and toxicity in one patient.

> Monitor digoxin effects and consider taking digoxin levels. Adjust the dose as necessary. Measurement of free digoxin levels or use of a chemiluminescent assay (CLIA) or turbidometric immunoassay for digoxin has been reported to mostly eliminate interference.

Digoxin + Herbal medicines or Dietary supplements

Liquorice (Kanzo) ❓

A patient taking digoxin developed symptomatic heart failure after taking a Chinese herbal laxative containing liquorice.

The general significance of this case is unclear.

Ginseng ❓

A man taking digoxin developed grossly elevated serum digoxin levels, without symptoms of toxicity, while taking Siberian ginseng. Both Chinese ginseng (*Panax ginseng*) and Siberian ginseng (*Eleutherococcus senticosus*) may interfere with some digoxin assays, including fluorescence polarisation immunoassay (FPIA) and microparticle enzyme immunoassay (MEIA).

Whether serum digoxin levels are actually affected is uncertain. Be aware that ginseng can possibly elevate serum digoxin levels or affect the assay of digoxin.

St John's wort (Hypericum perforatum) ✖

There is good evidence that St John's wort can reduce the levels of digoxin by roughly 30%. Digoxin toxicity has occurred in a patient taking digoxin when he stopped taking St John's wort.

Digoxin levels should be well monitored if St John's wort is either started or stopped and appropriate digoxin dosage adjustments made if necessary. The recommendation of the CSM in the UK is that St John's wort should not be taken by patients taking digoxin.

Chinese herbal medicines ⚠

Chinese medicines that contain bufalin, such as Chan Su, Lu-Shen-Wan and Kyushin, can interfere with some immunoassay methods of digoxin, particularly the fluorescence polarisation immunoassay. Similarly, a study found that a fluorescent polarization immunoassay method (Abbott Laboratories) for digoxin gave falsely high readings in the presence of danshen, whereas a microparticle enzyme immunoassay (Abbott Laboratories) gave falsely low readings.

It has been suggested that the false readings caused by bufalin could be eliminated by monitoring the free (i.e. unbound) digoxin concentrations or by using a chemiluminescent assay. Similarly, to reduce the interference from danshen, measure free digoxin levels or choose assay systems that are unaffected by the presence of danshen (said to be the Roche and Beckman systems or an enzyme linked chemiluminescent immunisorbent digoxin assay by Bayer HealthCare).

Ginkgo biloba ✔

A small study found that *Ginkgo biloba* leaf extract had no significant effects on the pharmacokinetics of a single dose of digoxin.

No action needed.

Other herbal medicines ❓

A digoxin level of 0.9 nanograms/mL was found in a patient taking an un-named herbal remedy, which contained black cohosh root *(Cimicifuga racemosa)*, cayenne pepper fruit *(Capsicum annuum)*, hops flowers *(Humulus lupulus)*, skullcap herb *(Scutellaria lateriflora)*, valerian root *(Valeriana officinalis)* and wood betony herb *(Pedicularis canadensis)*, all of which contain digoxin-like compounds which are detected by digoxin antibody immunoassays. Three packaged teas *(Breathe Easy*, blackcurrant, and jasmine) and 3 herbs (pleurisy root, chaparral, peppermint) have been found, in theory, to provide a therapeutic daily dose of digoxin, if 5 cups a day are drunk.

> It is apparent that if a patient taking digoxin also consumed these herbal remedies or teas they could develop symptoms of digoxin toxicity. However, theoretical interactions with herbal remedies are not always translated into practice. For example, hawthorn is used in cardiac disorders and the leaves and berries are reported to contain digoxin-like substances, but a study in healthy subjects found no pharmacokinetic or pharmacodynamic interaction between digoxin and an extract of hawthorn leaves and flowers *(Crataegus oxyacantha)*. Therefore although these predicted interactions should be borne in mind when using digoxin and herbal remedies they cannot be taken as total proof that an interaction will occur.

Digoxin + Levothyroxine ⚠

Hypothyroid subjects are relatively sensitive to the effects of digoxin and so need lower doses. As treatment with levothyroxine progresses, and they become euthyroid, the dosage of digoxin will need to be increased.

> Monitor the outcome of resolving hypothyroidism, checking for to ensure that the effects of digoxin are adequate. Monitor digoxin levels as necessary.

Digoxin + Lithium ❓

No pharmacokinetic interaction seems to occur between digoxin and lithium. However, the addition of digoxin to lithium possibly has a short-term detrimental effect on the control of mania. An isolated report describes severe bradycardia in one patient given both drugs.

> The probability of a clinically significant interaction occurring seems low, but bear these cases in mind if both drugs are given.

Digoxin + Macrolides ⚠

Clarithromycin markedly increases digoxin levels, and numerous cases of digoxin toxicity have been reported. Increases in serum digoxin levels also occur with telithromycin. Cases of rapid and marked two to fourfold increases in serum digoxin levels have also been reported for azithromycin, erythromycin, josamycin and roxithromycin.

> It is important to monitor all patients well for signs of increased digoxin effects (see digoxin, page 221) when any macrolide is first given. Measure digoxin levels and reduce the dosage as necessary. It has been suggested that the interaction between digoxin and clarithromycin may be dependent on the clarithromycin dosage, and may be more likely in the elderly, because of a reduction in renal function.

Digoxin + **Neomycin** ⚠️

The AUC of digoxin can be reduced by up to about 50% by the concurrent use of neomycin.

Separating administration does not prevent this interaction. Monitor the response to digoxin treatment and adjust the dose as necessary.

Digoxin + **NSAIDs**

Diclofenac, Etoricoxib, or Ibuprofen ❓

Studies have found that both diclofenac and etoricoxib can raise the serum digoxin levels by about one-third. Studies suggest that serum digoxin levels are unchanged by ibuprofen, although some reports suggest increases of up to 60% are possible.

Although rises of this extent (especially with ibuprofen) would be expected to be clinically significant, there appear to be no reports of an interaction in practice. Bear this interaction in mind in patients taking both drugs, and monitor digoxin levels if a problem is suspected.

Indometacin ⚠️

Rises in serum digoxin levels and digoxin toxicity have been reported in neonates given digoxin with indometacin. The picture is less clear in adults, as there are studies reporting either no change or increased digoxin levels. However, there seem to be no examples of a consistent interaction in practice.

In neonates, digoxin levels should be monitored if concurrent use is necessary, and the dose reduced accordingly. In adults, bear this interaction in mind if patients are given both drugs and monitor digoxin levels if a problem is suspected.

Digoxin + **Penicillamine** ⚠️

Serum digoxin levels can be reduced by 40 to 60% by penicillamine. This interaction was also reported to occur in children.

Patients taking digoxin should be checked for signs of under-dosing if penicillamine is added. Consider checking digoxin levels if an interaction is suspected.

Digoxin + **Phenytoin** ❓

Phenytoin moderately reduces digoxin levels, but the clinical significance of this is unknown. There are also isolated case reports of marked bradycardia in patients taking digoxin with phenytoin. Fatalities have been reported when phenytoin was used in cases of suspected digoxin toxicity.

It would seem sensible to monitor the effects of concurrent use and consider monitoring digoxin levels if an interaction is suspected. The use of phenytoin in digoxin toxicity appears to be obsolete.

Digoxin + **Propafenone** ⚠

Propafenone can increase serum digoxin levels by 30 to 90% or more (particularly in children).

Most patients appear to be affected and dosage reductions in the range of 15 to 70% were found necessary in one study. The extent of the rise may possibly depend on the propafenone level rather than on the propafenone dose. Monitor digoxin levels and adjust the dose accordingly.

Digoxin + **Protease inhibitors** ⚠

A woman had elevated serum digoxin levels and signs of toxicity after she was given ritonavir. Pharmacokinetic studies have shown that ritonavir and saquinavir with ritonavir cause modest to marked increases in single-dose digoxin levels.

It would seem prudent to closely monitor patients taking digoxin when ritonavir is started or stopped. Note that there appears to be a greater effect with intravenous digoxin than with oral digoxin. There do not appear to be any reports or studies of the interaction of digoxin with other protease inhibitors; however, most protease inhibitors are inhibitors and/or substrates for P-glycoprotein, so it would seem likely that they may all interact to a greater or lesser degree.

Digoxin + **Proton pump inhibitors** ✔

A small rise in serum digoxin levels may occur in patients also given omeprazole, pantoprazole, rabeprazole and possibly lansoprazole. However, these changes are thought to be within the normal variations of digoxin levels and so are not considered clinically significant. However, one patient developed digoxin toxicity 3 months after starting to take omeprazole.

No action needed. The isolated case of toxicity seems unlikely to be generally significant.

Digoxin + **Quinidine** ⚠

Quinidine, on average, doubles the serum levels of digoxin in most patients within 5 days of concurrent use.

Halve the digoxin dose, monitor digoxin levels and further adjust the dose as necessary. Patients with renal impairment may require larger dose reductions. Remember to increase the digoxin dose if quinidine is stopped.

Digoxin + **Quinine** ⚠

Some patients may show a rise of more than 60% in serum digoxin levels if they are given quinine.

Monitor the effects of concurrent use and reduce the digoxin dosage where necessary. Some patients may show a substantial increase in serum digoxin levels whereas others will show only a small or moderate rise. There appear to be no case reports of digoxin toxicity arising from this interaction.

Digoxin + Rifampicin (Rifampin) ❓

There is some evidence that digoxin levels may be approximately halved by rifampicin.

It would seem sensible to monitor the outcome of concurrent use and monitor digoxin levels if an interaction is suspected. It may be that renal impairment increases the extent of this interaction.

Digoxin + Salbutamol (Albuterol) and related bronchodilators ⚠

In one study, oral salbutamol slightly reduced digoxin levels, by 0.3 nanomol/L. Note that all beta$_2$ agonists (oral and inhaled) can cause a fall in serum potassium levels.

It may be prudent to monitor potassium levels if beta$_2$ agonists are started, particularly nebulised, oral or intravenous beta$_2$ agonists. If symptoms of digoxin toxicity occur on concurrent use (see digoxin, page 221) it may be prudent to recheck potassium levels.

Digoxin + Statins ✓

Atorvastatin, fluvastatin and simvastatin cause small but probably clinically unimportant increases in the serum levels of digoxin.

The increase in digoxin levels is apparently only small and therefore normally not likely to be clinically relevant.

Digoxin + Sucralfate ❓

Sucralfate causes only a small reduction in the absorption of digoxin, but an isolated report describes a marked reduction in one patient.

The reduction in digoxin levels is apparently only small and therefore normally not likely to be clinically relevant.

Digoxin + Sulfasalazine ⚠

Serum digoxin levels can be reduced by up to 50% by sulfasalazine. This interaction appears to be dose related.

Monitor to ensure that the effects of digoxin are adequate, and consider measuring digoxin levels if an interaction is suspected. Adjust the dose as necessary.

Digoxin + Tizanidine ⚠

The UK manufacturers say that the concurrent use of digoxin may potentiate the bradycardia caused by tizanidine alone.

Monitor heart rate and adjust the digoxin dose accordingly.

Digoxin + Topiramate ✅

Topiramate slightly reduces the maximum levels and AUC of digoxin by less than 20%.

> The manufacturer suggests good monitoring of digoxin if topiramate is added or withdrawn, but changes of this magnitude seem unlikely to be clinically relevant in most patients.

Digoxin + Trimethoprim ⚠️

Serum digoxin levels can be increased by about 22% by trimethoprim, but some individuals may show a much greater rise.

> Monitor the effects of digoxin if trimethoprim is given, and consider measuring digoxin levels, particularly in the elderly. Adjust the dose as necessary. Trimethoprim is a constituent of co-trimoxazole but it is not known whether prophylactic doses of co-trimoxazole (160 mg of trimethoprim a day from a 960-mg dose of co-trimoxazole) will interact to a clinically significant degree. An interaction would seem likely with high-dose co-trimoxazole, and care is needed in the elderly with any co-trimoxazole dose .

Dipyridamole

Dipyridamole + H₂-receptor antagonists ❓

The effective disintegration, dissolution and eventual absorption of dipyridamole in tablet or suspension form depends upon having a low pH in the stomach. Drugs that significantly raise the gastric pH are expected to reduce the bioavailability of dipyridamole tablets. This effect has been seen with famotidine.

> The clinical significance of this interaction is unknown. Bear it in mind if an H_2-receptor antagonist is given with dipyridamole. Note that modified-release preparations of dipyridamole (that are buffered) do not appear to be affected.

Dipyridamole + Proton pump inhibitors ❓

The effective disintegration, dissolution and eventual absorption of dipyridamole in tablet or suspension form depends upon having a low pH in the stomach. Drugs that significantly raise the gastric pH are expected to reduce the bioavailability of dipyridamole tablets. This effect has been seen with lansoprazole.

> The clinical significance of this interaction is unknown. Bear it in mind if a proton pump inhibitor is given with dipyridamole. Note that modified-release preparations of dipyridamole (that are buffered) do not appear to be affected.

Dipyridamole + **Warfarin and other oral anticoagulants**

Mild bleeding (epistaxis, bruising, haematuria) can sometimes occur if anticoagulants are given with dipyridamole. Note that prothrombin times remain stable and well within the therapeutic range.

> These effects would not be unexpected if an antiplatelet and an anticoagulant were used concurrently. Bear them in mind when considering the combination.

D Disopyramide

Disopyramide + **Macrolides** ❌

Case reports suggest that erythromycin increases disopyramide levels, and this has resulted in QT prolongation, cardiac arrhythmias and heart block. Similar effects have been seen when clarithromycin or azithromycin are given with disopyramide. Josamycin and telithromycin are expected to interact similarly. See also drugs that prolong the QT interval, page 237.

> Some of the manufacturers of disopyramide recommend avoiding the combination of disopyramide and macrolides that inhibit CYP3A, and this would certainly be prudent in situations where close monitoring is not possible.

Disopyramide + **Phenobarbital** ❌

Serum disopyramide levels are reduced by about 35% by phenobarbital. Note that primidone is metabolised to phenobarbital and therefore may interact similarly.

> The extent to which this interaction would reduce the antiarrhythmic effects of disopyramide is unknown, but monitor the effects and the serum levels of disopyramide (if possible) if phenobarbital is added or withdrawn. One manufacturer suggests avoiding the combination.

Disopyramide + **Phenytoin** ❌

Serum disopyramide levels are reduced by phenytoin and may fall below therapeutic levels. Loss of arrhythmic control may occur. Fosphenytoin, a prodrug of phenytoin, may interact similarly.

> Antiarrhythmic response and serum disopyramide levels (where possible) should be well monitored. Adjust the disopyramide dose as necessary. Serum disopyramide levels appear to return to normal within 2 weeks of withdrawing the phenytoin.

Disopyramide + **Rifampicin (Rifampin)** ⚠

The serum levels of disopyramide can be reduced by rifampicin.

It seems likely that the dosage of disopyramide will need to be increased in most patients taking rifampicin. Monitor the effects of concurrent use and adjust the dose as necessary.

Disopyramide + **Warfarin and other oral anticoagulants** ❓

Limited data suggests that warfarin requirements can be increased or decreased by disopyramide.

There is insufficient evidence to recommend monitoring all patients, but bear this interaction in mind if patients taking anticoagulants are given disopyramide.

D

Disulfiram

Disulfiram + **Isoniazid** ❓

In most patients the use of isoniazid with disulfiram is uneventful, but a number of patients have developed difficulties in co-ordination, changes in affect and behaviour, and drowsiness.

Concurrent use need not be avoided, but if marked changes in mental status occur, or if there is unsteady gait, the manufacturers recommend that the disulfiram should be withdrawn.

Disulfiram + **Metronidazole** ⚠

Acute psychoses and confusion can result from the use of metronidazole with disulfiram.

Concurrent use should be avoided or very well monitored.

Disulfiram + **Phenytoin** ⚠

Phenytoin serum levels are markedly and rapidly increased by the concurrent use of disulfiram. Phenytoin toxicity has been seen in 2 patients.

This interaction seems to occur in most patients and develops rapidly. Recovery may take 2 to 3 weeks after the disulfiram is withdrawn. Monitor phenytoin levels carefully during concurrent use. Phenytoin dosage reductions may be needed, but it may be difficult to maintain the balance required.

Disulfiram + **Theophylline** ⚠

The clearance of theophylline is slightly reduced by disulfiram. Higher doses of disulfiram appear to have a greater effect.

Monitor the effects of theophylline if disulfiram is added and consider monitoring serum levels. Theophylline dosage reductions may be needed.

Disulfiram + **Warfarin and other oral anticoagulants** ⚠

The anticoagulant effects of warfarin are increased by disulfiram, and in some cases bleeding has occurred.

It seems likely that most individuals will demonstrate this interaction. If concurrent use is thought appropriate, the effects of warfarin should be monitored and suitable dosage adjustments made when adding or withdrawing disulfiram. Care should be taken when starting warfarin in patients already taking disulfiram, and consideration should be given to using a smaller loading dose.

D

Diuretics

Diuretics + **Herbal medicines or Dietary supplements**

Germanium ❌

On two occasions severe oedema (12 to 13 kg weight gain) developed over 10 to 14 days in a patient taking furosemide after he also took a preparation containing ginseng and germanium.

The significance of this interaction is unclear. The effects were attributed to the germanium. Note that the patient did not respond to increased doses of oral furosemide, but did respond to intravenous furosemide. Also, it has been said that the use of germanium should be discouraged due to its potential to cause renal toxicity.

Liquorice ❓

A patient developed severe hypokalaemia after taking liquorice and hydrochlorothiazide. This interaction seems possible with liquorice (which can lower potassium levels) and any potassium-depleting diuretic (i.e. thiazides or loop diuretics).

The additive effects of these drugs may result in clinically significant hypokalaemia, but evidence is extremely sparse. Consider this interaction in a case of otherwise unexplained hypokalaemia.

St John's wort (Hypericum perforatum) ❌

St John's wort decreases the AUC of eplerenone by 30%.

Concurrent use is not recommended by the manufacturers.

Diuretics + Lithium

Amiloride ✓

Some manufacturers suggest that amiloride reduces the renal clearance of lithium, thereby increasing the risk of lithium toxicity. There appears to be no evidence to confirm this alleged interaction and two studies suggesting that no interaction occurs.

No action needed.

Eplerenone ⚠

Eplerenone and lithium have not been studied, but the manufacturers predict that eplerenone may raise lithium levels.

The UK manufacturers say avoid or closely monitor lithium levels. Patients taking lithium should be aware of the symptoms of lithium toxicity (see lithium, page 305) and told to report them immediately should they occur.

Loop diuretics ⚠

The concurrent use of lithium and furosemide can be safe and uneventful, but serious lithium toxicity has been described. Bumetanide interacts similarly. The risk of lithium toxicity with a loop diuretic is greatly increased during the first month of concurrent use.

It would be imprudent to give furosemide or bumetanide to patients stabilised on lithium unless the effects can be well monitored because some patients may develop serious toxicity. Patients taking lithium should be aware of the symptoms of lithium toxicity (see lithium, page 305) and told to report them immediately should they occur. Consider increased monitoring of lithium levels in patients newly started on this combination.

Spironolactone ❓

One study found that spironolactone caused the lithium levels to rise from 0.63 to 0.9 mmol/L. However, another study found no interaction.

Evidence for this interaction is sparse, no additional monitoring is necessary, but patients on lithium should be aware of the symptoms of lithium toxicity (see lithium, page 305) and told to report them immediately should they occur.

Thiazides ⚠

The thiazide and related diuretics can cause a rapid rise in lithium levels, which may lead to lithium toxicity. This interaction has been seen with bendroflumethiazide, chlorothiazide, chlortalidone, hydrochlorothiazide and indapamide, and potentially occurs with hydroflumethiazide. Other thiazides and related diuretics are expected to behave similarly.

Lithium levels should be closely monitored if a thiazide is started or stopped. One UK manufacturer recommends an initial lithium dose reduction, but this does not seem to be in line with most other recommendations. Patients taking lithium should be aware of the symptoms of lithium toxicity (see lithium, page 305) and told to report them immediately should they occur.

Triamterene ❓

Triamterene appears to increase lithium excretion.

> Information is sparse. The reports available do not give a clear indication of the outcome of concurrent use, but some monitoring would seem prudent.

Diuretics + Macrolides ⚠

Erythromycin increases the AUC of eplerenone 2.9-fold. The manufacturer predicts that clarithromycin and telithromycin will interact to a greater extent. Eplerenone reduced the AUC of erythromycin by 14%, which was not considered clinically relevant.

> The manufacturers recommend a maximum eplerenone dose of 25 mg daily in those taking erythromycin. Because they predict a greater effect with clarithromycin and telithromycin they contraindicate the concurrent use of these macrolides. Other macrolides seem less likely to interact, see macrolides, page 310.

Diuretics + NSAIDs

Potassium-sparing diuretics ⚠

The manufacturer advises caution on the concurrent use of NSAIDs and eplerenone because NSAIDs can cause renal impairment, especially in dehydrated or elderly patients. Several cases of acute renal failure have been seen when triamterene was given with NSAIDs.

> Patients should be well hydrated and have their renal function checked before starting this combination.

Loop diuretics ❓

The antihypertensive and diuretic effects of loop diuretics appear to be reduced by NSAIDs, although the extent of this interaction largely depends on the individual NSAID. Indometacin appears to cause the most significant effect. Note that diuretics increase the risk of NSAID-induced acute renal failure.

> Concurrent use need not be avoided but the effects should be checked and the diuretic dosage raised as necessary. Not all patients are affected. Patients at greatest risk are likely to be the elderly with cirrhosis, cardiac failure and/or renal impairment, and they may need to avoid NSAIDs.

Thiazides ❓

The antihypertensive effects of the thiazides can be reduced to some extent by indometacin, but it appears to be of only moderate clinical importance and may possibly only be a transient interaction.

> Monitor the effects of the concurrent use of indometacin and adjust the thiazide dosage or alter the NSAID if necessary. Other NSAIDs appear to interact to a lesser extent or not at all.

Diuretics + **Phenobarbital** ❌

St John's wort (Hypericum perforatum) decreases the AUC of eplerenone by 30%. The manufacturers therefore predict that more potent enzyme inducers, such as phenobarbital, may have a greater effect. Note that primidone is metabolised to phenobarbital and therefore may interact similarly.

Concurrent use is not recommended by the manufacturers.

Diuretics + **Phenytoin**

Furosemide ⚠

The diuretic effects of furosemide can be reduced as much as 50% if phenytoin is taken concurrently.

The clinical significance of this finding is unclear. However, it may be prudent to consider monitoring the diuretic effects if phenytoin is started. Fosphenytoin, a prodrug of phenytoin, may interact similarly.

Eplerenone ❌

St John's wort *(Hypericum perforatum)* decreases the AUC of eplerenone by 30%. The manufacturers therefore predict that more potent enzyme inducers, such as phenytoin, may have a greater effect. Fosphenytoin, a prodrug of phenytoin, may interact similarly.

Concurrent use is not recommended by the manufacturers.

Diuretics + **Potassium**

Eplerenone ❌

The manufacturers predict that if eplerenone is given with potassium severe hyperkalaemia will occur.

Concurrent use is contraindicated.

Spironolactone or Triamterene ⚠

The concurrent use of spironolactone or triamterene with potassium supplements can result in severe and even life-threatening hyperkalaemia. Amiloride is expected to interact similarly. Potassium-containing salt substitutes can be as hazardous as potassium supplements.

Concurrent use need not be avoided but close monitoring of potassium levels, both before and during treatment is necessary.

Diuretics + **Protease inhibitors** ❌

Saquinavir increases the AUC of eplerenone 2.1-fold. The manufacturer predicts that nelfinavir and ritonavir will interact to a greater extent.

The manufacturer recommends a maximum eplerenone dose of 25 mg daily in those taking saquinavir. Because they predict a greater effect with nelfinavir and ritonavir they contraindicate the concurrent use of these protease inhibitors.

Diuretics + Reboxetine ❓

Reboxetine may reduce potassium levels. Hypokalaemia is therefore possible if reboxetine is used with potassium-depleting diuretics (e.g. loop or thiazide diuretics).

Monitor potassium levels on concurrent use. Note that the onset of any interaction may be delayed.

Diuretics + Rifampicin (Rifampin) ✕

St John's wort (*Hypericum perforatum*) decreases the AUC of eplerenone by 30%. The manufacturers therefore predict that more potent enzyme inducers, such as rifampicin, may have a greater effect.

Concurrent use is not recommended by the manufacturers.

Diuretics + Sevelamer ⚠

Sevelamer abolished the diuretic effect of furosemide 250 mg twice daily in a haemodialysis patient. Urine output returned to the patient's normal levels 24 hours after sevelamer was stopped, and the reduction in urine output was not seen when the dosing frequency was altered so that furosemide was taken in the morning and sevelamer at lunch and dinnertime.

If the effect of furosemide seems less than expected, give the furosemide at least 1 hour before or 3 hours after sevelamer.

Diuretics + Tacrolimus ⚠

As tacrolimus may cause hyperkalaemia, the manufacturers say that concurrent use of potassium-sparing diuretics should be avoided. The manufacturers of eplerenone give similar advice.

If concurrent use is essential potassium levels should be monitored closely.

Diuretics + Theophylline ⚠

Furosemide is reported to increase, decrease or to have no effect on serum theophylline levels. Both theophylline and loop or thiazide diuretics can cause hypokalaemia, which may be additive.

If both drugs are used be aware for the potential for changes in theophylline levels. Consider measuring theophylline levels, and make appropriate dosage adjustments as necessary. It may be prudent to also monitor potassium levels.

Diuretics + Toremifene ❓

Hypercalcaemia is a recognised adverse effect of toremifene, and the manufacturers suggest that drugs such as the thiazides, which decrease renal calcium excretion, may increase the risk of hypercalcaemia.

This warning is based on theoretical considerations, and their clinical importance awaits confirmation.

Domperidone

D

Domperidone + Dopamine agonists ⚠

Domperidone would be expected to reduce the prolactin-lowering effect of bromocriptine.

It would be prudent to monitor the efficacy of bromocriptine if domperidone is required. Note that domperidone is the antiemetic of choice in Parkinson's disease.

Donepezil

Donepezil + SSRIs ❓

Two case reports suggest that paroxetine may increase donepezil levels and adverse effects. The manufacturers predict that fluoxetine will also interact, as, like paroxetine, it inhibits CYP2D6.

The manufacturers advise caution on concurrent use.

Dopamine agonists

Dopamine agonists + Ergot derivatives ✖

Bromocriptine and cabergoline are ergot dopamine agonists and although the manufacturers have no evidence of an interaction with other ergot derivatives, they do not recommend concurrent use.

Avoid concurrent use.

Dopamine agonists + H₂-receptor antagonists ⚠

Cimetidine may reduce the clearance of pramipexole by 35%. *Ciprofloxacin* increases the AUC of ropinirole by 84%. The manufacturers therefore predict that other CYP1A2 inhibitors (they name cimetidine) will interact similarly.

The clinical relevance of these interactions do not appear to have been assessed. The manufacturers recommend considering a dose reduction of the dopamine agonist if cimetidine is used.

Dopamine agonists + HRT ⚠

Population pharmacokinetic analysis of clinical study data showed that oestrogens (from HRT) reduced ropinirole clearance by one-third.

In women already receiving HRT, ropinirole treatment may be started using the usual dose titration. However, a reduction in the ropinirole dosage may be needed if HRT is started, and an increase if it is withdrawn.

Dopamine agonists + Macrolides ⚠

Erythromycin markedly increases bromocriptine plasma levels (by more than 4-fold), and a case of toxicity has been reported. Bromocriptine toxicity has also occurred in a patient given josamycin. Clarithromycin increases the bioavailability of cabergoline by about 2- to 4-fold.

Concurrent use should be well monitored if macrolides that affect CYP3A4 are given (e.g. clarithromycin, erythromycin, telithromycin, see macrolides, page 310, for further details). It has been suggested that the bromocriptine dose may need to be reduced by 50% to avoid toxicity.

Dopamine agonists + Metoclopramide ✗

Centrally-acting dopamine antagonists (such as metoclopramide) are expected to oppose the effects of the dopamine agonists. Metoclopramide would also be expected to reduce the prolactin-lowering effect of bromocriptine.

Concurrent use should be avoided, or monitored closely to ensure that the dopamine agonist remains effective. Domperidone is the antiemetic of choice in Parkinson's disease.

Dopamine agonists + Nasal decongestants ✗

Post-partum women taking bromocriptine have developed symptoms such as severe headache, marked hypertension, psychosis, or seizures with cerebral vasospasm after also taking isometheptene, phenylpropanolamine, or pseudoephedrine.

Direct information seems to be limited to these cases, but the severity of the reactions suggests that it might be prudent for postpartum patients to avoid these and related drugs while taking bromocriptine. Advise patients to also avoid non-prescription products containing these drugs (often cough and cold remedies).

Dopamine agonists + **Quinolones** ⚠

Ciprofloxacin increases the AUC of ropinirole by 84%.

> The clinical relevance of this pharmacokinetic interaction has not been assessed. The manufacturers suggest that an adjustment of the ropinirole dose may be required in the presence of ciprofloxacin. Other quinolones may also interact, see quinolones, page 382.

Dopamine agonists + **SSRIs** ⚠

Ciprofloxacin increases the AUC of ropinirole by 84%. The manufacturers therefore predict that other CYP1A2 inhibitors (they name fluvoxamine) will interact similarly.

> The clinical relevance of this pharmacokinetic interaction has not been assessed. The manufacturers suggest that the ropinirole dose may need to be adjusted in patients taking fluvoxamine.

D

Doxapram

Doxapram + **Theophylline** ❓

No pharmacokinetic interaction appears to occur between theophylline and doxapram in neonates. However, the manufacturers of doxapram say that clinical data suggests there may be an interaction (not confined to neonates), which is manifested by agitation and increased skeletal muscle activity.

> Although this reaction seems rare, it would be prudent to monitor concurrent use for any adverse outcome.

Drugs that prolong the QT interval

The consensus of opinion is that the concurrent use of two or more drugs that prolong the QT interval should generally be avoided because of the risk of additive effects, leading to the possible development of serious and potentially life-threatening torsade de pointes arrhythmias. It is thought that torsade de pointes is unlikely to develop until the corrected QT (QTc) interval exceeds 500 milliseconds, but this is not an exact figure and the risks are uncertain and unpredictable. Because of these uncertainties, many drug manufacturers and regulatory agencies now contraindicate the concurrent use of drugs known to prolong the QT interval, and a 'blanket' warning is often issued because the QT-prolonging effects of the drugs are expected to be additive. The extent of the drug-induced prolongation usually depends on the dosage of the drug and the particular drugs in question. For some drugs QT prolongation is a fairly frequent effect when the drug is used alone, and it is well accepted that use of these drugs requires careful monitoring (e.g. a number of the antiarrhythmics). Pairs of antiarrhythmics should therefore be avoided where possible. For other drugs, QT prolongation is rare, but because of the relatively benign indications for these drugs, the risk-benefit ratio is considered poor, and use of these drugs has been severely restricted or discontinued (e.g. astemizole, terfenadine, cisapride). For others there is less clear evidence of the risk of QT prolongation (e.g. tacrolimus, tamoxifen, tricyclic antidepressants) and therefore the associated risks of combinations of these types of drug are much lower. Drugs known to have a high risk of causing QT-prolongation include:

- Antiarrhythmics (class Ia: disopyramide, procainamide, quinidine)
- Antiarrhythmics (class III: amiodarone, sotalol)
- Antihistamines (astemizole, terfenadine, if levels raised, and possibly mizolastine)
- Antimalarials (artemether, present in co-artemether, and other artemisinin derivatives, halofantrine)
- Antipsychotics (amisulpride, droperidol, haloperidol (high dose and intravenous use), pimozide, sertindole, thioridazine)
- Arsenic trioxide
- Erythromycin (intravenous, but see also, below)
- Ranolazine
- Sparfloxacin (see also, below)

Drugs known to be associated with some risk of causing QT-prolongation include:

- Clomipramine (risk with other tricyclics appears to be mainly in overdose)
- Chlorpromazine
- Lithium (if levels raised)
- Macrolides (clarithromycin, oral erythromycin, (see also, above), spiramycin)
- Methadone (doses greater than 100 mg)
- Quinolones (gatifloxacin, levofloxacin, moxifloxacin, and see also, above)
- Pentamidine intravenous
- Quinine

Further, hypokalaemia increases the risks of torsade de pointes arrhythmias and so potassium levels should be closely monitored when drugs that can cause hypokalaemia are used with drugs that prolong the QT interval. However, there appear to be very few reports of this interaction. Drugs known to lower potassium levels include:

- Amphotericin B
- Corticosteroids
- Loop diuretics
- Salbutamol (Albuterol) and related bronchodilators
- Stimulant laxatives
- Theophylline
- Thiazide diuretics

Duloxetine

Duloxetine + Flecainide ⚠

Duloxetine (a moderate inhibitor of CYP2D6) may inhibit the metabolism of flecainide (a substrate for CYP2D6), increasing the risk of flecainide adverse effects.

The manufacturer advises caution.

Duloxetine + **Herbal medicines or Dietary supplements** ⚠

Concurrent use of duloxetine and St John's wort (*Hypericum perforatum*) may lead to serotonin syndrome, page 392. One possible case has been reported.

The manufacturers advise caution.

Duloxetine + **Lithium** ⚠

The concurrent use of duloxetine with lithium may lead to serotonin syndrome, page 392.

The manufacturers advise caution.

Duloxetine + **MAOIs** ✖

The concurrent use of MAOIs and duloxetine may lead to serotonin syndrome, page 392.

The manufacturers contraindicate the use of duloxetine with non-selective irreversible MAOIs, during and for 14 days after discontinuing an MAOI. At least 5 days should be allowed after stopping duloxetine before starting an MAOI.

Duloxetine + **Moclobemide** ✖

There is a possible risk of serotonin syndrome, page 392, if duloxetine is used with moclobemide; one case has been reported.

The manufacturer advises avoiding concurrent use.

Duloxetine + **Opioids** ⚠

The concurrent use of duloxetine with tramadol or pethidine (meperidine) may lead to serotonin syndrome, page 392.

The manufacturers advise caution.

Duloxetine + **Propafenone** ⚠

Duloxetine (a moderate inhibitor of CYP2D6) may inhibit the metabolism of propafenone (a substrate for CYP2D6), increasing the risk of propafenone adverse effects.

The manufacturer advises caution.

Duloxetine + Quinidine ⚠

Inhibitors of CYP2D6 are expected to increase duloxetine levels. This has been seen with fluoxetine and is predicted to occur with quinidine.

The manufacturer advises caution on concurrent use. Monitor for duloxetine adverse effects, which include nausea, dry mouth, and hot flushes.

Duloxetine + Quinolones ✖

Potent inhibitors of CYP1A2 are expected to increase duloxetine levels. This has been seen with *fluvoxamine* (see below) and is predicted to occur with quinolones (e.g. ciprofloxacin and enoxacin).

The manufacturer advises that concurrent use should be avoided. Note that the quinolones may interact to varying extents, see quinolones, page 382.

D

Duloxetine + SSRIs

Fluvoxamine ✖

The combined use of duloxetine with an SSRI may result in serotonin syndrome, page 392. Fluvoxamine increases duloxetine levels by up to 6-fold.

The manufacturers contraindicate the concurrent use of fluvoxamine with duloxetine.

Other SSRIs ⚠

The combined use of duloxetine and an SSRI may result in serotonin syndrome, page 392. Low-dose paroxetine caused a modest increase in the AUC of duloxetine, and fluoxetine is predicted to interact similarly.

The manufacturers of duloxetine advise caution on the concurrent use of SSRIs.

Duloxetine + Tricyclics ✖

Duloxetine markedly increases the AUC of desipramine. Other tricyclics metabolised by CYP2D6, such as nortriptyline, amitriptyline and imipramine, may interact similarly. The use of duloxetine with other serotonergic drugs, such as the tricyclics, may increase the risk of serotonin syndrome, page 392.

The manufacturer advises caution on concurrent use. Monitor for duloxetine adverse effects, and for signs of serotonin syndrome.

Duloxetine + Triptans ⚠

Concurrent use of duloxetine and the triptans (e.g. sumatriptan) may lead to serotonin syndrome, page 392.

The manufacturers advise caution.

Duloxetine + **Tryptophan** ⚠

Concurrent use of duloxetine and tryptophan may lead to serotonin syndrome, page 392.

The UK manufacturers advise caution with concurrent use, however the US manufacturer advises avoiding concurrent use.

Duloxetine + **Venlafaxine** ⚠

Concurrent use of duloxetine and venlafaxine may lead to serotonin syndrome, page 392.

The manufacturers advise caution.

D

Dutasteride

Dutasteride + **Protease inhibitors** ⚠

Moderate CYP3A4 inhibitors increase dutasteride levels by 60 to 80%, which, due to the wide safety margin of dutasteride, is not thought to be clinically significant. However, potent CYP3A4 inhibitors, such as the protease inhibitors, would be expected to have a larger effect, which may cause a clinically significant rise in dutasteride levels.

The manufacturers suggest reducing the dosing frequency if increased dutasteride adverse effects occur.

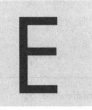

Entacapone or Tolcapone

Entacapone or Tolcapone + Inotropes and Vasopressors ❓

Entacapone potentiated the increase in heart rate and arrhythmogenic effects of isoprenaline (isoproterenol) and adrenaline (epinephrine) in a study in healthy subjects.

The manufacturers of entacapone and tolcapone suggest caution on the concurrent use of drugs such as adrenaline (epinephrine), dobutamine, dopamine, isoprenaline (isoproterenol) and noradrenaline (norepinephrine).

Entacapone or Tolcapone + Iron ⚠

Entacapone forms chelates with iron *in vitro*.

The manufacturer recommends that iron preparations and entacapone are given 2 to 3 hours apart.

Entacapone or Tolcapone + MAOIs ✖

The manufacturers of entacapone and tolcapone contraindicate the concurrent use of non-selective MAOIs.

Avoid concurrent use.

Entacapone or Tolcapone + Moclobemide ❓

In a single dose study, there was no adverse effect on heart rate or blood pressure when entacapone was given with moclobemide.

The manufacturers of entacapone and tolcapone recommend caution until further clinical experience is gained.

Entacapone or Tolcapone + **Tricyclics** ❓

Studies suggest that no important interaction occurs between entacapone and imipramine or between tolcapone and desipramine.

Despite these studies, the manufacturer of entacapone says there is limited clinical experience of the use of entacapone with tricyclic antidepressants, and they therefore recommend caution. Similarly, the manufacturers of tolcapone suggest that caution should be exercised if desipramine is taken concurrently.

Enteral feeds

Consider also the interactions of food.

E

Enteral feeds + **Phenytoin** ⚠

A 70% reduction in phenytoin absorption has been described when it is given with enteral feeds (e.g. *Isocal*, *Osmolite*) administered via nasogastric tubes.

This interaction has been managed by giving the phenytoin diluted in water 2 hours after stopping the feed, flushing with 60 mL of water, and waiting another 2 hours before restarting the feed. However, one study found this method unsuccessful. Other suggestions include waiting 6 hours after the phenytoin dose before restarting the feed, stopping continuous feed 1 hour rather than 2 hours before and after phenytoin administration, the use of twice daily phenytoin or the use of intravenous phenytoin. Monitor the outcome carefully. The same problem can also occur when enteral feeds are given by the jejunostomy tube but methods to manage this are not yet established.

Enteral feeds + **Quinolones** ⚠

The absorption of ciprofloxacin can be as much as halved by enteral feeds such as *Ensure*, *Jevity*, *Osmolite*, *Pulmocare* and *Sustacal*.

No treatment failures have been reported but this interaction is expected to be clinically important. Monitor the outcome of concurrent use carefully. Consider also food, page 258.

Enteral feeds + **Sucralfate** ⚠

Sucralfate can interact with the protein component of enteral feeds within the oesophagus to produce an obstructive plug (a bezoar).

The manufacturers recommend separating the administration of sucralfate suspension and enteral feeds given by nasogastric tube by one hour.

Enteral feeds + **Theophylline** ⚠

Enteral feeds can significantly affect theophylline levels (a reduction of 50% was seen in one case).

Avoiding giving enteral feeds for one hour either side of theophylline seems to be an effective way of managing this interaction, but it would still be prudent to monitor the outcome on theophylline levels. Not all preparations of theophylline are necessarily affected, but there is insufficient evidence to identify those that may be a problem.

Enteral feeds + **Warfarin and other oral anticoagulants** ❓

Enteral feeds may contain sufficient vitamin K1 (commonly about 4 to 10 micrograms per 100 mL) to antagonise the effects of warfarin. One study in children reported that those receiving enteral nutrition (mostly vitamin K-enriched formula) required 2.4-fold higher maintenance warfarin doses.

Starting or stopping enteral feeds might affect dose requirements of vitamin K antagonists (coumarins and indanediones). It is also possible that there is a local interaction in the gut, as in one case separating the administration of the warfarin and an enteral feed by 3 hours or more was effective. Patients should be advised not to add or substitute dietary supplements such as *Ensure* without increased monitoring of their coagulation status.

Ergot derivatives

Ergot derivatives + **Macrolides** ✖

Ergot toxicity can develop rapidly in patients taking ergotamine or dihydroergotamine if they are given erythromycin. However, in one case, the reaction occurred when erythromycin was started 3 days after the last dose of dihydroergotamine. Other cases have been reported with clarithromycin and josamycin. Toxicity is also predicted to occur with midecamycin and telithromycin.

The combination of ergot derivatives and macrolides that inhibit CYP3A4 is best avoided. Note that the macrolides differ in their ability to inhibit CYP3A4, see macrolides, page 310. No cases of toxicity appear to have been described with azithromycin, dirithromycin, or spiramycin, and none would be expected.

Ergot derivatives + **NNRTIs**

Delavirdine or Efavirenz ✖

Delavirdine and efavirenz are predicted to inhibit the metabolism of ergot derivatives, which may result in the development of ergotism.

The manufacturers generally contraindicate potent CYP3A4 inhibitors which would include delavirdine and efavirenz.

Nevirapine ⚠

Nevirapine is predicted to increase the metabolism of ergot derivatives, and might therefore be expected to reduce their efficacy.

Monitor the outcome of concurrent use to ensure the effects of ergot derivatives are adequate.

Ergot derivatives + Protease inhibitors ❌

A patient taking indinavir rapidly developed ergotism after taking usual doses of ergotamine. At least 6 other patients taking ritonavir with ergotamine have had the same reaction. A patient taking nelfinavir developed peripheral arterial vasoconstriction after taking ergotamine. Other ergot derivatives and protease inhibitors are predicted to interact similarly.

The manufacturers of many ergot derivatives generally contraindicate potent CYP3A4 inhibitors, which would include the protease inhibitors.

Ergot derivatives + Reboxetine ❓

The manufacturers suggest that concurrent use of reboxetine and ergot derivatives might result in increased blood pressure, although no clinical data are quoted.

The general significance of this interaction is unclear.

Ergot derivatives + Rifampicin (Rifampin) ⚠

Rifampicin is predicted to increase the metabolism of ergot derivatives, and might therefore be expected to reduce their efficacy. Note that rifampicin has been used as a potent enzyme inducer to reduce ergotamine levels in a patient with ergotism, and was said to play a key role in reducing ergotamine levels.

Monitor the outcome of concurrent use to ensure the effects of ergot derivatives are adequate.

Ergot derivatives + Sibutramine ❌

There are no reports of adverse reactions between sibutramine and dihydroergotamine but the manufacturers contraindicate the combination as it may theoretically lead to the potentially fatal serotonin syndrome, page 392. This has occurred with related drugs.

Avoid concurrent use.

Ergot derivatives + SSRIs ❓

Isolated cases of the serotonin syndrome have been seen in patients taking paroxetine (with imipramine), or sertraline, when they were also given dihydroergotamine.

> These appear to be isolated cases and not of general importance. Nevertheless they illustrate the potential for the development of serotonin syndrome, page 392, in patients given multiple drugs that affect serotonin receptors.

Ergot derivatives + Tetracyclines ⚠

Several patients taking ergotamine or dihydroergotamine developed ergotism when they were also given doxycycline or tetracycline. Liver impairment may have been a contributory factor.

> The general importance of this interaction is uncertain, but it seems likely to be small. However, note that one of the manufacturers of ergotamine actually recommends that the concurrent use of tetracycline should be avoided. Impaired liver function may possibly be a contributory factor in this interaction and it may be prudent to monitor patients with this risk factor more closely.

Ergot derivatives + Triptans ✖

The simultaneous use of ergot derivatives is contraindicated with all triptans because of the theoretical risk of additive vasoconstriction, although there is some evidence of safe use.

> In the UK the manufacturers of sumatriptan say that ergotamine should not be given less than 6 hours after taking sumatriptan, and recommend that sumatriptan should not be taken less than 24 hours after taking ergotamine. Similar recommendations are made by the manufacturers of almotriptan, rizatriptan, and zolmitriptan, whereas the manufacturers of eletriptan and frovatriptan recommend that ergot derivatives are not given for a minimum of 24 hours (not just 6 hours) after these triptans. In general, in the US, it is recommended that triptans and ergotamine or ergot-type medication should not be taken within 24 hours of each other.

Ertapenem

Ertapenem + Valproate ⚠

Ertapenem appears to dramatically and rapidly reduce valproate levels resulting in increased seizure frequency.

> It would be prudent to monitor valproate levels in any patient given carbapenems. The valproate dosage may need to be increased. Consider using another antibacterial, or an alternative to valproate. Limited evidence suggests that carbamazepine and phenytoin do not interact. Note that ertapenem should be used with caution in patients with a history of seizures.

Ethosuximide

Ethosuximide + Isoniazid ⚠️

A single report describes a patient who developed psychotic behaviour and signs of ethosuximide toxicity when concurrently treated with isoniazid.

The clinical importance of this interaction is unknown, but bear it in mind in case of an unexpected response to treatment. Indicators of ethosuximide toxicity include nausea, vomiting, anorexia and insomnia.

Ethosuximide + Phenobarbital ❓

Primidone lowers serum ethosuximide levels and possibly shortens its half-life. Similarly, phenobarbital has been reported both to reduce and not affect the half-life of ethosuximide. Phenobarbital levels (from primidone) do not appear to be affected by ethosuximide.

The clinical significance of these effects is unclear.

Ethosuximide + Phenytoin ❓

Three cases have occurred in which ethosuximide appeared to have been responsible for increasing phenytoin levels, leading to the development of phenytoin toxicity in 2 patients. Phenytoin may reduce the half-life of ethosuximide (by 50% in one study). Fosphenytoin, a prodrug of phenytoin, may interact similarly.

Warn the patient to monitor for indicators of phenytoin toxicity (blurred vision, nystagmus, ataxia or drowsiness). Take phenytoin levels as necessary, and monitor the effectiveness of ethosuximide treatment.

Ethosuximide + Valproate ⚠️

Sodium valproate has increased the serum levels of ethosuximide by about 50%. Sedation occurred and ethosuximide dose reductions were necessary. However, other studies have described no changes or even reduced ethosuximide levels when valproate was also given. Ethosuximide may also lower valproate serum levels.

Monitor the effects of concurrent use, adjusting the ethosuximide dose and increasing the valproate dose accordingly. Valproate levels may be helpful.

Etoposide

Etoposide + Herbal medicines or Dietary supplements ⚠

In vitro studies suggest that hypericin, a component of St John's wort (*Hypericum perforatum*) may antagonise the antineoplastic effects of etoposide. It may also stimulate the hepatic metabolism of etoposide by CYP3A4.

> Information is very limited but what is known suggests that it would be prudent to avoid St John's wort in patients taking etoposide.

E

Etoposide + Phenobarbital ⚠

Etoposide clearance appears to be increased by almost 80% by phenobarbital, and this may result in reduced efficacy. Note that primidone is metabolised to phenobarbital and therefore may interact similarly.

> Monitor the outcome of concurrent use and be alert for the possible need to give larger doses of etoposide.

Etoposide + Phenytoin ⚠

Etoposide clearance appears to be increased by almost 80% by phenytoin, and this may result in reduced efficacy. Fosphenytoin, a prodrug of phenytoin, may interact similarly.

> Monitor the outcome of concurrent use and be alert for the possible need to give larger doses of etoposide.

Etoposide + Warfarin and other oral anticoagulants ❓

Etoposide, as part of several different antineoplastic regimens, has been seen to increase the INR of patients taking warfarin. It is possible that all coumarins will interact similarly.

> Monitor the effect of concurrent use on the anticoagulant response to warfarin and adjust the dose as necessary.

Exemestane

Exemestane + HRT ⊗

HRT would be expected to oppose the effects of exemestane, so concurrent use is contraindicated.

Some information suggests that there need not be a complete restriction on their concurrent use, but this needs confirmation. Concurrent use should therefore be avoided.

Exemestane + Rifampicin (Rifampin) ⚠

Rifampicin reduces the AUC and maximum serum levels of exemestane by 54% and 41%, respectively.

It would seem prudent to monitor concurrent use for reduced exemestane efficacy.

Ezetimibe

Ezetimibe + Fibrates ⊗

Fenofibrate and gemfibrozil may modestly increase ezetimibe levels, although this is not thought to be clinically relevant. However, both fibrates and ezetimibe increase the secretion of cholesterol into the bile, which increases the risk of gallstone formation.

The manufacturers suggest that concurrent use should be avoided.

Ezetimibe + Rifampicin (Rifampin) ⚠

Multiple doses of rifampicin decrease ezetimibe levels and almost totally abolish its effects.

It would be prudent to monitor concurrent use to ensure that ezetimibe is effective.

Ezetimibe + Statins ⚠

No pharmacokinetic interaction appears to occur between ezetimibe and the statins, but the incidence of rhabdomyolysis may be increased on concurrent use. Note that the use of ezetimibe and a statin results in additive lipid-lowering effects, and combination preparations are available.

Patients taking statins should be counselled regarding myopathy (e.g. report any unexplained muscle pain, tenderness or weakness). This should be reinforced if they are also given ezetimibe.

Ezetimibe + Warfarin and other oral anticoagulants ⚠

No clinically significant interaction occurred between ezetimibe and warfarin in one study. However, raised INRs have been seen in patients taking warfarin after they were also given ezetimibe.

> The manufacturers advise monitoring the prothrombin time in any patients taking an oral anticoagulant and adjusting the dose as necessary.

E

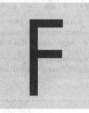

Famciclovir

Famciclovir + Probenecid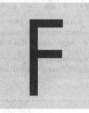

The renal excretion of drugs similar to famciclovir is reduced by probenecid. Therefore the manufacturers of famciclovir suggest that probenecid may increase levels of penciclovir, the active metabolite of famciclovir, possibly resulting in increased adverse effects.

As yet there seems to be no experimental or clinical evidence to show that this interaction occurs or that it is likely to be clinically important. Consider also aciclovir, page 11.

Felbamate

Felbamate + Gabapentin

There is some evidence to suggest that the half-life of felbamate may be prolonged by gabapentin.

The clinical importance of this interaction is unknown, but be alert for the need to reduce the felbamate dosage.

Felbamate + Phenobarbital

Felbamate normally causes a moderate increase of about 25 to 30% in serum phenobarbital levels (derived from phenobarbital or primidone). Phenobarbital toxicity has occurred in one patient when felbamate was added.

Warn the patient to monitor for indicators of phenobarbital toxicity (drowsiness, ataxia or dysarthria), and take levels if necessary.

Felbamate + **Phenytoin** ⚠

Felbamate causes a moderate increase in serum phenytoin levels. Phenytoin dosage reductions of 10 to 40% have been required to manage this interaction. Felbamate serum levels are reduced but the importance of this is uncertain.

Warn the patient to monitor for indicators of phenytoin toxicity (blurred vision, nystagmus, ataxia or drowsiness). Take phenytoin levels and adjust the dose as necessary.

Felbamate + **Valproate** ⚠

Felbamate can raise sodium valproate serum levels (by up to about 50% with a 2.4 g dose of felbamate), which may cause toxicity. Valproate may slightly decrease the clearance of felbamate.

Monitor the outcome of concurrent use. Monitor valproate levels if toxicity is suspected. Be aware that the felbamate dose may need to be decreased.

F · Fibrates

Fibrates + **Probenecid** ⚠

Plasma clofibrate levels can be approximately doubled by probenecid.

The outcome of this interaction does not appear to have been assessed, but it would seem prudent to be alert for an increase in clofibrate adverse effects.

Fibrates + **Rifampicin (Rifampin)** ⚠

Preliminary evidence shows that rifampicin can reduce the plasma levels of the active metabolite of clofibrate by about one-third.

Information is limited but it may be prudent to monitor concurrent use to ensure clofibrate is effective.

Fibrates + **Statins** ⚠

Gemfibrozil markedly increases levels of atorvastatin, pravastatin, rosuvastatin and simvastatin. Because of the increased risks of muscle toxicity (e.g. myopathy or rhabdomyolysis) it is generally accepted that use of a statin in conjunction with a fibrate should only be undertaken if the benefits outweigh the risks. The incidence of statin/fibrate interactions leading to myopathy may be up to 5%.

Creatine kinase levels should be measured before initiation. Patients taking statins should be counselled regarding myopathy (e.g. report any unexplained muscle pain, tenderness or weakness). This should be reinforced if they are also given a fibrate. The manufacturers of rosuvastatin contraindicate doses of 40 mg and above with fibrates, and the manufacturers of simvastatin contraindicate doses of above 10 mg daily with gemfibrozil. The manufacturers of simvastatin also suggest that doses of greater than 10 mg daily should only be used with other fibrates (except fenofibrate) if the benefits outweigh the risks of treatment.

Fibrates + Warfarin and other oral anticoagulants ⚠

The fibrates increase the effects of oral anticoagulants. This has been reported with: bezafibrate and acenocoumarol, phenprocoumon or warfarin; ciprofibrate and warfarin; clofibrate and phenindione or warfarin; fenofibrate and acenocoumarol or warfarin, and with gemfibrozil and warfarin. There have been fatalities as a result of this interaction.

With clofibrate, dosage reductions of one-third to one-half may be needed to avoid the risk of bleeding. Monitor the INR and adjust the dose accordingly. Less is known about fenofibrate and even less about bezafibrate, ciprofibrate and gemfibrozil but it would be prudent to follow the same precautions suggested for clofibrate if any of them is used with any oral anticoagulant.

Flecainide

F

Flecainide + H₂-receptor antagonists ❓

Cimetidine can increase flecainide plasma levels by about 30%.

The clinical importance of this interaction does not appear to have been assessed, but be alert for the need to reduce the flecainide dosage if cimetidine is added.

Flecainide + NSAIDs ❓

Because valdecoxib (the metabolite of parecoxib) increases *dextromethorphan* levels by about 3-fold the manufacturers predict that the levels of flecainide (which is similarly metabolised) will also be raised by valdecoxib.

The general importance of this interaction is unclear, but be aware that the effects of flecainide may be increased.

Flecainide + SSRIs ❓

Studies in patients and *in vitro* investigations have shown that fluoxetine and its metabolite, norfluoxetine, inhibits CYP2D6, the enzyme that metabolises flecainide. Paroxetine is expected to have similar effects and the manufacturers of escitalopram predict that it may also interact in this way.

There appear to be no reported interactions, but, given that fluoxetine interacts this way with other CYP2D6 substrates (such as propafenone, page 374), it would seem prudent to be alert for increased and prolonged effects if any of these SSRIs is given with flecainide.

Flecainide + Terbinafine ⚠

In vitro studies suggest that terbinafine is an inhibitor of CYP2D6. It may therefore be expected to increase the plasma levels of other drugs that are substrates of this enzyme, such as flecainide.

Until more is known it would seem wise to be aware of the possibility of an increase in adverse effects if flecainide is given with terbinafine and consider a dose reduction if necessary.

Flutamide

Flutamide + Warfarin and other oral anticoagulants ⚠

Case reports suggest that in some patients flutamide may increase the effects of warfarin. The interaction developed over 2 months in some cases but developed within 4 days in another.

It may be prudent to initially check the INR of any patient taking an oral anticoagulant within the first week of concurrent use.

Folates

Folates + Methotrexate ⚠

Folic acid or folinic acid are sometimes added if low-dose methotrexate is given for rheumatoid arthritis or psoriasis to reduce adverse effects. Folinic acid is frequently used to minimise toxicity with high-dose methotrexate in cancer therapy.

Patients taking methotrexate should avoid the inadvertent use of folates in multivitamin preparations.

Folates + Phenobarbital ⚠

If folic acid supplements are given to treat folate deficiency, which can be caused by the use of phenobarbital or primidone, the serum antiepileptic levels may fall, leading to decreased seizure control in some patients.

Monitor phenobarbital levels and adjust the dose accordingly.

Folates + Phenytoin ⚠

If folic acid supplements are given to treat folate deficiency, which can be caused by the use of phenytoin, the serum phenytoin levels may fall, leading to decreased seizure control in some patients. Reductions in serum phenytoin levels of 16 to 50% have been described with folic acid doses between 5 mg and 15 mg; doses as low as folic acid 1 mg may interact.

Monitor phenytoin levels and adjust the dose accordingly. Fosphenytoin is a prodrug of phenytoin. Although it does not appear to have been studied, it may interact similarly.

Folates + Sulfasalazine ❓

Sulfasalazine can reduce the absorption of folic acid by about 30%.

The clinical significance of this interaction is unclear. Note that sulfasalazine is itself associated with blood dyscrasias due to folate deficiency, and this may be treated with folic acid or folinic acid.

Food

Food + Furazolidone ✖

After 5 to 10 days of use furazolidone has MAO-inhibitory activity about equivalent to that of the antidepressant MAOIs. It may therefore be expected to interact with tyramine-rich foods.

It would seem prudent to warn patients given furazolidone not to take any of the foods or drinks that are prohibited with non-selective MAOIs. See MAOIs, page 256.

Food + Griseofulvin ❓

The absorption of griseofulvin is increased by food, especially high-fat meals.

Griseofulvin should be taken with or after food to ensure adequate absorption.

Food + Isoniazid ⚠

The absorption of isoniazid is reduced by food. Patients taking isoniazid who eat some foods, such as mature cheese and particularly fish from the scombroid family (e.g. tuna, mackerel, salmon) that are not fresh, may experience an exaggerated histamine poisoning reaction e.g. chills, diarrhoea, flushing and itching of the skin, headache, tachycardia, vomiting, wheeze.

For maximal absorption isoniazid should be taken without food, hence the manufacturer's guidance to take it at least 30 minutes before or 2 hours after food. There is no need to introduce general dietary restrictions, but if any of these reactions is experienced, examine the patient's diet and advise the avoidance of any probable offending foodstuffs.

Food + Isotretinoin ❓

The absorption of isotretinoin is approximately doubled by food.

> Isotretinoin should be taken with food to maximise absorption.

Food + Levodopa ❓

The fluctuations in response to levodopa experienced by some patients may be due to the timing of their meals and the type of diet, particularly the protein content. The effects of levodopa can be reduced by the amino acid methionine, and the blood levels of levodopa can be reduced by the amino acid tryptophan.

> If problems occur, a change in the pattern of drug and food administration on a trial-and-error basis may be helpful. Multiple small doses of levodopa and spreading out the intake of proteins may also diminish the effects of these interactions. Diets that conform to the recommended daily allowance of protein (said to be 800 mg/kg in one report) are reported to reduce this adverse drug-food interaction.

Food + Linezolid ⚠

Linezolid has weak MAOI effects and therefore modestly increases the blood pressure response to oral tyramine.

> Patients taking linezolid should not consume excessive amounts of tyramine-rich foods and drinks (100 mg of tyramine per meal is recommended by the manufacturers).

Food + Macrolides ⚠

Food reduces the absorption of azithromycin from capsules but does not affect the AUC of azithromycin from tablets or suspension.

> Azithromycin capsules should be taken at least one hour before or 2 hours after a meal. Azithromycin suspension and tablets may be taken without regard to food.

Food + MAOIs ❌

A potentially life-threatening hypertensive crisis can develop in patients taking non-selective MAOIs who eat tyramine-rich food (e.g. cheeses, salami, yeast extracts, pickled herrings) and drinks (e.g. some beers and wines) or young broad bean pods, which contain dopa. Fatalities have occurred.

> As little as 20 mg of tyramine can raise the blood pressure by 30 mmHg in patients taking tranylcypromine. However, because tyramine levels vary so much it is impossible to guess the amount of tyramine present in any food or drink. Old, over-ripe strong smelling cheeses with a salty, biting taste, or those with characteristic holes due to fermentation should be avoided, as they generally contain high levels of tyramine. Fresh cheeses made from pasteurised milk tend to have lower levels of tyramine. The tyramine-content can even differ significantly within a single cheese between the centre, with lowest levels of tyramine, and the

rind, containing the most. There is no guarantee that patients who have uneventfully eaten these hazardous foodstuffs on many occasions may not eventually experience a full-scale hypertensive crisis, if all the possible variables conspire together. Therefore tyramine-rich foods should be avoided. Fermented or aged foods, such as cheeses, sausages and beer, or smoked meats tend to be the most common tyramine-rich foods.

Food + Moclobemide ⚠

Tyramine 150 mg has been found to cause a 30 mmHg rise in systolic blood pressure when given with moclobemide. No reports of the potentially life-threatening hypertensive reactions seen with non-selective MAOIs appear to have been published for moclobemide.

Note that 150 mg of tyramine is equivalent to that found in about 200 g of Stilton cheese or 300 g of Gorgonzola cheese, which are really excessive amounts of cheese to be eaten in a few minutes. Most patients therefore do not need to follow the special dietary restrictions required with the non-selective MAOIs, but, to be on the safe side, the manufacturers of moclobemide advise all patients to avoid large amounts of tyramine-rich foods, because a few individuals may be particularly sensitive to its effects.

Food + NRTIs ⚠

Food decreases the absorption of didanosine by up to 50%. Food enhances the bioavailability of tenofovir.

Buffered didanosine should be taken at least 30 minutes before food. Enteric coated didanosine should be taken 2 hours before or after food. Advise patients to take tenofovir with meals.

Food + NSAIDs ✓

Food reduces the rate of absorption but has no or little effect on the extent of absorption of most NSAIDs. The extent of ketoprofen absorption is reduced by food.

The small changes seen will have no clinical relevance if these drugs are being used regularly to treat chronic pain and inflammation. However, if they are being used for the treatment of acute pain, administration on an empty stomach would be preferable in terms of onset of effect. However, it is usually recommended that NSAIDs (including ketoprofen) are given with or after food, in an attempt to minimise their gastrointestinal adverse effects.

Food + Penicillamine ⚠

Food can reduce the absorption of penicillamine by about 50%.

If maximal effects are required penicillamine should be taken at least 30 minutes before food.

Food + **Penicillins** ✅

Food can reduce the absorption of ampicillin by about 30%, and the peak levels and AUC of phenoxymethylpenicillin by about 50%. Limited evidence suggests that food has no significant effect on the bioavailability of flucloxacillin.

> Ampicillin and phenoxymethylpenicillin should be taken one hour before food or on an empty stomach. Despite the apparent lack of interaction with flucloxacillin, it is recommended that it should be taken one hour before food or on an empty stomach to optimise absorption.

Food + **Pirenzepine** ✅

Food reduces the bioavailability of pirenzepine by about 30%, but this is probably of little clinical importance.

> No action needed.

Food + **Protease inhibitors** ❓

Food increases the bioavailability of atazanavir, darunavir, lopinavir, nelfinavir, saquinavir, and tipranavir, but decreases that of indinavir. Food only minimally affects the bioavailability of amprenavir, fosamprenavir and ritonavir.

> Indinavir should be given one hour before or 2 hours after meals, or with light meals only. Atazanavir, darunavir, lopinavir, nelfinavir, and tipranavir should be taken with food to enhance bioavailability. Saquinavir (soft and hard capsules) should be taken up to 2 hours after a meal. The US manufacturers of amprenavir say that it should not be given with high-fat meals, but otherwise it may be given with or without food.

Food + **Proton pump inhibitors** ⚠

Food reduces the bioavailability of lansoprazole and esomeprazole by up to 50%.

> It is recommended that lansoprazole should not be given with food. Giving lansoprazole one hour before food is probably enough to avoid the interaction. Esomeprazole capsules and suspension should be taken one hour before meals, but food does not appear to alter the effects of esomeprazole tablets on gastric acidity.

Food + **Quinolones** ⚠

Dairy products reduce the bioavailability of ciprofloxacin (AUC reduced by about 30%) and norfloxacin (peak plasma levels reduced by about 50%), and to a minor extent, gatifloxacin (AUC reduced by 15%).

> The effect of these changes on the control of infection is uncertain but it would seem prudent to advise patients not to take these dairy products within one to 2 hours of either ciprofloxacin or norfloxacin. The slight reduction in gatifloxacin levels is probably not clinically relevant. Enoxacin, lomefloxacin, ofloxacin and probably fleroxacin do not appear to interact significantly. They therefore may

F

provide a useful alternative to the interacting quinolones. Consider also enteral feeds, page 243.

Food + Rifampicin (Rifampin) ⚠

Food delays and reduces the absorption of rifampicin.

Rifampicin should be taken on an empty stomach, 30 minutes before a meal, or 2 hours after a meal to ensure rapid and complete absorption.

Food + Strontium ❓

The manufacturer notes that food, milk and dairy products reduce the bioavailability of strontium by about 60 to 70%, when compared with administration 3 hours after a meal.

Strontium should not be taken within 2 hours of eating. The manufacturer recommends that it should be taken at bedtime, at least 2 hours after eating.

Food + Tetracyclines ⚠

The absorption of most tetracyclines can be markedly reduced (by up to 65%) by milk or other dairy products. Doxycycline and minocycline are less affected by dairy products (25 to 30% reduction).

It is usual to recommend that tetracyclines are taken one hour before food or 2 hours after food to avoid an interaction with all forms of dietary calcium.

Food + Warfarin and other oral anticoagulants

Cranberry juice ❌

In some patients the anticoagulant effects of warfarin were increased after they drank cranberry juice. One patient had a very marked increase and died from a haemorrhage, while a further patient had a reduction in his INR. However, subsequent controlled studies suggest that no interaction occurs.

The current recommendation of the CSM/MHRA in the UK is that patients taking warfarin should limit or avoid drinking cranberry juice. They also advise similar precautions with other cranberry products (such as capsules or concentrates).

Foods, general ❓

A number of foodstuffs have been implicated in interactions with warfarin. Some of these were not thought to be related to their vitamin K content. These include:

● antagonism of the effects of warfarin by ice cream, avocado, soybean protein, and soybean oil and other intravenous lipids
● an increase in prothrombin time with the use of aspartame or following the consumption of mango fruit

These reactions seem unlikely to be of general importance, although bear them in mind in case of an unexpected response to oral anticoagulants.

Foods containing vitamin K ❓

The effects of warfarin can be reduced or abolished by vitamin K, including that found in health foods, food supplements, enteral feeds or exceptionally large amounts of some green vegetables or green tea.

Patients should be counselled on the effects of dietary supplements or dramatic dietary alterations when started on warfarin.

Natto ❌

Natto, a Japanese food made from fermented soya bean, can reduce the effects of warfarin.

Patients should be advised to avoid natto until more is known about this interaction.

F

Foscarnet

Foscarnet + NRTIs ❌

The manufacturers say that the concurrent use of lamivudine and foscarnet is not recommended until further information becomes available.

Avoid concurrent use or seek specialist advice.

Furazolidone

Furazolidone + Nasal decongestants ❌

After 5 to 10 days of use, furazolidone has MAO-inhibitory activity about equivalent to that of the non-selective MAOIs. Concurrent use with drugs such as phenylpropanolamine or ephedrine, may be expected to result in a potentially serious rise in blood pressure.

Although reports of hypertensive crises with furazolidone appear lacking it would still seem prudent to warn patients to avoid any of the drugs, foods or drinks that are prohibited with MAOIs.

Fusidic acid

Fusidic acid + **Protease inhibitors** ⚠

A patient taking fusidic acid with saquinavir and ritonavir developed elevated fusidic acid levels with toxicity, and elevated saquinavir and ritonavir levels (roughly 4-fold increases).

The clinical significance of this case is unclear. It has been suggested that concurrent use should be avoided.

Fusidic acid + **Statins** ❓

Isolated cases of rhabdomyolysis have been described in patients given atorvastatin or simvastatin with fusidic acid. Fusidic acid was also a possible contributing factor in another case.

The general significance of this interaction is unclear. Patients given statins should be counselled regarding myopathy (e.g. report any unexplained muscle pain, tenderness or weakness). Reinforce this if fusidic acid is given.

F

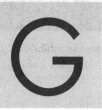

Galantamine

Galantamine + Quinidine ⚠

Paroxetine increases the risk of galantamine adverse effects (in particular nausea and vomiting) probably by inhibiting the metabolism of galantamine by CYP2D6. The manufacturers therefore predict that other CYP2D6 inhibitors (such as quinidine) will interact similarly.

> If the adverse effects of galantamine develop or worsen, reduce its dose.

Galantamine + SSRIs ⚠

Paroxetine increases the risk of galantamine adverse effects (in particular nausea and vomiting) probably by inhibiting the metabolism of galantamine by CYP2D6. The manufacturers therefore predict that other CYP2D6 inhibitors (such as fluoxetine) will interact similarly. They also name fluvoxamine but note that fluvoxamine is usually considered to be a *weak* inhibitor of this isoenzyme.

> If the adverse effects of galantamine develop or worsen, reduce its dose.

Ganciclovir

Valganciclovir is a prodrug of ganciclovir and therefore has the potential to interact similarly.

Ganciclovir + Imipenem ✖

The manufacturer notes that generalised seizures have been reported in patients who received ganciclovir with imipenem-cilastatin. Note that both ganciclovir and imipenem alone may cause seizures. Valganciclovir is a prodrug of ganciclovir and would therefore be expected to interact similarly.

The manufacturer recommends that ganciclovir and its prodrug valganciclovir should not be used concurrently with imipenem unless the benefits outweigh the risks.

Ganciclovir + Mycophenolate ❓

No clinically significant pharmacokinetic interaction appears to occur between ganciclovir and mycophenolate. However, the manufacturers say that in renal impairment there may be competition for tubular secretion and increased concentrations of both drugs may occur. There are reports of neutropenia in patients taking mycophenolate with ganciclovir.

No action is needed, but increased monitoring may be prudent in patients with reduced renal function. Both mycophenolate mofetil and ganciclovir and its prodrug, valganciclovir, have the potential to cause neutropenia and leucopenia, therefore patients should be closely monitored for additive toxicity.

Ganciclovir + NRTIs

Didanosine ⚠

In several studies ganciclovir has been found to raise the maximum serum levels and AUC of didanosine by roughly 70%, even when the drugs are given 2 hours apart. Other studies have suggested that the efficacy of ganciclovir may be reduced by didanosine. Valganciclovir is a prodrug of ganciclovir and would therefore be expected to interact similarly.

The manufacturers say that the implications of these pharmacokinetic changes is unclear. Until more is known it would seem prudent to monitor concurrent use for didanosine toxicity. Also monitor for ganciclovir efficacy.

Lamivudine ✖

The manufacturers say that the concurrent use of lamivudine and intravenous ganciclovir (and therefore probably valganciclovir) is not recommended until further information becomes available.

Avoid concurrent use or seek specialist advice.

Tenofovir ⚠

The manufacturers say that tenofovir (which may cause renal impairment) has not been evaluated with nephrotoxic drugs such as ganciclovir (and therefore probably valganciclovir).

The manufacturers advise that if concurrent use is essential renal function should be monitored at least weekly.

Zidovudine ⚠

Anaemia, neutropenia, leucopenia and gastrointestinal disturbances were seen when zidovudine and ganciclovir were used concurrently. The dose of zidovudine had to be reduced to 300 mg daily in many patients. Ganciclovir appears to moderately increase

G

the levels of zidovudine. Valganciclovir is a prodrug of ganciclovir and would therefore be expected to interact similarly.

The UK manufacturer of ganciclovir suggests that zidovudine should not be given during ganciclovir induction treatment, and patients should be closely monitored for neutropenia when maintenance ganciclovir is used with zidovudine.

Ganciclovir + Probenecid ⚠️

Probenecid reduces the renal excretion of ganciclovir and increases its AUC by about 50%.

The clinical importance of this interaction is uncertain. Be alert for increased ganciclovir effects and toxicity if probenecid is used concurrently with ganciclovir or its prodrug, valganciclovir. Ganciclovir eye drops are unlikely to interact.

Gestrinone

G

Gestrinone + Phenobarbital ❓

The manufacturers warn that phenobarbital (and therefore probably primidone) may increase the metabolism of gestrinone and thereby reduce its effects.

The clinical significance of this warning is unclear. There appear to be no reports of an interaction in practice.

Gestrinone + Phenytoin ❓

The manufacturers warn that phenytoin (and therefore probably fosphenytoin) may increase the metabolism of gestrinone and thereby reduce its effects.

The clinical significance of this warning is unclear. There appear to be no reports of an interaction in practice.

Gestrinone + Rifampicin (Rifampin) ❓

The manufacturers warn that rifampicin may increase the metabolism of gestrinone and thereby reduce its effects.

The clinical significance of this warning is unclear. There appear to be no reports of an interaction in practice.

Glucagon

Glucagon + Warfarin and other oral anticoagulants ⚠

The anticoagulant effects of warfarin are rapidly and markedly increased by glucagon in large doses (62 to 362 mg over 3 to 8 days), and bleeding can occur. This interaction did not occur in patients given, in total, less than 30 mg of glucagon over 1 to 2 days.

It has been suggested that if glucagon 25 mg per day or more is given for two or more days, the dosage of warfarin should be reduced in anticipation of the interaction, and prothrombin times closely monitored. Information about other anticoagulants is lacking, but it would be prudent to assume that all coumarins will interact similarly.

Gold

Gold + Leflunomide ✗

The manufacturers say that the concurrent use of leflunomide and gold has not yet been studied but it would be expected to increase the risk of serious adverse reactions (haematological toxicity or hepatotoxicity).

The manufacturers advise avoiding concurrent use. As the active metabolite of leflunomide has a long half-life of 1 to 4 weeks a washout with colestyramine or activated charcoal should be given if patients are to be switched to other DMARDs.

Gold + Penicillamine ✗

Gold appears to increase the risk of penicillamine toxicity.

Avoid concurrent use. Increased penicillamine monitoring should be considered in those with previous adverse effects to gold, as these patients are likely to experience increased adverse effects to penicillamine.

Grapefruit juice

In general, grapefruit juice inhibits intestinal CYP3A4, and only slightly affects hepatic CYP3A4. This is demonstrated by the fact that intravenous preparations of drugs that are metabolised by CYP3A4 are not much affected, whereas oral preparations of the same drugs are, and their levels are increased by grapefruit juice. Some drugs that are not metabolised by CYP3A4 show decreased levels with grapefruit juice. This is probably because grapefruit juice is an inhibitor of some drug transporters, such as

P-glycoprotein. The active constituent of grapefruit juice is uncertain. However, grapefruit contains naringin, which degrades during processing to naringenin, a substance known to inhibit CYP3A4. Because of this, it has been assumed that whole grapefruit will not interact, but that processed grapefruit juice will. However, subsequently some reports have implicated the whole fruit. Other possible active constituents in the whole fruit include bergamottin and dihydroxybergamottin.

Grapefruit juice + **Phosphodiesterase type-5 inhibitors** ✗

Grapefruit juice can affect the pharmacokinetics of sildenafil (AUC increased by 23%), probably by inhibiting the metabolism on sildenafil by CYP3A4. Tadalafil and vardenafil are predicted to interact similarly.

> It has been suggested that although the pharmacokinetic changes are unlikely to be clinically significant, the combination is best avoided because concurrent use results in an increased variability in sildenafil pharmacokinetics. However, this seems over-cautious, as reduced doses of sildenafil can be given with more potent CYP3A4 inhibitors. The manufacturers of tadalafil and vardenafil advise caution and avoidance, respectively, in those who drink grapefruit juice.

Grapefruit juice + **Sirolimus** ✗

G

The manufacturers of sirolimus predict that grapefruit juice may raise its serum levels, probably because *ketoconazole* has been shown to do so (both ketoconazole and grapefruit juice can inhibit CYP3A4 by which sirolimus is metabolised).

> The extent of any change in sirolimus levels is uncertain. The manufacturers suggest that concurrent use should be avoided.

Grapefruit juice + **Statins** ✗

Large amounts of grapefruit juice markedly increase the plasma levels of lovastatin (up to 12-fold) and simvastatin (up to 9-fold).

> Large increases in the serum levels of lovastatin and simvastatin are potentially hazardous because elevated statin levels carry the risk of toxicity (muscle damage and the possible development of rhabdomyolysis). As even small quantities of grapefruit juice can significantly affect simvastatin levels the manufacturer says that concurrent use should be avoided. No clinically significant interaction appears to occur with atorvastatin and pravastatin.

Grapefruit juice + **Tacrolimus** ✗

Grapefruit juice can markedly increase the serum levels of tacrolimus (by up to 400% in one study).

> Tacrolimus levels and effects (e.g. on renal function) should be monitored as a matter of routine, but it is advisable to increase monitoring if grapefruit juice is started or stopped, or avoid the combination.

Griseofulvin

Griseofulvin + Phenobarbital ⚠

The antifungal effects of griseofulvin can be reduced (serum levels reduced by about one-third) or even abolished by the concurrent use of phenobarbital. Note that primidone is metabolised to phenobarbital and may therefore interact similarly.

Concurrent use should be well monitored to confirm that griseofulvin is effective. If appropriate, a non-interacting antiepileptic such as sodium valproate may be considered.

Griseofulvin + Warfarin and other oral anticoagulants ❓

The anticoagulant effects of warfarin can be reduced by griseofulvin in some patients. In one patient a 41% increase in the dose of warfarin was needed.

Monitor the anticoagulant effect if griseofulvin is added or withdrawn in patients taking warfarin. Note that in one patient the interaction took 12 weeks to develop.

Guanethidine

Guanethidine + Inotropes and Vasopressors ❌

The pressor effects of noradrenaline (norepinephrine), metaraminol and other related drugs can be increased in the presence of guanethidine.

The pressor effects of drugs such as noradrenaline (norepinephrine) can be grossly exaggerated and so caution is warranted if concurrent use is considered essential. It would seem prudent to stop the guanethidine.

Guanethidine + Methylphenidate ❌

The antihypertensive effects of guanethidine can be reduced or abolished by methylphenidate.

The concurrent use of guanethidine and methylphenidate should be avoided.

Guanethidine + Nasal decongestants ❌

The antihypertensive effects of guanethidine can be reduced or abolished by ephedrine. Other related drugs, such as pseudoephedrine, that are used as cough and cold remedies, may also interact in this way.

Concurrent use should be avoided.

G

Guanethidine + Tricyclics ⚠

The antihypertensive effects of guanethidine are reduced or abolished by amitriptyline, desipramine, imipramine, nortriptyline and protriptyline. Doxepin in doses of 300 mg or more daily interacts similarly, but in smaller doses appears not to do so, although one case is reported with doxepin 100 mg daily.

Not every combination of guanethidine and a tricyclic antidepressant has been studied but all are expected to interact similarly. Concurrent use should be avoided unless the effects are very closely monitored and the interaction balanced by raising the dosage of the antihypertensive.

G

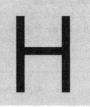

H₂-receptor antagonists

Cimetidine is a non-specific enzyme inhibitor and therefore interacts with a number of cytochrome P450 substrates. Other H$_2$-receptor antagonists do not have enzyme-inhibitory effects and therefore do not interact in this way. They may therefore provide useful alternatives to cimetidine. However, note that if an interaction occurs due to an alteration in gastric pH, all H$_2$-receptor antagonists would be expected to interact similarly.

H$_2$-receptor antagonists + Lidocaine ⚠

Cimetidine modestly reduces the clearance of intravenous lidocaine and raises its serum levels (by about 30% within 6 hours in one study). Lidocaine toxicity may occur if the dosage is not reduced. However, not all patients are affected.

> Monitor all patients closely for evidence of toxicity and, if possible, consider checking serum lidocaine levels regularly. A reduced infusion rate may be needed. Ranitidine does not interact and so would appear to be a suitable alternative to cimetidine.

H$_2$-receptor antagonists + Macrolides ⚠

Cimetidine can almost double the serum levels of erythromycin, although this has only been seen in a single dose study. A single case report describes reversible deafness attributed to this interaction.

> Evidence for this interaction is very limited. However, it may be prudent to be alert for erythromycin adverse effects (nausea, vomiting, diarrhoea, abdominal discomfort). Ranitidine is a possible non-interacting alternative, as are azithromycin and clarithromycin.

H$_2$-receptor antagonists + Mirtazapine ⚠

Cimetidine increases the AUC and peak plasma levels of mirtazapine by 54% and 22%, respectively. Mirtazapine does not appear to affect the pharmacokinetics of cimetidine.

> The manufacturers advise that the mirtazapine dosage may need to be reduced during concurrent use and increased if cimetidine is stopped. Monitor for an increase in adverse effects when starting cimetidine.

H₂-receptor antagonists + **Moclobemide** ⚠

Cimetidine increases the plasma levels of moclobemide by almost 40%.

> It has been recommended that if moclobemide is added to treatment with cimetidine it should be started at the lowest therapeutic dose, and titrated as required. If cimetidine is added to treatment with moclobemide, the dosage of the moclobemide should initially be reduced by 50% and later adjusted as necessary.

H₂-receptor antagonists + **NNRTIs** ❌

Antacids roughly halve the AUC of delavirdine, and H₂-receptor antagonists would be expected to interact similarly. This is because delavirdine is poorly soluble at pHs greater than 3.

> Long-term concurrent use is not recommended.

H₂-receptor antagonists + **NRTIs** ❓

The concurrent use of didanosine and ranitidine results in a minor increase in the serum levels of didanosine, and a minor decrease in the serum levels of ranitidine. Cimetidine raises serum zalcitabine levels. Cimetidine reduces the renal secretion of zidovudine, but does not have a significant effect on zidovudine serum levels.

> None of these changes are expected to be clinically significant.

H₂-receptor antagonists + **Opioids** ⚠

Cimetidine increases the plasma levels of alfentanil, and some preliminary observations suggest that cimetidine may increase the effects of fentanyl. Isolated reports describe adverse reactions in patients taking methadone, morphine, or mixed opium alkaloids when cimetidine was also given, or morphine when ranitidine was also given.

> The clinical relevance of these effects on alfentanil and fentanyl are unknown. The case reports are not expected to be of general significance.

H₂-receptor antagonists + **Pentoxifylline** ❓

Cimetidine moderately increases plasma pentoxifylline levels and adverse effects such as headache and nausea are more common.

> Be aware that adverse effects may be increased, but otherwise no action is needed.

H₂-receptor antagonists + **Phenytoin** ⚠

Phenytoin serum levels are raised by cimetidine (maximum rise of 280% over 3 weeks). Very rarely bone marrow depression develops on concurrent use. Limited evidence suggests that low (non-prescription) doses of cimetidine may not interact. Fosphenytoin, a prodrug of phenytoin, may interact similarly.

> Monitor phenytoin levels and adjust the dose accordingly. Alternatively other H₂-receptor antagonists (ranitidine, famotidine, nizatidine) do not usually interact, although isolated cases have been reported. Be alert for signs of phenytoin toxicity (e.g. blurred vision, nystagmus, ataxia or drowsiness) when these H₂-receptor antagonists are first given.

H₂-receptor antagonists + **Phosphodiesterase type-5 inhibitors** ⚠

Cimetidine increases the AUC of sildenafil by 56%.

> The UK manufacturer of sildenafil suggests that a low starting dose of 25 mg should be used if cimetidine is given, although the modest increase in levels seems unlikely to cause particular problems. The US manufacturers do not recommend any additional precautions.

H₂-receptor antagonists + **Procainamide** ⚠

Cimetidine can increase procainamide levels by more than 50%, which may lead to procainamide toxicity.

> Patients, particularly the elderly, should be closely monitored for signs of procainamide toxicity, and a dose reduction should be considered. Ranitidine and famotidine appear to interact only minimally or not at all.

H₂-receptor antagonists + **Propafenone** ✓

Cimetidine raised the mean peak and steady-state plasma propafenone levels by 24% and 22%, respectively, but these did not reach statistical significance.

> No action thought to be needed.

H₂-receptor antagonists + **Protease inhibitors** ⚠

Atazanavir and fosamprenavir levels are reduced by H₂-receptor antagonists such as ranitidine, probably by affecting gastric acidity. Amprenavir is predicted to be similarly affected. Not all H₂-receptor antagonists have been studied, but they would be expected to interact similarly. Saquinavir levels may be markedly increased by cimetidine.

> To avoid any interaction the manufacturers suggest that atazanavir/ritonavir should be given once daily with food, 2 hours before and at least 10 hours after the dose of the H₂-receptor antagonist. The UK manufacturer suggests that no fosamprenavir dose adjustment is needed with ranitidine or other H₂-receptor

H

antagonists; however, the US manufacturer says the combination should be used with caution because fosamprenavir may be less effective. Increased monitoring should be considered to check for saquinavir adverse effects if cimetidine is given.

H₂-receptor antagonists + **Quinidine** ⚠

Cimetidine can raise quinidine serum levels and toxicity may develop in some patients.

Be alert for changes in the response to quinidine if cimetidine is started or stopped. Ideally the quinidine serum levels should be monitored and the dosage reduced as necessary. Reductions of 25 to 35% have been suggested.

H₂-receptor antagonists + **Quinine** ⚠

The clearance of quinine is reduced by cimetidine, resulting in a 42% increase in the AUC of quinine.

The clinical importance of this is uncertain, but be particularly alert for any evidence of quinine adverse effects during concurrent use. Note that ranitidine appears not to interact.

H₂-receptor antagonists + **Sirolimus** ⚠

The manufacturers of sirolimus predict that its serum levels will be increased by cimetidine.

Sirolimus levels and/or effects (e.g. on renal function) should be monitored as a matter of routine, but it may be prudent to increase monitoring if cimetidine is started or stopped.

H₂-receptor antagonists + **SSRIs** ⚠

Citalopram, escitalopram, paroxetine and sertraline levels are moderately increased by cimetidine.

Initial dosage reductions are not needed, but be aware that some patients may have an increase in SSRI adverse effects (dry mouth, nausea, diarrhoea, dyspepsia, tremor, ejaculatory delay, sweating), in which case dose reductions may be appropriate. Although not proven, it is thought that ranitidine and famotidine are unlikely to interact.

H₂-receptor antagonists + **Tacrine** ⚠

Cimetidine increases the plasma levels of tacrine by up to about 50%.

An increase in the effects and possibly adverse effects of tacrine (nausea, vomiting, diarrhoea) seems possible. In one interaction study, a patient had to be withdrawn due to nausea and vomiting caused by this combination. Monitor concurrent use for adverse effects.

H₂-receptor antagonists + **Theophylline** ⚠

Cimetidine raises theophylline serum levels (by about one-third) and toxicity has been seen. The interaction is unlikely to be clinically relevant in most patients with low-dose (non-prescription) cimetidine.

Monitor theophylline levels if cimetidine is added or withdrawn. The peak effect appears to occur after 3 days. Alternatively, use ranitidine or famotidine, which appear not to interact.

H₂-receptor antagonists + **Tricyclics** ⚠

The concurrent use of cimetidine can raise the plasma levels of amitriptyline, desipramine, doxepin, imipramine and nortriptyline. Severe adverse effects have occurred in a few patients. Other tricyclic antidepressants are expected to interact similarly.

Patients taking tricyclics and cimetidine should be monitored for evidence of increased toxicity (dry mouth, urinary retention, blurred vision, constipation, tachycardia, postural hypotension). Reduce the tricyclic dose if necessary. Ranitidine does not appear to interact.

H₂-receptor antagonists + **Triptans** ⚠

Cimetidine raises the AUC of zolmitriptan by almost 50%.

The UK manufacturer recommends a zolmitriptan dose reduction to a maximum of 5 mg in 24 hours if patients are also taking cimetidine. The US manufacturer does not suggest a dose adjustment.

H

H₂-receptor antagonists + **Warfarin and other oral anticoagulants** ⚠

The anticoagulant effects of warfarin can be increased by cimetidine. Severe bleeding has occurred in a few patients but some show no interaction at all. Acenocoumarol and phenindione seem to interact similarly.

Monitor the INR if cimetidine is added or withdrawn. The interaction is rapid and may occur within days and even as early as after 24 hours. Famotidine, nizatidine and ranitidine usually appear to be non-interacting alternatives, although isolated cases of bleeding have been seen.

Heparin

Heparin + **Nitrates** ✓

Some studies claim that the effects of heparin are reduced by the concurrent infusion of nitrates, but others have failed to confirm this interaction.

Given that heparin is routinely monitored, it is likely that if any interaction occurs, it will be rapidly detected and compensated for.

Heparin + **NSAIDs**

Ketorolac ❌

The risk of bleeding seems to be particularly high if ketorolac is used with anticoagulants.

The CSM in the UK and the manufacturer of ketorolac says that it is contraindicated with anticoagulants, including low doses of heparin.

NSAIDs, general ⚠

An increased risk of bleeding occurs when NSAIDs (that have antiplatelet actions) are given with heparin or low molecular weight heparins. Anticoagulants can exacerbate gastrointestinal bleeding caused by NSAIDs.

Concurrent use is not uncommon, but prescribers should be aware that there is an increased risk of bleeding and monitor appropriately.

Heparin + **Ticlopidine** ⚠

Concurrent use of ticlopidine with heparin increases haemorrhagic risk.

If concurrent use is undertaken, there should be close clinical and laboratory monitoring.

H

Herbal medicines or Dietary supplements

There seem to be few clinical reports of interactions and so recommendations are difficult to make. An additional problem in interpreting these interactions, is that the interacting constituent of the herb is usually not known and is therefore not standardised. It could vary widely between different products, and batches of the same product. Bear this in mind.

Herbal medicines or Dietary supplements + HRT ❓

The hormones in HRT are similar to those used in hormonal contraceptives, and so may be affected by enzyme-inducing drugs, such as St John's wort (*Hypericum perforatum*), in the same way as contraceptives, page 202. Reduced effects are therefore possible.

Any interaction would be most likely to be noticed where HRT is prescribed for menopausal vasomotor symptoms, but might be difficult to detect where the indication is osteoporosis. Further study is needed to confirm the importance of this possible interaction.

Herbal medicines or Dietary supplements +
Imatinib ⚠

In one study the AUC and maximum plasma levels of imatinib were decreased by 30% and 15% by St John's wort (*Hypericum perforatum*).

Subtherapeutic levels of imatinib may occur. It is generally recommended that concurrent should be avoided.

Herbal medicines or Dietary supplements + Lithium
Herbal diuretic ⚠

A woman developed lithium toxicity after taking a herbal diuretic containing corn silk, *Equisetum hyemale*, juniper, ovate buchu, parsley and bearberry.

This interaction is similar to that seen with prescription diuretics, page 231. Concurrent use needs monitoring, and patients should be encouraged to seek advice before self-medicating.

St John's wort (Hypericum perforatum) ❓

A case report describes mania in a patient taking St John's wort and lithium.

The general importance of this interaction is unclear. Bear it in mind in case of an unexpected response to treatment.

Herbal medicines or Dietary supplements + MAOIs ❓

Two patients developed headache, insomnia, and in one case hallucinations, when they took phenelzine with ginseng.

The clinical significance of this interaction is unclear. Bear it in mind in case of an unexpected response to treatment.

Herbal medicines or Dietary supplements +
Metronidazole ✅

Silymarin (an active constituent of milk thistle) reduces metronidazole levels by a modest 30%.

The clinical significance of this interaction is unclear, but other interactions that result in a 30% reduction in metronidazole levels are not considered to be clinically significant.

H

Herbal medicines or Dietary supplements +
NNRTIs ✖

There is evidence to suggest that St John's wort (*Hypericum perforatum*) may decrease blood levels of nevirapine (clearance increased by 35%). Similar interactions are possible with delavirdine and efavirenz.

This supports the advice issued by the CSM in the UK, that St John's wort may decrease blood levels of the NNRTIs with possible loss of HIV suppression. Combined use should be avoided.

Herbal medicines or Dietary supplements + NSAIDs

Ginkgo biloba ⚠

Case reports describe fatal intracerebral bleeding in a patient taking *Ginkgo biloba* with ibuprofen, and prolonged bleeding and subdural haematomas in a patient taking *Ginkgo biloba* with rofecoxib.

The evidence from these reports is too slim to forbid patients taking aspirin or NSAIDs and *Ginkgo biloba* concurrently, but some do recommend caution. Medical professionals should be aware of the possibility of increased bleeding tendency with *Ginkgo biloba* and monitor patients appropriately.

Tamarindus indica ⚠

Tamarindus indica fruit extract caused a 2-fold increase in the AUC of ibuprofen.

The clinical relevance of this interaction is unknown, but large rises in the ibuprofen levels may result in toxicity.

H

Herbal medicines or Dietary supplements +
Opioids ✖

St John's wort (*Hypericum perforatum*) decreased methadone levels by up to 60% in one study, and withdrawal symptoms have been reported. Some herbal teas may contain opioids such as morphine.

Advise patients taking methadone to avoid St John's wort. Additive CNS depressant effects may occur if herbal teas containing opioids are taken with prescribed opioid preparations.

Herbal medicines or Dietary supplements +
Penicillins ⚠

Chewing khat reduces the absorption of ampicillin, and to a lesser extent amoxicillin, but the effects are minimal 2 hours after khat chewing stops.

Khat (the leaves and stem tips of *Catha edulis*) is chewed in some African and Arabian countries for its stimulatory properties. The authors of one of the studies concluded that both ampicillin and amoxicillin should be taken 2 hours after khat chewing to ensure that maximum absorption occurs.

Herbal medicines or Dietary supplements + Phenobarbital ❌

St John's wort (*Hypericum perforatum*) is predicted to reduce the blood levels of phenobarbital.

> The CSM in the UK advise that St John's wort should be stopped and that the phenobarbital dosage should be adjusted. However, note that this prediction also covered carbamazepine, which has subsequently been found not to interact, so a clinically significant interaction with phenobarbital now seems less likely.

Herbal medicines or Dietary supplements + Phenytoin

Ayurvedic medicines ❌

A case report, and an *animal* study, indicate that an antiepileptic Ayurvedic herbal preparation, SRC (*Shankhapushpi*), can markedly reduce serum phenytoin levels, leading to an increased seizure frequency if the phenytoin dosage is not raised. SRC is a syrup prepared from *Convolvulus pluricaulis* leaves, *Nardostachys jatamansi* rhizomes, *Onosma bracteatum* leaves and flowers, and the whole plant of *Centella asiatica*, *Nepeta hindostana* and *Nepeta elliptica*.

> *Shankhapushpi* (SRC) is given because it has some antiepileptic activity but there is little point in combining it with phenytoin if the outcome is a fall in serum phenytoin levels, accompanied by an increase in seizure frequency. For this reason concurrent use should be avoided. It would seem prudent to be similarly cautious with the use of fosphenytoin, a prodrug of phenytoin.

St John's wort (*Hypericum perforatum*) ❌

St John's wort is predicted to reduce the blood levels of phenytoin. Fosphenytoin, a prodrug of phenytoin, may interact similarly.

> The CSM in the UK advise that St John's wort should be stopped and that the phenytoin dosage should be adjusted. However, note that this prediction also covered carbamazepine, which has subsequently been found not to interact, so a clinically significant interaction with phenytoin now seems less likely.

H

Herbal medicines or Dietary supplements + Phosphodiesterase type-5 inhibitors ❓

St John's wort is predicted to reduce the levels of phosphodiesterase type-5 inhibitors, because other inducers of CYP3A4 have been shown to do so. For example, the AUC of sildenafil is reduced by about 70% by *bosentan* and the AUC of tadalafil is reduced by 88% by *rifampicin*. Vardenafil is also metabolised by CYP3A4, and therefore its levels may possibly be lowered by St John's wort.

> If these phosphodiesterase type-5 inhibitors are not effective in patients taking St John's wort, consider reviewing the need for concurrent use. If concurrent use is necessary, a dose increase in the phosphodiesterase type-5 inhibitor may be required.

Herbal medicines or Dietary supplements + **Protease inhibitors**

Garlic ✖

A garlic supplement reduced the plasma levels of saquinavir by 50%.

> All garlic supplements should probably be avoided if saquinavir is ever given as the sole protease inhibitor (not recommended). The clinical relevance of this interaction with boosted saquinavir is unclear, but note that no significant interaction appears to occur with ritonavir.

St John's wort (Hypericum perforatum) ✖

St John's wort causes a marked reduction in the serum levels of indinavir, which may result in HIV treatment failure. Other protease inhibitors are predicted to interact similarly.

> The advice of the CSM in the UK is that patients taking protease inhibitors should avoid St John's wort, and that anyone already taking both should stop the St John's wort and have their HIV RNA viral load measured. The manufacturers also note that protease inhibitor levels may increase on stopping St John's wort, and the dose may need adjusting. They note that the inducing effect may persist for up to 2 weeks after stopping treatment with St John's wort.

Herbal medicines or Dietary supplements + **Proton pump inhibitors** ❓

Both *Gingko biloba* and St John's wort (*Hypericum perforatum*) induce the metabolism of omeprazole, and this might result in reduced efficacy. Other proton pump inhibitors are likely to be similarly affected.

> There is insufficient evidence to suggest that these herbs should be avoided in patients taking proton pump inhibitors. However, the potential reduction in their efficacy should be borne in mind, particular where the consequences may be serious, such as in patients with healing ulcers. Note that rabeprazole seems less likely to be affected.

Herbal medicines or Dietary supplements + **Rimonabant** ❓

The manufacturers predict that potent inducers of CYP3A4 such as St John's wort (*Hypericum perforatum*) may lower the serum levels of rimonabant. This is based on the fact that potent *inhibitors* of CYP3A4 *increase* rimonabant levels (see under azoles, page 122).

> Caution is recommended with concurrent use of St John's wort and rimonabant. Patients should be monitored to ensure rimonabant remains effective.

Herbal medicines or Dietary supplements +
Sirolimus ⚠

The manufacturers of sirolimus predict that St John's wort (*Hypericum perforatum*) may lower its serum levels, probably because rifampicin (rifampin), another CYP3A4 inducer, has been shown to do so.

> The extent of any change in sirolimus levels is uncertain, but if concurrent use cannot be avoided it would seem prudent to increase the frequency of monitoring of sirolimus levels.

Herbal medicines or Dietary supplements + SSRIs

Ayahuasca ❓

A man taking fluoxetine experienced symptoms of the serotonin syndrome after ingesting the psychoactive beverage ayahuasca (also known as caapi, daime, hoasca, natema, yage), which is characteristically derived from the vine *Banisteriopsis caapi*.

> This appears to be the only report of an interaction. However as ayahuasca contains monoamine oxidase-inhibiting harmala alkaloids concurrent use may potentially cause serotonin syndrome, page 392.

St John's wort (Hypericum perforatum) ✖

Several patients taking sertraline developed symptoms diagnosed as serotonin syndrome, page 392, after also taking St John's wort. Another patient taking St John's wort developed severe sedation after taking a single dose of paroxetine. Isolated cases of mania have also been reported when SSRIs were taken with St John's wort.

> The incidence of an interaction is probably small, but because of the potential severity of the reaction it would seem prudent to avoid the concurrent use of any SSRI and St John's wort. The CSM in the UK advise that St John's wort should be stopped if patients are taking an SSRI.

H

Herbal medicines or Dietary supplements +
Statins ❓

St John's wort (*Hypericum perforatum*) appears to reduce the levels of simvastatin and its active metabolite.

> The significance of this interaction is unclear but it may be prudent to check that simvastatin remains effective in the presence of St John's wort.

Herbal medicines or Dietary supplements +
Tacrolimus ⚠

St John's wort (*Hypericum perforatum*) has been found, on average, to decrease the maximum serum concentration of tacrolimus by 65% and the AUC by 32%. However, the decrease in AUC ranged from 15% to 64%, with one patient having a 31% *increase* in AUC.

> Given the unpredictability of the interaction (and the variability in content of St John's wort products) it would seem prudent to avoid St John's wort in transplant patients, and possibly patients taking tacrolimus for other indications. If St John's wort is withdrawn monitor tacrolimus levels and adjust the dose accordingly.

Herbal medicines or Dietary supplements +
Ticlopidine ⚠

Ginkgo biloba has been associated with platelet, bleeding and clotting disorders and there are isolated reports of serious adverse reactions after its concurrent use with ticlopidine.

> Caution should be exercised if *Ginkgo biloba* is used with any drug that affects platelet aggregation.

Herbal medicines or Dietary supplements +
Trazodone ❓

Coma developed in an elderly patient with Alzheimer's disease after she took trazodone with *Ginkgo biloba*. She later recovered.

> This appears to be an isolated case, from which no general conclusions can be drawn.

H

Herbal medicines or Dietary supplements +
Tricyclics ⚠

The plasma levels of amitriptyline can be reduced by St John's wort (*Hypericum perforatum*) and nortriptyline seems to be similarly affected. Other tricyclics are also expected to interact.

> Both the tricyclics and St John's wort are antidepressants, but whether the final sum of this interaction is more or less antidepressant activity is not known. Monitor antidepressant efficacy if St John's wort is given with any tricyclic.

Herbal medicines or Dietary supplements +
Triptans ✖

The CSM in the UK noted that pharmacodynamic interactions have been identified between triptans and St John's wort (*Hypericum perforatum*) leading to an increased risk of adverse effects. This has been seen with other drugs with serotonergic effects, such as the SSRIs, page 279.

> The CSM suggest that patients taking triptans should not take St John's wort preparations: the manufacturers generally advise caution, which seems prudent, see serotonin syndrome, page 392.

Herbal medicines or Dietary supplements +
Venlafaxine

Jujube ❓

An isolated report describes an acute serotonin reaction when venlafaxine was given with a Chinese herbal remedy, jujube (sour date nut; suanzaoren; *Ziziphus jujuba*).

Patients should be asked about the use of herbal remedies and advised to discontinue them before prescribing antidepressant drugs if there is any possibility of an interaction.

St John's wort (Hypericum perforatum) ⚠

A possible case of serotonin syndrome, page 392, have been reported in a patient taking venlafaxine and St John's wort.

Caution is advised if venlafaxine is given with other drugs that affect the serotonergic neurotransmitter systems, such as St John's wort.

Herbal medicines or Dietary supplements + **Warfarin**
and other oral anticoagulants

Boldo ❓

A report describes a woman on warfarin whose INR rose modestly when she began to take boldo and fenugreek. She was eventually restabilised with a 15% dose reduction.

If patients taking warfarin also take boldo/fenugreek it may be prudent to check the INR after 1 to 2 weeks.

Chamomile ❓

A single case describes a woman taking warfarin who developed a marked increase in her INR with bleeding complications 5 days after she started drinking chamomile tea and using a chamomile-based skin lotion.

Note that there appear to be no reports of chamomile alone causing anticoagulation, which might suggest that the risk of an additive effect is small.

Cucurbita ❓

The INR of a patient taking warfarin increased from 2.4 to 3.5 after he took curbicin, which contains saw palmetto (*Serenoa repens*) and *Cucurbita pepo*.

The clinical importance of this interaction is unknown, but bear it in mind in case of an increased response to anticoagulant treatment.

Danshen ❌

Several case reports indicate that danshen (the root of *Salvia miltiorrhiza*), a Chinese herbal remedy, can increase the effects of warfarin resulting in bleeding.

Avoid concurrent use where possible, although with very careful monitoring and warfarin dosage adjustments, safe concurrent use might be possible.

H

Dong quai ✕

Two case reports describe a very marked increase in the anticoagulant effects of warfarin when dong quai was added.

Patients taking warfarin should be warned of the potential risks of also taking dong quai. Until more information is available, dong quai should be avoided unless the effects on anticoagulation can be monitored.

Fenugreek ❓

A report describes a woman taking warfarin whose INR rose modestly when she began to take boldo and fenugreek. She was eventually restabilised with a 15% dose reduction.

If patients on warfarin take boldo/fenugreek it may be prudent to check the INR after 1 to 2 weeks.

Fish oils ⚠

The manufacturers say that high doses of omega-3 marine triglycerides (4 capsules) increase bleeding time.

The manufacturers recommend that patients taking anticoagulants should be monitored for increased anticoagulant effects (such as bruising or bleeding), and the doses adjusted as necessary.

Garlic ❓

Two patients taking warfarin developed increased INRs after the addition of garlic capsules. One patient developed haematuria. However, a controlled study suggests no interaction occurs.

This interaction seems rare, but bear it in mind in case of unexpected bleeding. It is worth noting that there have been cases of spontaneous bleeding attributed to garlic alone.

Ginkgo biloba ❓

An isolated report describes intracerebral haemorrhage associated with the use of *Ginkgo biloba* and warfarin. Other evidence suggests that no interaction occurs.

The clinical importance of this interaction is unknown, but bear it in mind in case of a increased response to anticoagulant treatment.

Ginseng ⚠

One pharmacological study found that American ginseng (*Panax quinquefolius*) modestly decreased the effect of warfarin, whereas another study found that *Panax ginseng* did not alter the effect of warfarin. Two case reports describe decreased warfarin effects, one with thrombosis, attributed to the use of ginseng (probably *Panax ginseng*). Note that there have been reports of spontaneous bleeding with ginseng alone, and *Panax ginseng* has been found to contain antiplatelet components.

Until further information becomes available it would seem prudent to be alert for decreased effects of coumarins in patients using ginseng, particularly American ginseng. However, the possibility of an increased risk of bleeding due to the antiplatelet component of *Panax ginseng* cannot entirely be ruled out.

Glucosamine +/- Chondroitin ✗

A couple of reports suggest that glucosamine with or without chondroitin may increase the INR in patients taking warfarin. In contrast, one case of a decreased INR has been reported when glucosamine was taken with acenocoumarol.

There do not appear to have been any controlled studies of this interaction. The cases described suggest it would be prudent to monitor the INR more closely if glucosamine is started. If a patient shows an unexpected change in INR, bear in mind the possibility of self-medication with supplements such as glucosamine.

Lycium barbarum L. ❓

One patient developed a raised INR after taking a tea made from the fruits of *Lycium barbarum* L. (also known as Chinese wolfberry, gou qi zi, Fructus Lycii Chinensis, or *Lycium chinense*).

The clinical importance of this interaction is unknown, but bear it in mind in case of an increased response to anticoagulant treatment.

Quilinggao ❓

A single case report describes a man taking warfarin who had a marked increase in his INR with bleeding complications, 9 days after he switched the brand of quilinggao (a Chinese herbal product made from a mixture of herbs) he was using.

The clinical importance of this interaction is unknown, but bear it in mind in case of an increased response to anticoagulant treatment.

Saw palmetto ❓

The INR of a patient taking warfarin increased from 2.4 to 3.5 after he took curbicin, which contains saw palmetto and cucurbita.

The clinical importance of this interaction is unknown, but bear it in mind in case of an increased response to anticoagulant treatment.

St John's wort (Hypericum perforatum) ✗

St John's wort can cause a moderate reduction in the anticoagulant effects of warfarin.

The CSM in the UK advise that if St John's wort is being taken by patients also taking anticoagulants the herb should be stopped and the anticoagulant dosage adjusted as necessary.

Ubidecarenone (Coenzyme Q10) ✔

The anticoagulant effects of warfarin have been either reduced, or transiently, increased by ubidecarenone. However, no interaction was found in a study.

The clinical importance of this interaction is unknown, but bear it in mind in case of a reduced response to anticoagulant treatment.

H

HRT

As HRT contains many of the same hormones as the contraceptives, studies with contraceptives, page 199, may be applicable to HRT and *vice versa*, although the relative doses should be borne in mind.

HRT + Letrozole ❌

HRT would be expected to diminish the effects of letrozole (which has anti-oestrogenic effects), so concurrent use is contraindicated.

Some information suggests that there need not be a complete restriction on their concurrent use, but this needs confirmation. Until then, concurrent use should be avoided.

HRT + Levothyroxine ⚠

Oral HRT appears to increase the requirement for levothyroxine in some patients.

It would be prudent to monitor thyroid function several months after starting or stopping oral HRT to check levothyroxine requirements. Transdermal HRT would not be expected to interact, but this needs confirmation.

HRT + MAO-B inhibitors ⚠

In a controlled study, the AUC of selegiline was modestly increased by HRT (60%), but this was not considered to be clinically significant.

One UK manufacturer of selegiline advises that the concurrent use of HRT should be avoided.

HRT + Modafinil ❓

The hormones in HRT are similar to those used in oral contraceptives, and so may be affected by enzyme-inducing drugs in the same way as contraceptives, page 204. Reduced effects are therefore possible if modafinil is also given.

Any interaction would be most likely to be noticed where HRT is prescribed for menopausal vasomotor symptoms. Further study is needed to confirm the importance of this possible interaction.

HRT + NNRTIs ❓

The hormones in HRT are similar to those used in oral contraceptives, and so may be affected by enzyme-inducing drugs, such as nevirapine and efavirenz, in the same way as contraceptives, page 204. Reduced effects are therefore possible if either of these drugs is also given.

Any interaction would be most likely to be noticed where HRT is prescribed for menopausal vasomotor symptoms. Further study is needed to confirm the importance of this possible interaction.

HRT + Phenobarbital ❓

The hormones in HRT are similar to those used in oral contraceptives, and so may be affected by enzyme-inducing drugs in the same way as contraceptives, page 205. Reduced effects are therefore possible if phenobarbital or primidone is also given.

Any interaction would be most likely to be noticed where HRT is prescribed for menopausal vasomotor symptoms. Further study is needed to confirm the importance of this possible interaction.

HRT + Phenytoin ❓

The hormones in HRT are similar to those used in oral contraceptives, and so may be affected by enzyme-inducing drugs in the same way as contraceptives, page 206. Reduced effects are therefore possible if phenytoin or fosphenytoin is also given.

Any interaction would be most likely to be noticed where HRT is prescribed for menopausal vasomotor symptoms. Further study is needed to confirm the importance of this possible interaction.

HRT + Protease inhibitors ❓

The hormones in HRT are similar to those used in oral contraceptives, and so may be affected by enzyme-inducing drugs in the same way as contraceptives, page 206. Reduced effects are therefore possible if a protease inhibitor is also given.

Any interaction would be most likely to be noticed where HRT is prescribed for menopausal vasomotor symptoms. Further study is needed to confirm the importance of this possible interaction.

H

HRT + Rifabutin ❓

The hormones in HRT are similar to those used in oral contraceptives, and so may be affected by enzyme-inducing drugs in the same way as contraceptives, page 207. Reduced effects are therefore possible if rifabutin is also given.

Any interaction would be most likely to be noticed where HRT is prescribed for menopausal vasomotor symptoms. Further study is needed to confirm the importance of this possible interaction.

HRT + Rifampicin (Rifampin) ❓

The hormones in HRT are similar to those used in oral contraceptives, and so may be affected by enzyme-inducing drugs in the same way as contraceptives, page 207. Reduced effects are therefore possible if rifampicin is also given.

Any interaction would be most likely to be noticed where HRT is prescribed for menopausal vasomotor symptoms. Further study is needed to confirm the importance of this possible interaction.

HRT + Tacrine ❓

HRT increases the AUC of tacrine by 60% (and even up to 3-fold in one individual) and reduces the clearance by about 30%.

> The importance of this interaction is unclear. Increased tacrine levels may increase both the efficacy and adverse effects of tacrine. Monitor patients for signs of tacrine toxicity and consider a tacrine dose reduction if indicated.

HRT + Tamoxifen ✖

HRT would be expected to diminish the effects of tamoxifen and other anti-oestrogens, so concurrent use is contraindicated.

> Some information suggests that there need not be a complete restriction on their concurrent use, but this needs confirmation. Until then, concurrent use should be avoided.

HRT + Topiramate ❓

The hormones in HRT are similar to those used in oral contraceptives, and so may be affected by enzyme-inducing drugs in the same way as contraceptives, page 208. Reduced effects are therefore possible if topiramate is also given.

> Any interaction would be most likely to be noticed where HRT is prescribed for menopausal vasomotor symptoms. Further study is needed to confirm the importance of this possible interaction.

HRT + Toremifene ✖

HRT would be expected to diminish the effects of toremifene (which has anti-oestrogenic effects), so concurrent use is contraindicated.

> Some information suggests that there need not be a complete restriction on their concurrent use, but this needs confirmation. Until then, concurrent use should be avoided.

HRT + Warfarin and other oral anticoagulants ❓

A report describes a woman who needed more acenocoumarol when her HRT treatment with oral conjugated oestrogens was changed to transdermal estradiol. A retrospective analysis of women starting HRT found that three needed warfarin dose increases of about 10 to 30%.

> Direct information is limited. Note that, because of the increased risk of developing venous thromboembolism with HRT, the use of HRT in women already on anticoagulant therapy requires careful consideration of the risks and benefits. If the combination is used be aware that the anticoagulant response may be affected.

H

5-HT₃-receptor antagonists

5-HT₃-receptor antagonists + **Drugs that prolong the QT interval** ⚠

All available 5-HT₃-receptor antagonists (dolasetron, granisetron, ondansetron, palonosetron, tropisetron) have caused small increases (generally not exceeding 15 milliseconds) in the QTc interval. Some consider that these changes are not clinically relevant. Nevertheless, many of the manufacturers give various cautions about using 5-HT₃-receptor antagonists together with other drugs that prolong the QT interval, page 237.

> The UK manufacturer of dolasetron contraindicates the concurrent use of class I or class III antiarrhythmics, whereas the US manufacturer advises caution with all drugs that may prolong the QT interval. The UK manufacturer of ondansetron recommends caution in patients treated with antiarrhythmics or beta blockers (presumably sotalol) whereas the US manufacturer does not issue any cautions regarding QT-prolongation. The UK and US manufacturers of tropisetron recommend caution with other drugs that increase the QT interval.

5-HT₃-receptor antagonists + **Opioids** ⚠

Ondansetron reduces the analgesic efficacy of tramadol and at least double the dose was required in one clinical study. This resulted in more vomiting despite the ondansetron.

> It would seem prudent to use alternative analgesics if ondansetron is required.

5-HT₃-receptor antagonists + **SSRIs** ❓

Symptoms similar to serotonin syndrome have been reported in two patients receiving paroxetine and ondansetron or sertraline and dolasetron.

> It has been suggested that that a variant of serotonin syndrome, page 392, may rarely be seen when 5-HT₃-receptor antagonists and SSRIs are given together, and clinicians should consider this possibility if both drugs are given.

H

Hydralazine

Hydralazine + **NSAIDs** ❓

Indometacin abolished the hypotensive effects of intravenous hydralazine in one study, but did not affect it in another.

> Although information is limited various NSAIDs have been reported to reduce the efficacy of other antihypertensive drug classes. It would be prudent to monitor the concurrent use of hydralazine and NSAIDs.

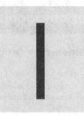

Imatinib

Imatinib + Macrolides ❓

Ketoconazole increases the AUC of imatinib by 40%. Macrolides such as erythromycin and clarithromycin are, like ketoconazole, inhibitors of CYP3A4. The manufacturers of imatinib therefore predict that the macrolides will raise imatinib levels.

It is not clear what action should be taken as information about the effects of increased imatinib levels is limited. Other macrolides may also interact, although it seems unlikely that they all will, see macrolides, page 310.

Imatinib + Phenobarbital ⚠

Rifampicin decreases the AUC of imatinib by 74%. The manufacturers suggest that phenobarbital (and therefore probably primidone) will interact similarly.

The manufacturers suggest that concurrent use should be avoided. However, if this is not possible it would be prudent to monitor the outcome of concurrent use, and increase the imatinib dose as necessary.

Imatinib + Phenytoin ❓

Rifampicin decreases the AUC of imatinib by 74%. The manufacturers suggest that phenytoin (and therefore possibly fosphenytoin) will interact similarly.

The manufacturers suggest that concurrent use should be avoided. However, if this is not possible it would be prudent to monitor the outcome of concurrent use, and increase the imatinib dose as necessary.

Imatinib + Rifampicin (Rifampin) ⚠

Rifampicin decreases the AUC of imatinib by 74%.

The manufacturers suggest that concurrent use should be avoided. However, if this is not possible it would be prudent to monitor the outcome of concurrent use, and increase the imatinib dose as necessary.

Imatinib + **Statins** ⚠️

Imatinib increased the maximum serum levels of simvastatin 2-fold and the AUC 3.5-fold in one study.

> These rises increase the risk of simvastatin toxicity (most notably myopathy and rhabdomyolysis), for which reason the simvastatin dosage should be reduced appropriately. Patients should be counselled regarding myopathy (e.g. report any unexplained muscle pain, tenderness or weakness).

Imatinib + **Warfarin and other oral anticoagulants** ❌

The manufacturers suggest that imatinib may inhibit the metabolism of warfarin. This suggestion seems to be based on an observation in one patient, and on *in vitro* studies that show that imatinib can inhibit CYP2C9, which is involved in the metabolism of warfarin. There seems to be no other evidence that a clinically relevant interaction is likely to occur.

> The manufacturers say that patients needing anticoagulation should be given low-molecular-weight or standard heparin.

Imipenem

Imipenem + **Valproate** ⚠️

Case reports describe reduced valproate levels after imipenem was given. This has led to seizures.

> Although evidence is limited this is in line with the way other carbapenems interact. It would be prudent to monitor valproate levels in any patient given carbapenems. The valproate dosage may need to be increased. Consider using another antibacterial, or an alternative to valproate. Limited evidence suggests that carbamazepine and phenytoin are not affected. Note that imipenem should be used with caution in patients with a history of seizures.

Inotropes and Vasopressors

Inotropes and Vasopressors + **Linezolid** ❌

Because of its weak MAO-inhibitory properties, the manufacturers of linezolid caution its use with adrenaline (epinephrine), dopamine, dobutamine, and noradrenaline (norepinephrine) unless there are facilities available for close observation of the patient and monitoring of blood pressure. However, the evidence available suggests that blood pressure rises are only very moderate and certainly unlikely to be of the hypertensive crisis proportions seen with the antidepressant MAOIs.

> If any of these drugs is prescribed with linezolid patients should be monitored for a rise in blood pressure.

Inotropes and Vasopressors + **MAO-B inhibitors** ✖

A case report describes a hypertensive reaction attributed to the concurrent use of dopamine and selegiline. Rasagiline is expected to interact like selegiline.

The manufacturers of selegiline recommend that dopamine should be used cautiously, if at all, in patients who are chronically receiving selegiline or who have received selegiline in the 2 weeks prior to dopamine therapy. However, note that, in general, an interaction would not be expected, see MAOIs, below.

Inotropes and Vasopressors + **MAOIs**

Metaraminol or Phenylephrine ✖

Metaraminol and phenylephrine are vasopressors with both direct and indirect sympathomimetic actions. This means that it may cause serious and potentially fatal hypertensive reactions in patients taking MAOIs.

Avoid the use of metaraminol or phenylephrine in patients who are either taking MAOIs or who have stopped taking them in the previous 2 weeks.

Other inotropes and vasopressors ❓

The pressor effects of inotropes and vasopressors with indirect sympathomimetic actions, such as adrenaline (epinephrine), isoprenaline (isoproterenol), noradrenaline (norepinephrine) and methoxamine may be unchanged or only moderately increased in patients taking MAOIs. The increase may be somewhat greater in those who show a significant hypotensive response to the MAOI.

No immediate action needed, but bear these potential moderate reactions in mind if using the combination.

Inotropes and Vasopressors + **Tricyclics** ⚠

Patients taking tricyclic antidepressants show a grossly exaggerated response (hypertension, cardiac arrhythmias, etc.) to parenteral noradrenaline (norepinephrine), adrenaline (epinephrine), and to a lesser extent, to phenylephrine.

It has been suggested that these drugs should be introduced cautiously until the full effects are known. Anecdotal evidence suggests that local anaesthetics containing these vasoconstrictors are commonly used in patients taking tricyclic antidepressants with no problems. However there have been a few case reports of adverse effects occurring during dental treatment. Felypressin may be a safe alternative. The effects of phenylephrine given orally or as nasal drops does not appear to have been studied.

Iron

Iron + Levodopa ⚠️

The absorption of levodopa can be reduced by 30 to 50% by ferrous sulfate due to levodopa chelation. Therefore all iron compounds are expected to act similarly. Carbidopa levels are also reduced. There is some evidence that this interaction causes a decrease in symptom control.

Separating the administration of the iron as much as possible is likely to be an effective way of managing this interaction.

Iron + Levothyroxine ⚠️

Ferrous sulfate (and therefore probably other iron compounds) causes a reduction in the effects of levothyroxine in patients treated for hypothyroidism.

Monitor the effects of concurrent use and consider separating the doses by 2 hours or more, on the assumption that reduced absorption accounts for this interaction.

Iron + Methyldopa ⚠️

The antihypertensive effects of methyldopa can be reduced by ferrous sulfate or ferrous gluconate. Other iron compounds are expected to interact similarly.

Monitor the effects of concurrent use and increase the methyldopa dosage as necessary. Separating the dosages by up to 2 hours apparently only partially reduces the effects of this interaction.

Iron + Mycophenolate ✅

Therapeutic doses of ferrous sulfate (105 mg or 210 mg from modified-release tablets) did not alter the pharmacokinetics of mycophenolate in two studies. However, one study found that a single 1050-mg dose of ferrous sulfate (210 mg of elemental iron) reduced the AUC and maximum levels of mycophenolate by more than 90%. Other iron compounds would be expected to interact similarly.

No action needed with usual therapeutic doses of iron.

Iron + Penicillamine ⚠️

The absorption of penicillamine can be reduced as much as two-thirds by oral iron.

For maximal absorption give the iron at least 2 hours after the penicillamine. Do not stop iron suddenly as the marked increase in absorption that follows may precipitate penicillamine toxicity.

Iron + **Proton pump inhibitors** ❓

Omeprazole may impair the absorption of oral iron preparations and vegetable sources of iron.

> Many factors and disease states can affect oral iron absorption. However bear these reports in mind should a patient taking any proton pump inhibitor fail to respond to oral iron therapy

Iron + **Quinolones** ⚠

Ferrous fumarate, gluconate, sulfate and other iron compounds can reduce the absorption of ciprofloxacin, gatifloxacin, levofloxacin, norfloxacin, ofloxacin and sparfloxacin. Serum levels of the antibacterial may become subtherapeutic as a result.

> Most quinolones should not be taken at the same time as iron. Since the quinolones are rapidly absorbed, taking them 2 hours before the iron should largely avoid this interaction. The exceptions are fleroxacin, which appears not to interact, and lomefloxacin, which seems to interact only minimally.

Iron + **Tetracyclines** ⚠

The absorption of both tetracyclines and iron compounds is markedly reduced by concurrent use. The tetracycline serum levels are reduced by 30 to 90% and their therapeutic effectiveness may be reduced or even abolished.

> The extent of the reductions depends on a number of factors.
> - the particular tetracycline used: tetracycline and oxytetracycline were affected the least in one study.
> - the time interval between the administration of the two drugs: giving the iron 3 hours before or 2 to 3 hours after the antibacterial is satisfactory with tetracycline, but one study found that even 11 hours was inadequate for doxycycline.
> - the particular iron compound used: with tetracycline the reduction in serum levels with ferrous sulfate was 80 to 90%, with ferrous fumarate, succinate and gluconate, 70 to 80%; with ferrous tartrate, 50%; and with ferrous sodium edetate, 30%. This was with doses containing equivalent amounts of elemental iron.
> Therefore separate administration by as much as possible and consider adjusting the choice of iron compound or tetracycline.

Isoniazid

Isoniazid + **Levodopa** ⚠

Levodopa-induced dyskinesias are improved by isoniazid, but the control of Parkinson's disease is worsened. This may take several weeks to develop.

> The combination need not be avoided, but be aware that an adjustment in treatment may be needed if parkinsonism deteriorates.

Isoniazid + NRTIs ⚠

The clearance of isoniazid is approximately doubled by zalcitabine, and there is a theoretical increased risk of peripheral neuropathy.

Monitor concurrent use carefully to ensure isoniazid is effective, and because of the potential for additive peripheral neuropathy.

Isoniazid + Paracetamol (Acetaminophen) ❓

Hepatotoxicity has been seen with the combination of isoniazid and paracetamol, usually in patients who have taken more than 4 g of paracetamol daily, but occasionally in those taking normal doses.

The ultra-cautious may wish to limit paracetamol intake, but information is very limited and more study is needed to confirm any interaction.

Isoniazid + Phenytoin ⚠

Phenytoin serum levels can be raised by isoniazid and some patients may develop toxicity. If both rifampicin (rifampin) and isoniazid are given, serum phenytoin levels may fall in patients who are fast acetylators of isoniazid, but may occasionally rise in those who are slow acetylators (said to be about 50% of the population).

It is unlikely that the acetylator status of the patient will be known. Therefore monitor phenytoin levels and adjust the dose accordingly. In some patients the interaction has taken several weeks to develop.

Isoniazid + Theophylline ❓

Two short-term studies found that theophylline serum levels were slightly increased by isoniazid and a case of theophylline toxicity supports this finding. However, another short-term study found that isoniazid slightly increased theophylline clearance.

The outcome of concurrent use is uncertain but it would be prudent to be alert for any evidence of increased theophylline levels and toxicity if isoniazid is given. It may take 3 to 4 weeks for this interaction to develop.

Isotretinoin

Isotretinoin + Tetracyclines ✖

The development of 'pseudotumour cerebri' (benign intracranial hypertension) has been associated with the concurrent use of isotretinoin and tetracyclines.

The manufacturers of isotretinoin contraindicate its use with tetracyclines.

Isotretinoin + Vitamin A ⚠

A condition similar to vitamin A (retinol) overdosage may occur if isotretinoin and vitamin A are given concurrently.

> The manufacturers of isotretinoin say that high doses of vitamin A (more than 4000 to 5000 units daily, the recommended daily allowance) should be avoided.

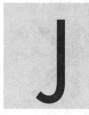

J

No interactions have been included for drugs beginning with the letter J.

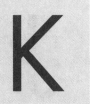

K

Kaolin

Kaolin + Quinidine ⚠

Limited evidence from single-dose studies suggests that kaolin-pectin may reduce the absorption of quinidine and lower its serum levels (salivary concentration reduced by about 50%).

Be alert for the need to increase the quinidine dosage if kaolin-pectin is used concurrently.

Kaolin + Tetracyclines ⚠

Kaolin-pectin reduces the absorption of tetracycline by about 50%.

If these two drugs are given together, consider separating the dosages by at least 2 hours to minimise admixture in the gut. It may even then be necessary to increase the tetracycline dosage. Information about other tetracyclines is lacking, but be alert for them to interact similarly.

Lamotrigine

Lamotrigine + **Oxcarbazepine**

Oxcarbazepine appears to lower lamotrigine levels by about 15 to 75%. Lamotrigine appears to increase the levels of the active metabolite of oxcarbazepine.

The clinical relevance is uncertain, but it would seem likely that some patients will have significantly reduced lamotrigine levels. Monitor concurrent use carefully, being aware that dosage adjustments may be necessary. The importance of the increase in oxcarbazepine metabolite levels is less clear.

Lamotrigine + **Phenobarbital**

Phenobarbital has been associated with reduced lamotrigine serum levels (reduction of about 50% in one study). Lamotrigine does not appear to affect phenobarbital or primidone levels.

Phenobarbital induces the metabolism of lamotrigine, and the recommended starting dose and long-term maintenance dose of lamotrigine in patients already taking phenobarbital or primidone is twice that of patients receiving lamotrigine monotherapy. However, note that if they are also taking valproate in addition to phenobarbital, the lamotrigine dose should be reduced.

Lamotrigine + **Phenytoin**

Phenytoin has been associated with reduced lamotrigine serum levels (by almost two-thirds in one study). Lamotrigine has no effect on phenytoin levels.

Phenytoin (and therefore probably fosphenytoin) induces the metabolism of lamotrigine, and the recommended starting dose and long-term maintenance dose of lamotrigine in patients already taking phenytoin is twice that of patients receiving lamotrigine monotherapy. However, note that if they are also taking valproate in addition to phenytoin, the lamotrigine dose should be reduced.

Lamotrigine + **Protease inhibitors** ⚠

Lopinavir/ritonavir halved lamotrigine plasma levels, whereas the protease inhibitor levels did not appear to be altered. Saquinavir/ritonavir had similar effects in another patient and therefore reduced lamotrigine levels should be anticipated with any ritonavir-boosted regimen.

> Lamotrigine efficacy should be monitored in patients taking lopinavir/ritonavir, and probably any ritonavir-boosted regimen. Anticipate the need to increase the lamotrigine dose.

Lamotrigine + **Rifampicin (Rifampin)** ❓

Rifampicin increases the clearance of lamotrigine and reduces its AUC by 97% and 44%, respectively. A lamotrigine dose increase was required in one case report.

> Information is limited but rifampicin could reduce the efficacy of lamotrigine. Monitor the patient and increase the lamotrigine dose if required.

Lamotrigine + **Valproate** ⚠

The serum levels of lamotrigine can be increased by sodium valproate. Small increases, decreases or no changes in sodium valproate levels have been seen with lamotrigine. Concurrent use has been associated with skin rashes and other toxic reactions.

> Monitor the outcome of concurrent use. In patients already taking valproate, the manufacturer of lamotrigine recommends a lamotrigine starting dose that is half that of lamotrigine monotherapy, irrespective of whether they are also receiving enzyme-inducing antiepileptics, and a very gradual dose-escalation rate. The development of rashes should be investigated promptly.

Leflunomide

Leflunomide + **Methotrexate** ⚠

Although no pharmacokinetic interaction appears to occur between methotrexate and leflunomide elevated liver enzyme levels have been seen.

> The UK manufacturers say that concurrent use is not advisable. The US manufacturers say that if concurrent use is undertaken, monitoring should be increased to monthly intervals. Close liver enzyme monitoring is also recommended if switching between these drugs, and colestyramine or activated charcoal washout should be performed when switching from leflunomide to methotrexate.

Leflunomide + **Penicillamine** ✖

The manufacturers say that the concurrent use of leflunomide and penicillamine has not yet been studied but it would be expected to increase the risk of serious adverse reactions (haematological toxicity or hepatotoxicity).

The manufacturers advise avoiding concurrent use. As the active metabolite of leflunomide has a long half-life of 1 to 4 weeks, a washout of colestyramine or activated charcoal should be given if patients are to be switched to other DMARDs.

Leflunomide + Phenytoin ⚠

In vitro studies have found that the active metabolite of leflunomide (A771726) is an inhibitor of CYP2C9, the isoenzyme concerned with the metabolism of phenytoin and fosphenytoin.

Although no cases of phenytoin toxicity appear to have been reported as a result of this interaction, caution would be advisable on concurrent use, especially as leflunomide has, in practice, been seen to inhibit the metabolism of other CYP2C9 substrates.

Leflunomide + Rifampicin (Rifampin) ❓

Rifampicin increases the levels of the active metabolite of leflunomide (A771726) by 40%.

There would seem to be no reason for avoiding concurrent use, but the manufacturers advise caution as levels may build up over time. It may be prudent to increase the frequency of leflunomide monitoring if these two drugs are used together.

Leflunomide + Vaccines ✖

The body's immune response is suppressed by leflunomide. The antibody response to vaccines may be reduced and the use of live attenuated vaccines may result in generalised infection.

For many inactivated vaccines even the reduced response seen is considered clinically useful. If a vaccine is given, it may be prudent to monitor the response, so that alternative prophylactic measures can be considered where the response is inadequate. Note that even where effective antibody titres are produced, these may not persist as long as in healthy subjects, and more frequent booster doses may be required. The use of live vaccines is generally considered to be contraindicated.

Leflunomide + Warfarin and other oral anticoagulants ⚠

Leflunomide appears to raise the INR of patients taking warfarin. Case reports describe bleeding, and INRs as high as 6 and 11.

It would seem prudent to closely monitor the INR of any patient taking warfarin who is started on leflunomide.

L

Levodopa

Levodopa + MAOIs ❌

A rapid, serious and potentially life-threatening hypertensive reaction can occur in patients taking MAOIs if they are also given levodopa.

An interaction with levodopa given with carbidopa or benserazide is unlikely. Even so, the manufacturers continue to list the MAOIs among their contraindications and say that patients should not be given levodopa during treatment with MAOIs, nor for a period of 2 to 3 weeks after their withdrawal.

Levodopa + Methyldopa ⚠

Methyldopa can increase the effects of levodopa. This has allowed a dosage reduction of about 30 to 70% in some patients taking levodopa alone, but it can also worsen dyskinesias in others. A small increase in the hypotensive actions of methyldopa may also occur.

This interaction is expected to be minimised in the presence of carbidopa or benserazide and so it seems unlikely that a dose reduction of levodopa would usually be required. The increased hypotensive effects seem to be small, but be aware they are possible.

Levodopa + Metoclopramide ⚠

Metoclopramide is a centrally-acting dopamine antagonist, which can oppose the effects of levodopa and worsen Parkinson's disease. It also stimulates gastric emptying and this may lead to a small increase in the bioavailability of levodopa.

Concurrent use should generally be avoided. Domperidone is the antiemetic of choice in Parkinson's disease.

Levodopa + Penicillamine ❓

Penicillamine can raise plasma levodopa levels in some patients. This may improve the control of the parkinsonism but the adverse effects of levodopa may also be increased.

Concurrent use need not be avoided, but monitor for an increase in the adverse effects of levodopa.

Levodopa + Phenytoin ❓

The therapeutic effects of levodopa can be reduced by phenytoin.

Evidence is limited (effects in 5 patients only). If concurrent use is necessary be aware that some patients may experience a worsening of symptoms. It seems possible that fosphenytoin, a prodrug of phenytoin, could have similar effects.

Levodopa + Pyridoxine ⊗

The effects of levodopa are reduced or abolished by pyridoxine, but this interaction does not occur when levodopa is given with the dopa-decarboxylase inhibitors carbidopa or benserazide, as is usual clinical practice.

In the rare cases that levodopa is used alone, pyridoxine in doses as low as 5 mg daily can reduce the effects of levodopa and should therefore be avoided. Warn patients about proprietary pyridoxine-containing preparations such as multivitamins and supplements. There is no evidence to suggest that a low-pyridoxine diet is desirable.

Levodopa + SSRIs ⚠

The use of an SSRI is often beneficial in patients with Parkinson's disease taking levodopa. However, sometimes parkinsonian symptoms are worsened.

Although the information is limited, it seems that in some cases parkinsonism can be worsened by SSRIs. Concurrent use is valuable and need not be avoided, but monitor the outcome and withdraw the SSRI if necessary.

Levothyroxine

Levothyroxine + Phenobarbital ❓

An isolated report describes a reduction in the response to levothyroxine in a patient also given secobarbital with amobarbital. It seems possible that all barbiturates may interact in this way. Note that phenobarbital has been shown to reduce the serum levels of endogenous thyroid hormones in some studies.

The general importance of this interaction is almost certainly small, but be alert for any evidence of changes in thyroid status if barbiturates are added or withdrawn from patients taking levothyroxine.

Levothyroxine + Phenytoin ❓

An isolated report describes a patient, previously well maintained on levothyroxine, who developed clinical hypothyroidism when also given phenytoin. Phenytoin can reduce endogenous serum thyroid hormone levels, but clinical hypothyroidism caused by an interaction seems to be rare.

The general importance of this interaction seems small, but be alert for any evidence of changes in thyroid status if phenytoin is added or withdrawn from patients taking levothyroxine.

L

Levothyroxine + **Protease inhibitors** ❓

A man needed to have his levothyroxine dosage doubled when he took ritonavir/
saquinavir, and a woman possibly had a similar reaction when she took indinavir then
nelfinavir. Hypothyroidism was unable to be corrected in another woman while she
was taking lopinavir/ritonavir and then nelfinavir. Another woman needed a
markedly *reduced* dose of levothyroxine when given indinavir.

Direct information is limited and the presence of an interaction seems to depend
on the individual protease inhibitor, how it affects glucuronidation, and how
much remaining thyroid function a patient has. Until more is known about this
interaction it would seem prudent to monitor thyroid function more closely if a
protease inhibitor is given to a patient with pre-existing thyroid dysfunction.

Levothyroxine + **Rifampicin (Rifampin)** ❓

Two case reports suggest that rifampicin might possibly reduce the effects of thyroid
hormones.

The evidence for this interaction is by no means conclusive. Bear this interaction
in mind if rifampicin is given to a patient taking levothyroxine.

Levothyroxine + **Sevelamer** ⚠

Sevelamer decreases levothyroxine absorption and appears to increase levothyroxine
requirements.

It would be prudent to monitor levothyroxine requirements in patients requiring
sevelamer. Whether separation of administration would minimise any interaction
remains to be demonstrated, but, where absorption is a problem, the manufacturers generally recommend avoiding giving other drugs at least 1 hour before or
3 hours after sevelamer.

Levothyroxine + **SSRIs** ❓

The effects of levothyroxine can be opposed (TSH levels became elevated) in some
patients by the concurrent use of sertraline.

These cases draw attention to the need to monitor the effects of giving sertraline to
patients taking thyroid hormones, the dosage of which may need to be increased.
However, note that this interaction seems relatively rare.

Levothyroxine + **Sucralfate** ❓

An isolated report describes a marked reduction in the effects of levothyroxine in a
patient taking sucralfate. A subsequent study found no interaction.

The general importance of this interaction is unknown, but bear it in mind in case
of an unexpected response to treatment. Consider avoiding taking sucralfate until
several hours after the levothyroxine dose.

Levothyroxine + **Theophylline** ⚠

Thyroid status may affect the rate at which theophylline is metabolised: in hypothyroidism it is decreased. As thyroid function is corrected with e.g. levothyroxine, metabolism increases and so larger doses of theophylline are needed.

Monitor the outcome of resolving hypothyroidism, checking that the effects of theophylline are adequate. Monitor theophylline levels as necessary.

Levothyroxine + **Tricyclics** ❓

The antidepressant response to imipramine, amitriptyline and possibly other tricyclics can be accelerated by the use of thyroid hormones. Isolated cases of paroxysmal atrial tachycardia, thyrotoxicosis and hypothyroidism due to concurrent therapy have been described.

These apparent interactions remain unexplained. Unless problems arise there would seem to be no good reason for avoiding concurrent use.

Levothyroxine + **Warfarin and other oral anticoagulants** ⚠

The anticoagulant effects of acenocoumarol, dicoumarol, phenindione, and warfarin are increased by thyroid hormones and bleeding has been seen. This is largely due to alteration of thyroid function, rather than a direct drug-drug interaction.

Hypothyroid patients taking an anticoagulant who are subsequently given thyroid hormones as replacement therapy will need a downward adjustment of the anticoagulant dosage as treatment proceeds. Monitor the INR and adjust the warfarin as necessary.

Lidocaine

Lidocaine + **Phenobarbital** ⚠

Plasma lidocaine levels, following slow intravenous injection, may be up to about 30% lower in patients who are taking phenobarbital. It seems likely that other barbiturates will interact similarly.

It may be necessary to increase the dosage of lidocaine to achieve the desired therapeutic response in patients taking barbiturates.

Lidocaine + **Phenytoin** ❓

The incidence of central adverse effects may be increased following the concurrent use of lidocaine and phenytoin. Sinoatrial arrest has been reported in one patient receiving the combination. Lidocaine levels may be reduced by phenytoin. Fosphenytoin, a prodrug of phenytoin, may interact similarly.

The clinical significance of this interaction is most likely to be small. However, the arrest emphasises the need to exercise caution when giving two drugs that have cardiodepressant actions.

Linezolid

Linezolid is a non-selective reversible inhibitor of MAO, and it therefore shares some of the interactions of the MAOIs. However, its effects are weak, and serious adverse interactions of the magnitude seen with the MAOIs do not seem to occur. However, some caution is prudent on the concurrent use of drugs that interact with MAOIs.

Linezolid + MAO-B inhibitors ⊗

The manufacturers contraindicate the use of linezolid with, and within 2 weeks of taking any other drug that inhibits MAO-B, because their MAO-inhibitory activities are predicted to be additive.

Avoid concurrent use.

Linezolid + MAOIs ⊗

The manufacturers contraindicate the use of linezolid with any other drug that inhibits either MAO-A or MAO-B, or within 2 weeks of taking either drug, because their MAO-inhibitory activities are predicted to be additive.

Avoid concurrent use.

Linezolid + Moclobemide ⊗

The manufacturers contraindicate the use of linezolid with any other drug that inhibits either MAO-A or MAO-B, or within 2 weeks of taking either drug, because their MAO-inhibitory activities are predicted to be additive.

Avoid concurrent use.

Linezolid + Nasal decongestants ⊗

Because of its weak MAO-inhibitory properties, the manufacturers of linezolid caution its use with drugs such as phenylpropanolamine and pseudoephedrine unless there are facilities available for close observation of the patient and monitoring of blood pressure. However, the evidence available suggests that blood pressure rises are only very moderate and certainly unlikely to be of the hypertensive crisis proportions seen with the antidepressant MAOIs.

If linezolid and drugs such as these are prescribed patients should be monitored for any rise in blood pressure. Patients should be warned about cough and cold remedies containing these and related drugs.

Linezolid + Opioids ❌

The use of pethidine (meperidine) with MAOIs has resulted in a potentially life-threatening reaction in a few patients. Excitement, muscle rigidity, hyperpyrexia, flushing, sweating and unconsciousness occur very rapidly. Respiratory depression and hypotension have also been seen. Because linezolid has weak MAOI properties the manufacturers predict it may interact similarly.

Avoid concurrent use.

Linezolid + SSRIs ⚠

Several case reports describe the development of serotonin syndrome in patients given linezolid with SSRIs (citalopram, fluoxetine, paroxetine and sertraline are implicated).

The interaction is probably rare. The manufacturers of linezolid say that patients taking SSRIs should have their blood pressure monitored and be closely observed (presumably for symptoms of serotonin syndrome e.g. agitation, diarrhoea, fever, hyperreflexia) if given linezolid. They say that if this is not possible, concurrent use should be avoided. See also serotonin syndrome, page 392.

Linezolid + Tricyclics ⚠

Serotonin syndrome, page 392, is predicted to occur when linezolid is used with tricyclics.

The manufacturers of linezolid say that patients taking tricyclics should have their blood pressure monitored and be closely observed if given linezolid. They say that if this is not possible, concurrent use should be avoided.

Linezolid + Venlafaxine ⚠

In theory the use of venlafaxine and linezolid may result in serotonin syndrome, page 392. One patient developed symptoms similar to serotonin syndrome while taking these drugs.

The interaction is probably rare. The manufacturers of linezolid say that patients taking serotonergic drugs should have their blood pressure monitored and be closely observed (presumably for symptoms of the serotonin syndrome) if given linezolid. They say that if this is not possible, concurrent use should be avoided.

Lithium

L

Lithium is given under close supervision with regular monitoring of serum concentrations because there is a narrow margin between therapeutic concentrations and those that are toxic. The dosage of lithium is adjusted to give therapeutic serum concentrations of 0.4 to 1 mmol/L, although it should be noted that this is the range used in the UK, and other ranges have been quoted. Initially weekly monitoring is advised, dropping to every 3 months for those on stable regimens. It is usual to take serum lithium samples about 10 to 12 hours after the last oral dose. Adverse effects that are not usually considered serious include nausea, weakness, fine tremor, mild polydipsia and polyuria. If serum concentrations rise into the 1.5 to 2 mmol/L range, toxicity usually occurs, and may present as lethargy, drowsiness, coarse hand tremor, lack of coordination, muscular weakness, increased nausea and vomiting, or diarrhoea. Higher levels result in neurotoxicity, which manifests as ataxia, giddiness, tinnitus, confusion, dysarthria, muscle twitching, nystagmus, and even coma or seizures. Cardiovascular symptoms may also develop and include ECG changes and circulatory problems, and there may be a worsening of polyuria. Virtually all of the reports are concerned with the carbonate, but sometimes lithium is given as other compounds. There is no reason to believe that these lithium compounds will interact any differently to lithium carbonate.

Lithium + Maprotiline ⚠

The concurrent use of *tricyclic antidepressants* and lithium has been successful but some patients may develop adverse effects. Serotonin syndrome, page 392, and neuroleptic malignant syndrome have been reported. One study suggests that maprotiline interacts similarly.

> If both drugs are used be alert for any evidence of neurotoxicity.

Lithium + Methyldopa ⚠

Symptoms of lithium toxicity, not always associated with raised lithium levels, have been described in 4 patients and 4 healthy subjects when they were also given methyldopa.

> Avoid concurrent use whenever possible, but if concurrent use is essential the effects should be closely monitored. Serum lithium monitoring may be unreliable because symptoms of toxicity can occur even though the levels remain within the normally accepted therapeutic range.

Lithium + Metronidazole ❓

The lithium levels of 3 patients were raised following the use of metronidazole. However, 2 of these patients had evidence of renal impairment, and one other report describes safe concurrent use.

> The general importance of this interaction is uncertain but bear it in mind in case of an unexpected response to treatment.

Lithium + NSAIDs ⚠

NSAIDs may increase serum lithium levels leading to toxicity, but there is great variability between different NSAIDs and also between individuals taking the same NSAID. For example, studies have found that celecoxib causes a modest 17% increase in lithium levels, yet case reports describe increases of up to about 350%. Similar effects occur with other NSAIDs, and it seems likely that all NSAIDs will interact similarly. However, note that sulindac seems unique in that it is the only NSAID that has been reported to also cause a *decrease* in lithium levels.

Factors such as advanced age, impaired renal function, decreased sodium intake, volume depletion, renal artery stenosis, and heart failure increase the risk of this interaction. NSAIDs should preferably be avoided, especially if other risk factors are present, unless serum lithium levels can be very well monitored (initially every few days) and the lithium dosage reduced appropriately. Patients taking lithium should be aware of the symptoms of lithium toxicity (see lithium, page 305) and told to report them immediately should they occur. This should be reinforced when they are given an NSAID.

Lithium + Phenytoin ❓

Lithium toxicity has been seen in patients concurrently treated with phenytoin. Note that symptoms of toxicity have developed even with lithium levels within the normal range.

The interaction is not well established. Patients taking lithium should be aware of the symptoms of lithium toxicity (see lithium, page 305) and told to immediately report them should they occur. This should be reinforced when they are given phenytoin.

Lithium + Sibutramine ✖

It has been suggested that lithium should not be given with sibutramine because of the risks of the potentially fatal serotonin syndrome.

Serotonin syndrome appears to occur rarely with other serotonergic drugs and lithium. If concurrent use is considered necessary, monitor closely for symptoms of serotonin syndrome, page 392. If these symptoms occur treatment should be withdrawn.

Lithium + SSRIs ⚠

The concurrent use of lithium and SSRIs can be advantageous and uneventful, but various kinds of neurotoxicities have occurred. Isolated reports describe the development of symptoms similar to those of serotonin syndrome in patients taking lithium with fluoxetine, fluvoxamine, paroxetine and possibly citalopram. In addition, fluoxetine appears to have caused increases and decreases in serum lithium levels.

If lithium is used with an SSRI be alert for any evidence of toxicity (see serotonin syndrome, page 392). If these symptoms occur treatment should be withdrawn.

Lithium + Theophylline ❓

Serum lithium levels are reduced by 20 to 30% by theophylline, which in some cases caused patients to relapse. However, these fluctuations are considered small.

Consider monitoring lithium levels if theophylline or aminophylline is also given.

L

Lithium + Tricyclics ⚠

The concurrent use of a tricyclic antidepressant and lithium can be beneficial in some patients. However, some patients may rarely develop adverse effects, a few of them severe. Cases of neurotoxicity, serotonin syndrome and neuroleptic malignant syndrome have been reported.

> If both drugs are used be alert for any evidence of neurotoxicity (see under serotonin syndrome, page 392). Additive QT-prolonging effects also possible, see drugs that prolong the QT interval, page 237.

Lithium + Triptans ⚠

Case resports describe the development of serotonin syndrome in patients taking sumatriptan and lithium. This is in line with the known effects of lithium and the triptans.

> If lithium is used with any triptan be alert for any evidence of toxicity (see serotonin syndrome, page 392). If these symptoms occur treatment should be withdrawn.

Lithium + Venlafaxine ⚠

No clinical pharmacokinetic interaction appears to occur if venlafaxine is given with lithium. However, serotonin syndrome has been reported in some patients.

> If both drugs are used be alert for any evidence of neurotoxicity (see under serotonin syndrome, page 392).

Low-molecular-weight heparins

Low-molecular-weight heparins + NSAIDs ⚠

The use of an NSAIDs and a low-molecular-weight heparin increases bleeding time, although one study found that this did not adversely affect factors such as intra-operative blood loss and bruising in those undergoing hip replacement. Concurrent use is considered to be a contributing factor in the development of spinal or epidural haematoma occurring after lumbar puncture. Anticoagulants can exacerbate gastro-intestinal bleeding caused by NSAIDs.

> Concurrent use is not uncommon, but prescribers should be aware that there is an increased risk of bleeding and monitor appropriately.

Low-molecular-weight heparins + Ticlopidine ⚠

Concurrent use of ticlopidine with a low-molecular-weight heparin increases haemorrhagic risk.

If concurrent use is undertaken, there should be close clinical and laboratory monitoring.

Loperamide

Loperamide + **Protease inhibitors** ❓

Loperamide reduces the bioavailability of saquinavir by about 50%, and saquinavir increases the bioavailability of loperamide by about 40%. Tipranavir alone, and in combination with ritonavir, reduces the bioavailability and plasma levels of loperamide and its metabolites.

Monitor patients to ensure that saquinavir remains effective. The increase in loperamide bioavailability is not expected to be clinically significant in the case of saquinavir, but the decrease with tipranavir may be of relevance, and loperamide may become less effective.

Loperamide + **Quinidine** ⚠

Quinidine increases penetration of loperamide into the brain resulting in respiratory depression.

Be alert for the CNS adverse effects of loperamide if quinidine is given. If adverse effects are troublesome consider reducing the dose of loperamide.

L

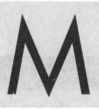

Macrolides

The macrolides are generally considered to be inhibitors of CYP3A4; however, it should be noted that they vary in the strength of their effect. Macrolides that are more potent inhibitors of CYP3A4 are likely to have greater effects on substrates of this isoenzyme, and therefore their use seems more likely to be associated with greater clinical consequences. Clarithromycin, erythromycin and telithromycin have the greatest effects, josamycin, midecamycin and roxithromycin have moderate effects, while azithromycin, dirithromycin and spiramycin only inhibit CYP3A4 to a small or clinically irrelevant extent. Note that clarithromycin is often predicted to have a more potent effect on CYP3A4 than erythromycin, but in many clinical studies this has not been shown to be the case, for example, see under phosphodiesterase type-5 inhibitors, page 311.

Macrolides + Mirtazapine ▲

The macrolides are predicted to inhibit the metabolism of mirtazapine by CYP3A4. Other CYP3A4 inhibitors (such as some azoles) have been shown to have this effect.

The manufacturers advise caution on concurrent use. Monitor for adverse effects (e.g. sedation). Note that the macrolides differ in their ability to inhibit CYP3A4, see above.

Macrolides + NNRTIs ▲

Delavirdine may increase clarithromycin exposure (AUC doubled), whereas efavirenz and nevirapine may reduce clarithromycin levels (by about 30 to 40%) and increase the levels of the active metabolite of clarithromycin. A neuropsychiatric reaction was attributed to the use of clarithromycin in a man taking nevirapine.

The manufacturer of delavirdine recommends that when clarithromycin is used concurrently the dose of clarithromycin should be reduced only in patients with renal impairment. Further study and experience of the use of efavirenz or nevirapine with clarithromycin is needed. Until then, caution is warranted.

Macrolides + **Opioids** ⚠

Macrolides are predicted to increase the levels of buprenorphine. Note that the macrolides differ in their ability to inhibit CYP3A4, see macrolides, page 310.

> It has been suggested that macrolides should be avoided when buprenorphine is used parenterally or sublingually as an analgesic. If concurrent use is essential in opioid addiction the manufacturers suggest that the buprenorphine dose should be halved. This interaction does not apply to azithromycin. Note that additive QT-prolonging effects may occur in predisposed individuals taking macrolides and high-dose methadone, see drugs that prolong the QT interval, page 237.

Macrolides + **Phenytoin**

Clarithromycin ❓

Preliminary evidence suggests that clarithromycin may raise serum phenytoin levels. Fosphenytoin, a prodrug of phenytoin, may interact similarly.

> The clinical importance of this interaction is unknown, but bear it in mind in case of an unexpected response to treatment. Indicators of phenytoin toxicity include blurred vision, nystagmus, ataxia or drowsiness. Note that erythromycin does not appear to interact.

Telithromycin ❌

Phenytoin possibly reduces telithromycin levels, which may reduce its efficacy. Fosphenytoin, a prodrug of phenytoin, may interact similarly.

> The manufacturers say to avoid telithromycin use during and up to 2 weeks after phenytoin treatment. Note that erythromycin does not appear to interact.

Macrolides + **Phosphodiesterase type-5 inhibitors**

Sildenafil or Vardenafil ⚠

Erythromycin and clarithromycin increase the AUC of sildenafil by 2- to 3-fold. It seems likely that telithromycin will interact similarly. Erythromycin increases the AUC of vardenafil 4-fold; it seems likely that clarithromycin and telithromycin will interact similarly.

> Dosing guidance is given as follows:
> Sildenafil for erectile dysfunction – consider a starting dose of 25 mg.
> Sildenafil for pulmonary hypertension – with erythromycin 20 mg twice daily erythromycin (UK advice. US states no dose reduction necessary). Recommended dose with clarithromycin or telithromycin 20 mg once daily. However, note that erythromycin had a greater effect than clarithromycin in the studies.
> Vardenafil – the dose of vardenafil should not exceed 5 mg in 24 hours with erythromycin (UK and US). The dose of vardenafil should not exceed 2.5 mg in 24 hours with clarithromycin (US).

Tadalafil ❓

Erythromycin and clarithromycin (and therefore probably telithromycin) are predicted to raise tadalafil levels by inhibiting its metabolism by CYP3A4. This effect has

M

been seen with other inhibitors of CYP3A4 (up to 4-fold rise with ketoconazole). Other macrolides have less effect on CYP3A4, see macrolides, page 310, and therefore seem less likely to interact.

The adverse effects of tadalafil may be increased in some patients. The manufacturers advise caution.

Macrolides + Protease inhibitors

Azithromycin with Nelfinavir ⚠

The pharmacokinetics of nelfinavir are minimally affected by azithromycin, but the AUC and maximum serum levels of azithromycin are roughly doubled by nelfinavir.

The clinical significance of this interaction has not been established. Monitor for increased effects and adverse effects of azithromycin.

Clarithromycin with Atazanavir ⚠

Atazanavir almost doubled the AUC of clarithromycin, and reduced the AUC of its active metabolite by 70%, while clarithromycin increased the AUC of atazanavir by 28%.

Reducing the dose of clarithromycin to avoid high levels may result in subtherapeutic levels of the active metabolite. The US manufacturer says that, other than for *Mycobacterium avium* complex infections, an alternative to clarithromycin should be considered. If the combination is used they suggest a 50% dose reduction for the clarithromycin. The UK manufacturer recommends caution.

Clarithromycin with Darunavir ❓

Clarithromycin levels were increased by 174%, but the level of the active metabolite were undetectable when darunavir was also given.

Clarithromycin dosage reductions are only expected to be needed for those with renal impairment.

Clarithromycin with Ritonavir ❓

Although no clinically significant effects were noted when clarithromycin was given with ritonavir, the clarithromycin became more dependent on renal clearance and so it was suggested that there may be a significant interaction in patients with renal failure.

The manufacturers of ritonavir and clarithromycin suggest that no dosage reductions should be needed in those with normal renal function, but they recommend reductions for those with reduced creatinine clearances. They also advise avoidance of clarithromycin dosages exceeding 1 g daily.

Clarithromycin with Saquinavir ✔

Clarithromycin raises saquinavir levels by about 180%, and saquinavir raises clarithromycin levels by 40%. However, the only data available is with the *soft capsules*.

M

For ritonavir boosted regimens, see ritonavir, above.

Clarithromycin with Tipranavir ❓

Clarithromycin levels were increased by about 70%, but the levels of the active metabolite were undetectable when given tipranavir was given. Tipranavir minimum levels were more than doubled.

For ritonavir boosted regimens, see ritonavir, above.

Erythromycin with Amprenavir or Fosamprenavir ⚠

The manufacturers say that both amprenavir and erythromycin levels may be increased on concurrent use. Fosamprenavir is predicted to interact similarly.

Monitor the outcome carefully. Advise patients to be alert for erythromycin and amprenavir or fosamprenavir adverse effects (e.g. gastrointestinal effects, tremors).

Erythromycin with Ritonavir ⚠

The manufacturers predict that ritonavir will greatly elevate erythromycin levels.

Concurrent use should not be undertaken unless the benefits outweigh the risks. Monitor for erythromycin adverse effects (e.g. gastrointestinal effects). Note that high levels of erythromycin can cause temporary hearing loss.

Telithromycin with Ritonavir ⚠

Ketoconazole increases the AUC of telithromycin 2-fold. Because ritonavir is a more potent enzyme inhibitor than ketoconazole the manufacturers predict that the exposure to telithromycin may be greater than 2-fold in the presence of ritonavir.

The manufacturers advise caution on concurrent use. Monitor for telithromycin adverse effects (such as diarrhoea, dizziness and headache).

Macrolides + **Proton pump inhibitors** ✔

Clarithromycin almost doubles the serum levels of esomeprazole, lansoprazole and omeprazole. A small rise in the serum levels of clarithromycin also occurs, which may be therapeutically useful. Some very limited evidence indicates that erythromycin causes a larger rise in serum omeprazole levels, without improving its gastric acid lowering effect.

Given the wide use of *Helicobacter pylori* eradication regimens containing these drugs it seems unlikely that this interaction is detrimental.

Macrolides + **Reboxetine** ✖

The manufacturers predict that macrolides will decrease the clearance of reboxetine by inhibiting CYP3A4. Other CYP3A4 inhibitors have been shown to have this effect.

The manufacturers recommend that macrolides (they specifically name erythromycin) should not be given with reboxetine. Note that the macrolides differ in their ability to inhibit CYP3A4, see macrolides, page 310.

M

Macrolides + **Rifabutin**

Azithromycin ⚠

Rifabutin and azithromycin seem not to affect the serum levels of each other, but in one study a very high incidence of neutropenia and leucopenia was seen.

> Until more information is available it would seem wise to monitor white cell counts during concurrent use.

Clarithromycin ⚠

Rifabutin markedly reduces the serum levels of clarithromycin, and clarithromycin increases the serum levels of rifabutin. There is an increased risk of uveitis with the combination.

> Monitor the outcome of concurrent use to ensure treatment is effective. Because of the increased risk of uveitis the CSM in the UK says that consideration should be given to reducing the dosage of rifabutin to 300 mg daily. If uveitis occurs the CSM recommends that rifabutin should be stopped and the patient should be referred to an ophthalmologist.

Macrolides + **Rifampicin (Rifampin)**

Clarithromycin ⚠

Limited evidence suggests that rifampicin markedly reduces the serum levels of clarithromycin (90% in one study), but it is not clear whether this results in treatment failure.

> Monitor the outcome of concurrent use to ensure treatment is effective.

Telithromycin ✖

Rifampicin reduces the AUC and maximum serum levels of telithromycin by 86% and 79% respectively.

> The UK manufacturers recommend that telithromycin should not be given during and for 2 weeks after the use of rifampicin.

Macrolides + **Rimonabant** ⚠

Ketoconazole doubles the AUC of rimonabant. Other drugs that are potent inhibitors of CYP3A4, such as clarithromycin and telithromycin, are predicted to interact similarly. Note that the macrolides differ in their ability to inhibit CYP3A4, see macrolides, page 310.

> The manufacturers of rimonabant recommend caution. Monitor for signs of increased rimonabant adverse effects.

M

Macrolides + Sirolimus ❌

Two patients had large elevations in their sirolimus levels following the addition of erythromycin.

> This interaction is in line with the manufacturer's prediction. They also predict that other inhibitors of CYP3A4 (they name clarithromycin and telithromycin) will interact similarly, and should be avoided. Note that the macrolides differ in their ability to inhibit CYP3A4, see macrolides, page 310. Other macrolides seem less likely to interact.

Macrolides + Statins

Atorvastatin ⚠️

Clarithromycin and erythromycin moderately raise the levels of atorvastatin. Note that the macrolides differ in their ability to inhibit CYP3A4, see macrolides, page 310; other macrolides may interact similarly.

> If concurrent use is necessary it would seem wise to warn the patient to be on the look out for symptoms of myopathy (e.g. muscle pain or weakness). Be especially cautious in patients also taking other drugs that interact with statins (e.g. fibrates and diltiazem). Note that the manufacturers of telithromycin suggest avoiding concurrent use (see guidance under simvastatin below).

Simvastatin or Lovastatin ❌

The levels of simvastatin and lovastatin are increased by clarithromycin, erythromycin, telithromycin and other macrolides that inhibit CYP3A4 (see macrolides, page 310). Rhabdomyolysis has been seen.

> It has been recommended that simvastatin and lovastatin should be stopped during short courses of these macrolides.

Other statins ❓

No interaction of note would be expected between fluvastatin, pravastatin or rosuvastatin and macrolides.

> Although no interaction would generally be expected to occur note that there have been case reports of rhabdomyolysis in patients taking statin/macrolide combinations that have been predicted not to interact. Any patient taking a statin should be advised to look out for symptoms of myopathy (e.g. muscle pain or weakness). It may be prudent to reinforce this when macrolides are given.

Macrolides + Tacrolimus ⚠️

Several patients have had marked increases in serum tacrolimus levels accompanied by evidence of renal toxicity when they also took erythromycin. The same interaction has been seen in patients given clarithromycin, and is predicted with josamycin.

> Tacrolimus levels and/or effects (e.g. on renal function) should be monitored as a matter of routine, but it may be prudent to increase monitoring if these macrolides are started or stopped. Note that the macrolides differ in their ability to inhibit

M

CYP3A4, see macrolides, page 310. Azithromycin has been predicted not to interact and in general case reports seem to confirm this, although one patient has experienced increased tacrolimus levels when also taking azithromycin.

Macrolides + **Theophylline**

Erythromycin

Theophylline levels can be increased by erythromycin and toxicity may develop. The onset may be delayed for 2 to 7 days. Erythromycin levels may be reduced by theophylline.

Monitor theophylline levels after 48 hours and adjust the dose accordingly. Monitor the effects of erythromycin to ensure that they are adequate.

Other macrolides ❓

Azithromycin, clarithromycin, dirithromycin, josamycin, midecamycin, rokitamycin, spiramycin, and telithromycin normally only cause modest changes in theophylline levels or do not interact at all. However, there are unexplained and isolated case reports of theophylline toxicity with josamycin and clarithromycin. Roxithromycin usually has no relevant interaction but a significant increase in theophylline levels was seen in one study.

The situation with roxithromycin is uncertain since only one study has suggested an interaction, but it would be prudent to be alert for the need to reduce the theophylline dosage. It would also seem prudent to monitor the outcome of the use of the other macrolides because a few patients, especially those with theophylline levels at the high end of the therapeutic range, may need some small theophylline dosage adjustments. In the case of azithromycin, care should be taken in adjusting the dose based on theophylline levels taken after about 5 days of concurrent use, as they may only be a reflection of a transient drop. In addition, acute infection *per se* may alter theophylline pharmacokinetics.

Macrolides + **Tolterodine** ⚠

The manufacturers of tolterodine warn that potent CYP3A4 inhibitors (they name clarithromycin and erythromycin) increase the risk of tolterodine toxicity. Other macrolides may also interact, see macrolides, page 310.

Based on the interactions of other CYP3A4 inhibitors with tolterodine it may be prudent to monitor for adverse effects and to bear in mind the possibility of an interaction if antimuscarinic effects (dry mouth, constipation, drowsiness) are increased. However, note that the UK manufacturers advise avoiding concurrent use, whereas the US manufacturers suggest reducing the tolterodine dose to 1 mg twice daily.

Macrolides + **Toremifene** ⚠

Based on theoretical considerations, the manufacturers advise care when toremifene is given with inhibitors of CYP3A such as the macrolides (they specifically name erythromycin, see macrolides, page 310, for more detail).

It would seem prudent to monitor for toremifene adverse effects (e.g. hot flushes, uterine bleeding, fatigue, nausea, dizziness) on concurrent use with the macrolides.

Macrolides + Trazodone ⚠

Clarithromycin impaired the clearance of trazodone and enhanced its sedative effects in healthy subjects.

The UK manufacturer of trazodone recommends that a lower dose of trazodone should be considered if it is given with a CYP3A4 inhibitor such as erythromycin, but that concurrent use should be avoided where possible. Note that other macrolides may also interact, see macrolides, page 310.

Macrolides + Triptans ⊗

Erythromycin increased the maximum serum levels of eletriptan 2-fold and the AUC 3.6-fold in one study.

The manufacturers suggest that concurrent use of erythromycin and other macrolide inhibitors of CYP3A4 (such as clarithromycin and telithromycin) should be avoided. Other macrolides seem less likely to interact, see macrolides, page 310.

Macrolides + Warfarin and other oral anticoagulants ⚠

A marked increase in the effects of warfarin, sometimes accompanied by bleeding, has been seen in a small number of patients also given azithromycin, clarithromycin, erythromycin, or roxithromycin, but most patients seem unlikely to develop a clinically important interaction. This interaction has also been seen in a few patients taking acenocoumarol or phenprocoumon with either clarithromycin, erythromycin, or roxithromycin.

Very few patients appear to have a clinically significant interaction. Any interaction appears to develop over the first 7 days (so note interactions may occur after an antibacterial treatment course has finished). It has been suggested that those taking relatively low doses of anticoagulant are most at risk. Consider increasing the frequency of INR monitoring.

Macrolides + Zafirlukast ✓

Erythromycin reduces the mean plasma levels of zafirlukast by about 40%, which may reduce its anti-asthma effects.

If these drugs are given concurrently, be alert for a reduced response.

M

MAO-B inhibitors

MAO-B inhibitors + MAOIs ⚠

Severe hypotension has been seen in patients given selegiline with MAOIs.

Avoid concurrent use wherever possible. If both drugs are used, monitor initial doses very carefully so hypotension can be rapidly managed. Note that one of the manufacturers of selegiline actually contraindicates concurrent use. The manufacturers of rasagiline contraindicate concurrent use, presumably because of the way selegiline interacts.

MAO-B inhibitors + Moclobemide ⚠

The combination of an MAO-A inhibitor (moclobemide) with an MAO-B inhibitor (selegiline or rasagiline) causes MAO inhibition similar to that seen with the non-selective MAOIs.

Patients should be given the same dietary restrictions about tyramine-rich foods and drinks (cheese, some wines and beers, etc.), which relate to the non-selective MAOIs, although the risks are less. See food, page 256. It is suggested that if selegiline is replaced by moclobemide, the dietary restrictions can be relaxed after a wash-out period of about 2 weeks. If switching from moclobemide to selegiline, a wash-out period of 1 to 2 days is sufficient. Similar advice would seem prudent with rasagiline. Note that all of the interactions of the non-selective MAOIs, are likely to apply to patients taking this combination.

MAO-B inhibitors + Nasal decongestants ✗

An isolated report describes a hypertensive crisis, which was attributed to an interaction between selegiline, ephedrine, and maprotiline. Rasagiline is expected to interact like selegiline.

In general, if selegiline is used at recommended doses it is selective for MAO-B and no restrictions are required. Nevertheless, this report suggests that, rarely, interactions are still possible, and some consider that patients taking selegiline should try to avoid pseudoephedrine. The manufacturers of rasagiline recommend against concurrent use of nasal decongestants that are indirectly-acting sympathomimetics, such as ephedrine and pseudoephedrine, due to the risk of hypertensive crises.

MAO-B inhibitors + Opioids ✗

A case report describes a patient who fluctuated between stupor and agitation, and developed muscle rigidity, sweating and a raised temperature when given pethidine (meperidine) with selegiline. This case is similar to cases reported with the older non-selective MAOIs.

On the basis of this evidence the manufacturers of selegiline contraindicate concurrent use with pethidine (meperidine). The manufacturers of rasagiline similarly contraindicate pethidine (meperidine), and also suggest that pethidine

M

(meperidine) should be avoided in the 14 days after rasagiline has been stopped. One manufacturer of selegiline also cautions tramadol, which seems prudent, but another contraindicates concurrent use with all opioids, which is probably unnecessary, based on the evidence with non-selective MAOIs.

MAO-B inhibitors + Quinolones ⚠

Ciprofloxacin increases the AUC of rasagiline by 83%.

The clinical relevance of this pharmacokinetic interaction has not been assessed. The manufacturers suggest that caution is warranted on concurrent use. Other quinolones may also interact, see quinolones, page 382.

MAO-B inhibitors + SSRIs ✖

Although safe concurrent use of selegiline and SSRIs has been reported in a number of patients, there are also documented cases of serotonin syndrome, page 392. Rasagiline is expected to interact similarly.

The manufacturers of rasagiline recommend avoiding combined use with fluoxetine and fluvoxamine. Rasagiline should not be started for 5 weeks after stopping fluoxetine or 2 weeks after starting fluvoxamine, and fluoxetine should not be started for 2 weeks after stopping rasagiline. They recommend caution with other SSRI antidepressants because of this risk. The manufacturers of selegiline contraindicate the concurrent use of SSRIs. In addition, selegiline should not be started for 5 weeks after stopping fluoxetine, 2 weeks after stopping sertraline, and one week after stopping other SSRIs. SSRIs should not be started for 2 weeks after stopping selegiline.

MAO-B inhibitors + Tricyclics ⚠

Rare cases of serotonin syndrome, page 392, and other CNS disturbances have been seen when selegiline is given with tricyclics. Rasagiline is expected to interact similarly.

If the combination is used the outcome should be well monitored, but the likelihood of problems seems to be small. Nevertheless, some manufacturers of selegiline advise avoiding the combination of tricyclic antidepressants and selegiline. The manufacturers of rasagiline advise caution if it is given with antidepressants.

MAO-B inhibitors + Venlafaxine ⚠

Serotonin syndrome, page 392, has been reported when selegiline was given with venlafaxine. This is in line with the manufacturers' prediction and the way that other serotonergic drugs behave with selegiline. Rasagiline is expected to interact similarly.

The manufacturers of selegiline suggest that the concurrent use of venlafaxine should be avoided. A 2-week washout period would seem appropriate when switching from one of these drugs to the other. The manufacturers of rasagiline advise caution on the concurrent use of antidepressants.

M

MAOIs

This section covers the non-selective MAOIs. Other drugs with MAO-inhibitory properties, such as linezolid, moclobemide, selegiline, and rasagiline, are discussed in their own sections.

MAOIs + Maprotiline ⊗

Toxic and sometimes fatal reactions (similar to or the same as serotonin syndrome, page 392) have very occasionally occurred in patients taking both MAOIs and *tricyclic antidepressants*. Maprotiline would be expected to interact similarly.

Avoid concurrent use. Maprotiline should not be started for 2 weeks after treatment with MAOIs has been stopped and an MAOI should not be started until at least 7 to 14 days after maprotiline has been stopped. If concurrent use is thought necessary it has been suggested that it should only be undertaken by those well aware of the problems and who can undertake adequate supervision.

MAOIs + Methyldopa ⊗

Theoretically hypertension may occur when non-selective MAOIs are taken with methyldopa, although additive blood-pressure lowering effects are also a possibility. The concurrent use of antidepressant MAOIs and methyldopa may not be desirable because methyldopa can sometimes cause depression.

It would seem prudent to avoid the combination wherever possible.

MAOIs + Mianserin ⊗

Toxic and sometimes fatal reactions (similar to or the same as serotonin syndrome, page 392) have very occasionally occurred in patients taking both MAOIs and *tricyclic antidepressants*. Case reports suggest that mianserin can interact similarly.

Avoid concurrent use. Mianserin should not be started for 2 weeks after treatment with MAOIs has been stopped and an MAOI should not be started until at least 7 to 14 days after mianserin has been stopped. If concurrent use is thought necessary it has been suggested that it should only be undertaken by those well aware of the problems and who can undertake adequate supervision.

MAOIs + Mirtazapine ⊗

No data seem to be available about the concurrent use of mirtazapine with MAOIs.

The manufacturers say that the concurrent use of mirtazapine and the MAOIs should be avoided both during and within 2 weeks of stopping treatment. This is a general warning that most of the manufacturers of antidepressants issue.

MAOIs + Nasal decongestants ❌

The concurrent use of a number of nasal decongestants with indirect sympathomimetic actions, such as ephedrine, phenylpropanolamine, and pseudoephedrine, and non-selective MAOIs can result in a potentially fatal hypertensive crisis.

Avoid concurrent use. These amines are found in many proprietary cough, cold and influenza preparations, or are used as appetite suppressants. Counsel patients accordingly.

MAOIs + Nefopam ❌

Nefopam has sympathomimetic activity, which theoretically may cause severe hypertension in those taking MAOIs.

Concurrent use should be avoided. With other drugs that interact in the manner predicted it is usually advised that concurrent use should also be avoided for 2 weeks after the MAOI has been stopped.

MAOIs + Opioids ❌

The concurrent use of pethidine (meperidine) and an MAOI has resulted in a serious and potentially life-threatening reaction in several patients. Excitement, muscle rigidity, hyperpyrexia, flushing, sweating and unconsciousness can occur very rapidly. Respiratory depression and hypertension or hypotension have also been seen. Similar interactions have been seen if tramadol is taken with MAOIs. Isolated cases of adverse reactions (e.g. hypertension, hypotension, hyperthermia and tachycardia) have been reported after fentanyl or morphine were given to patients taking MAOIs.

The interaction with pethidine is serious and potentially fatal, but the incidence is probably quite low. It may therefore be an idiosyncratic reaction. Nevertheless, it would be imprudent to give pethidine (meperidine) to any patient taking an MAOI. Bear in mind that the non-selective MAOIs are all essentially irreversible so that an interaction is possible for many days after their withdrawal (at least 2 weeks is the official advice). The manufacturers of tramadol contraindicate its use with MAOIs because of the risks of this reaction. Evidence for an interaction between other opioids and MAOIs is limited, and some of the cases appear to represent a different type of reaction to that seen with pethidine. Indeed, with some opioids there is evidence of safe concurrent use. Nevertheless, the manufacturers of many opioids contraindicate the use of MAOIs. These include alfentanil, codeine, diamorphine, fentanyl, hydromorphone, methadone, and oxycodone.

MAOIs + Phenobarbital ❓

Although the MAOIs can enhance and prolong the activity of barbiturates in *animals*, only a few isolated cases of adverse responses attributed to an interaction have been described in man.

There is no well-documented evidence showing that concurrent use should be avoided, although some caution is clearly appropriate because of the case reports.

M

MAOIs + **Reboxetine** ⊗

No data seem to be available about the concurrent use of reboxetine with MAOIs. However, the manufacturers predict that a hypertensive reaction is possible.

Concurrent use should be avoided. With other drugs that interact in the manner predicted it is usually advised that concurrent use should also be avoided for 2 weeks after the MAOI has been stopped.

MAOIs + **Salbutamol (Albuterol) and related bronchodilators** ❓

An isolated case of tachycardia and apprehension has also been described after an asthmatic taking phenelzine also took salbutamol (albuterol).

This appears to be isolated cases, and are possibly not of general importance. Bear them it mind in the event of an unexpected response to treatment.

MAOIs + **Sibutramine** ⊗

Sibutramine inhibits serotonin reuptake, and because the serious serotonin syndrome, page 392, can occur when MAOIs and SSRIs are used together, concurrent use is contraindicated.

The manufacturers state that 14 days should elapse between stopping either drug and starting the other.

MAOIs + **SSRIs** ⊗

A number of case reports describe serotonin syndrome, page 392, in patients given SSRIs with MAOIs: some have been fatal.

Direct information about the interaction between MAOIs and SSRIs is limited, and given that concurrent use is contraindicated, further reports seem unlikely. The manufacturers say that citalopram, escitalopram, fluvoxamine, paroxetine or sertraline should not be given within 14 days of discontinuing an irreversible MAOI nor should any type of MAOI be added until sertraline has been stopped for 14 days, or citalopram, escitalopram, fluvoxamine or paroxetine have been stopped for 7 days, (14 days in the US). The manufacturers of fluoxetine recommend that at least 5 weeks should elapse between stopping the fluoxetine and starting the MAOI and 2 weeks between stopping an MAOI and starting fluoxetine. A longer interval is suggested if long-term or high-dose fluoxetine has been used.

MAOIs + **Trazodone** ⊗

Toxic and sometimes fatal reactions (similar to or the same as serotonin syndrome, page 392) have very occasionally occurred in patients taking both MAOIs and *tricyclic antidepressants*. A case report suggests that trazodone may interact similarly.

Trazodone should not be started for 2 weeks after treatment with MAOIs has been

M

stopped, and an MAOI should not be started until 1 week after trazodone has been stopped. If concurrent use is thought necessary it has been suggested that it should only be undertaken by those well aware of the problems and who can undertake adequate supervision. The US manufacturers suggest starting at low doses, and increasing cautiously.

MAOIs + Tricyclics ⊗

Because of the very toxic and sometimes fatal reactions (similar to or the same as serotonin syndrome, page 392) that have very occasionally occurred in patients taking both MAOIs and tricyclic antidepressants, concurrent use is regarded as contra-indicated.

Avoid concurrent use. Tricyclic antidepressants should not be started for 2 weeks after treatment with MAOIs has been stopped (3 weeks if starting clomipramine or imipramine), and an MAOI should not be started until at least 7 to 14 days after a tricyclic or related antidepressant has been stopped (3 weeks in the case of clomipramine or imipramine). If concurrent use is thought necessary it has been suggested that it should only be undertaken by those well aware of the problems and who can undertake adequate supervision.

MAOIs + Triptans ⚠

The manufacturers of rizatriptan and sumatriptan contraindicate the concurrent use of MAOIs. The US manufacturer contraindicates the use of zolmitriptan both during, and for 2 weeks after, the use of *moclobemide*, whereas the UK manufacturer restricts the dose of zolmitriptan to 5 mg in 24 hours. In the absence of any direct information it would seem prudent to apply these warnings to the use of non-selective MAOIs.

Avoid use during and for 2 weeks after stopping an MAOI or restrict the dose of zolmitriptan.

MAOIs + Tryptophan ⚠

A number of patients have developed severe behavioural and neurological signs of toxicity (some similar to serotonin syndrome, page 392) after taking MAOIs with tryptophan, and fatalities have occurred.

It has been recommended that patients taking MAOIs should start treatment with a low dose of tryptophan (500 mg). This should be gradually increased while monitoring the patient for changes suggesting hypomania, and neurological changes, including ocular oscillations and upper motor neurone signs.

MAOIs + Venlafaxine ⊗

Serious and potentially life-threatening reactions (serotonin syndrome, page 392) can develop if venlafaxine and non-selective, irreversible MAOIs are given concurrently, or even sequentially if insufficient time is left in between.

The manufacturers of venlafaxine recommend that one week should elapse

M

between stopping the venlafaxine and starting an MAOI, and 2 weeks between stopping an MAOI and starting venlafaxine.

Maprotiline

Maprotiline + Moclobemide ❌

A number of studies suggest that no interaction, or only a moderate non-significant rise in *tricyclic antidepressant* levels occurs when they are given with moclobemide. However, several case reports describe serotonin syndrome, page 392, in patients receiving the combination. It seems likely that maprotiline will interact similarly.

Concurrent use should be avoided. Moclobemide has a short duration of action so no treatment free period is required before starting a tricyclic or related antidepressant. However, some recommend waiting 24 hours. Moclobemide should not be started until at least one week after a tricyclic or related antidepressant has been stopped.

Mebendazole

Mebendazole + Phenobarbital ⚠

Carbamazepine lowers the plasma levels of mebendazole. Phenobarbital and primidone are expected to interact similarly.

When treating systemic worm infections it may be necessary to increase the mebendazole dosage in patients taking phenobarbital or primidone. Monitor the outcome of concurrent use. This interaction is of no importance when mebendazole is used for intestinal worm infections where its action is a local effect on the worms in the gut.

Mebendazole + Phenytoin ⚠

Phenytoin lowers the plasma levels of mebendazole. Fosphenytoin is expected to interact similarly.

When treating systemic worm infections it may be necessary to increase the mebendazole dosage in patients taking phenytoin or fosphenytoin. Monitor the outcome of concurrent use. This interaction is of no importance when mebendazole is used for intestinal worm infections where its action is a local effect on the worms in the gut.

M

Medroxyprogesterone

For the interactions of medroxyprogesterone used as a contraceptive, see contraceptives, page 199.

Medroxyprogesterone + Warfarin and other oral anticoagulants ⚠

High-dose medroxyprogesterone acetate (1 g daily) increases the half-life and reduces the clearance of warfarin by about 70% and 35%, respectively.

Monitor the effect of concurrent use on the anticoagulant response and adjust the warfarin dose as necessary.

Mefloquine

Mefloquine + Rifampicin (Rifampicin) ✖

Rifampicin reduces the AUC of mefloquine by almost 70%.

The clinical relevance of this is uncertain, but some suggest that simultaneous use should be avoided to prevent treatment failure and the risk of *Plasmodium falciparum* resistance to mefloquine. Until more is known, this would seem a sensible precaution.

Mefloquine + Warfarin and other oral anticoagulants ⚠

The effects of warfarin and an unnamed coumarin were increased in two patients who took mefloquine.

Patients taking mefloquine should have their warfarin effects checked before travel to allow for monitoring of any changes in anticoagulant effects.

Meropenem

Meropenem + Probenecid ⚠

Probenecid increases the AUC of meropenem by about 50%.

The manufacturers say that because the potency and duration of meropenem are adequate without probenecid, they do not recommend concurrent use.

M

Meropenem + **Valproate** ⚠

Meropenem and other carbapenems appear to dramatically and rapidly reduce valproate levels resulting, in some cases, in increased seizure frequency.

It would be prudent to monitor valproate levels in any patient given carbapenems. The valproate dosage may need to be increased. Consider using another antibacterial, or an alternative to valproate. Limited evidence suggests that carbamazepine and phenytoin are not affected.

Methotrexate

Methotrexate + **Neomycin** ✅

The gastrointestinal absorption of methotrexate can be reduced by neomycin.

The significance of this interaction is unclear, but bear it in mind in case of an unexpected response to treatment.

Methotrexate + **NSAIDs** ⚠

Increased methotrexate toxicity, sometimes life-threatening, has been seen in a few patients also taking an NSAID, whereas other patients have taken NSAIDs with methotrexate uneventfully. The mechanism of this interaction suggests that all NSAIDs have the potential to interact similarly. The pharmacokinetics of methotrexate can also be changed by some NSAIDs.

Concurrent use need not be avoided but close monitoring is necessary. The risk appears to be lowest in those taking low-dose methotrexate for psoriasis or rheumatoid arthritis, with normal renal function. Patients must be counselled regarding non-prescription NSAIDs.

Methotrexate + **Penicillins** ⚠

Reduced clearance and acute methotrexate toxicity has been attributed to the concurrent use of various penicillins (amoxicillin, benzylpenicillin, carbenicillin, dicloxacillin, flucloxacillin, mezlocillin, oxacillin, phenoxymethylpenicillin, piperacillin, and ticarcillin) in a small number of case reports.

Serious interactions between methotrexate and penicillins are uncommon. Risk factors are as yet unknown and even patients taking low doses of methotrexate have been affected. Given the current evidence monitoring is advisable. One recommendation is to carry out twice-weekly platelet and white cell counts for 2 weeks initially, with the measurement of methotrexate levels if toxicity is suspected.

M

Methotrexate + **Probenecid** ⚠️

Probenecid markedly increases serum methotrexate levels (3- to 4-fold).

A marked increase in both the therapeutic and toxic effects of methotrexate can occur, apparently even with low doses if other risk factors are present (e.g. renal impairment, concurrent NSAIDs). Anticipate the need to reduce the dosage of the methotrexate and monitor the effects well if probenecid is also taken. If this is not possible, avoid the combination.

Methotrexate + **Proton pump inhibitors** ❓

Two reports describe a reduction in the excretion of methotrexate in 2 patients taking omeprazole. However, similar elevations in methotrexate levels in another patient taking omeprazole were independent of omeprazole use. One patient had myalgia and elevated 7-hydroxymethotrexate levels when treated with methotrexate and pantoprazole, and in 3 patients lansoprazole appeared to reduce methotrexate clearance and increase its levels.

The general significance of this interaction is unclear, but until more is known it would be prudent to bear this interaction in mind as a potential cause of methotrexate toxicity.

Methotrexate + **Quinolones** ❓

A report describes methotrexate toxicity in 2 patients also taking ciprofloxacin.

Full blood count should be monitored when methotrexate is used. If any abnormalities arise, consider this interaction as a possible cause.

Methotrexate + **Tetracyclines** ❓

Two case reports describe the development of methotrexate toxicity in patients also taking tetracycline or doxycycline.

The significance of this interaction is unclear, but bear it in mind in case of an unexpected response to treatment.

Methotrexate + **Theophylline** ⚠️

In one study theophylline clearance was reduced by 19% after 6 weeks of treatment with intramuscular methotrexate 15 mg weekly. A few patients complained of nausea and the theophylline dosage had to be reduced in one.

The clinical significance of this interaction is unclear as reductions of this magnitude are rarely significant. It seems most likely to affect those patients with theophylline levels at the top of the therapeutic range.

M

Methotrexate + Trimethoprim ⚠

The concurrent use of low-dose methotrexate and co-trimoxazole or trimethoprim has resulted in several cases of severe bone marrow depression, some of which were fatal.

> Full blood count should be monitored when methotrexate is used. If any abnormalities arise, consider this interaction as a possible cause.

Methotrexate + Vaccines ⚠

The immune response of the body is suppressed by cytotoxic antineoplastics. The effectiveness of vaccines may be poor and generalised infection may occur in patients immunised with live vaccines. In one study the antibody response to pneumococcal vaccination was reduced by 60% in patients receiving antineoplastics, and suboptimal responses to influenza and measles vaccines have been reported.

> Extreme care should be taken when considering vaccinating immunosuppressed patients, especially with live vaccines, which should generally be avoided. Monitor the immune response to other types of vaccine. Consider whether vaccination can be carried out prior to or following methotrexate use.

Methylphenidate

Methylphenidate + Phenytoin ❓

Raised serum phenytoin levels and phenytoin toxicity have been seen in 3 patients also given methylphenidate, but it is an uncommon reaction and two studies suggest that most patients do not experience an interaction.

> This interaction is unlikely to be generally significant, but bear it in mind in case of an unexpected response to treatment. Indicators of phenytoin toxicity include blurred vision, nystagmus, ataxia or drowsiness.

Methylphenidate + SSRIs ❓

Isolated reports describe delirium in one patient and a seizure in another when methylphenidate was taken with sertraline.

> The clinical significance of this interaction is unknown, but bear it in mind in case of an unexpected response to treatment. Note that the use of methylphenidate with SSRIs (fluoxetine, paroxetine, sertraline) has been reported to be beneficial and without significant adverse effects.

Methylphenidate + Tricyclics ❓

Several studies have reported an increase in imipramine or desipramine levels following the addition of methylphenidate, which takes several days to occur, and several days to wear off. Isolated cases of behavioural problems have been seen, but a large review indicates the absence of a clinically significant interaction.

This interaction is of unknown importance, but tricyclic antidepressant toxicity could theoretically occur. Bear this in mind in case of an unexpected response to treatment.

Metoclopramide

Metoclopramide + Paracetamol (Acetaminophen) ✓

Metoclopramide increases the rate of absorption of paracetamol and raises its maximum plasma levels.

As the total amount of paracetamol absorbed was unchanged this interaction is unlikely to be clinically significant, although a more rapid onset of action may be advantageous.

Metoclopramide + SSRIs ❓

Case reports describe serotonin syndrome, page 392, in patients taking SSRIs with metoclopramide. Extrapyramidal symptoms have occurred in patients given fluoxetine, fluvoxamine or sertraline with metoclopramide.

Information seems to be limited to these reports, but they highlight the fact that care should be taken if two drugs with the potential to cause the same adverse effects are used together. Some monitoring for increased adverse effects would be advisable if an SSRI is taken with metoclopramide.

Metronidazole

Metronidazole + Phenobarbital ⚠

Phenobarbital markedly increases the metabolism of metronidazole, and treatment failure as a result of this interaction has been reported in both adults and children. Other barbiturates are expected to interact similarly.

Monitor the effects of concurrent use and anticipate the need to increase the metronidazole dosage by 2- to 3-fold.

Metronidazole + Phenytoin ❓

A small and usually clinically unimportant rise in phenytoin levels may occur if metronidazole is given with phenytoin, although a few patients have developed phenytoin toxicity. Fosphenytoin, a prodrug of phenytoin, may interact similarly.

M

This interaction is unlikely to be generally significant, but bear it in mind in case of an unexpected response to treatment. Indicators of phenytoin toxicity include blurred vision, nystagmus, ataxia or drowsiness.

Metronidazole + **Warfarin and other oral anticoagulants** ⚠

The anticoagulant effects of warfarin are markedly increased by metronidazole and bleeding has been seen.

Monitor the INR when both drugs are used and adjust the warfarin dose accordingly. Nothing seems to be documented about other anticoagulants but it would be prudent to expect the coumarins to behave similarly.

Mexiletine

Mexiletine + **Opioids** ⚠

The absorption of mexiletine is reduced in patients following a myocardial infarction, and very markedly reduced and delayed if opioids (diamorphine or morphine) are given concurrently.

The delay and reduction in the absorption would seem to limit the value of oral mexiletine during the first few hours after a myocardial infarction, particularly if opioid analgesics are used. The manufacturer suggests that a higher loading dose of oral mexiletine may be preferable in this situation. Alternatively, an intravenous dose of mexiletine may be given.

Mexiletine + **Phenytoin** ⚠

Phenytoin halves the AUC of mexiletine. Fosphenytoin, a prodrug of phenytoin, may interact similarly.

It seems likely that the fall in mexiletine levels will be clinically important in at least some individuals. Monitor for mexiletine efficacy, and where possible monitor mexiletine levels. Raise the dosage if necessary.

Mexiletine + **Rifampicin (Rifampin)** ⚠

The clearance of mexiletine is increased by rifampicin. The mexiletine AUC was reduced by 40% in one study.

It seems likely that the fall in mexiletine levels will be clinically important in some individuals. Monitor for mexiletine efficacy, and where possible monitor mexiletine levels. Raise the dosage if necessary.

M

Mexiletine + SSRIs ❓

Studies in patients and *in vitro* investigations have shown that fluoxetine and its metabolite, norfluoxetine, inhibit CYP2D6, the enzyme that metabolises mexiletine. Paroxetine would be expected to interact similarly. Fluvoxamine increases the AUC of mexiletine by 55% due to its effects on CYP1A2.

There appear to be no reported interactions with fluoxetine, but given the way it interacts with other CYP2D6 substrates it would seem prudent to be alert for increased and prolonged effects if it is given with mexiletine. Similar caution seems warranted with fluvoxamine.

Mexiletine + Terbinafine ⚠

In vitro studies suggest that terbinafine is an inhibitor of CYP2D6. It may therefore be expected to increase the plasma levels of other drugs that are substrates of this enzyme, such as mexiletine.

Until more is known it would seem wise to be aware of the possibility of an increase in adverse effects if mexiletine is given with terbinafine and consider a dose reduction if necessary.

Mexiletine + Theophylline ⚠

Serum theophylline levels are increased by mexiletine and toxicity may occur.

Monitor concurrent use and reduce the theophylline dosage as necessary. It has been suggested that 50% dose reductions may be required.

Mianserin

Mianserin + Moclobemide ✖

A number of studies suggest that no interaction, or only a moderate non-significant rise in *tricyclic antidepressant* levels occurs when they are given with moclobemide. However, several case reports describe serotonin syndrome, page 392, in patients receiving the combination. There is little evidence regarding mianserin, but it seems likely that it could interact similarly.

Concurrent use should be avoided. Moclobemide has a short duration of action so no treatment free period is required before starting a tricyclic or related antidepressant. However, some recommend waiting 24 hours. Moclobemide should not be started until at least one week after a tricyclic or related antidepressant has been stopped.

M

Mianserin + Phenobarbital ⚠

Plasma levels of mianserin can be markedly reduced by phenobarbital. Note that primidone is metabolised to phenobarbital and therefore may interact similarly.

It seems likely that the dose of mianserin will need to be increased. Monitor the response to mianserin and increase the dose as necessary.

Mianserin + Phenytoin ⚠

Plasma levels of mianserin can be markedly reduced by phenytoin. Fosphenytoin, a prodrug of phenytoin, may interact similarly.

It seems likely that the dose of mianserin will need to be increased. Monitor the response to mianserin and increase the dose as necessary.

Mianserin + Warfarin and other oral anticoagulants ❓

Mianserin may occasionally cause bleeding in patients taking warfarin. However on the whole concurrent use seems uneventful.

The general significance of the case reports is unknown, but bear it in mind in case of an excessive response to anticoagulant treatment.

Mifepristone

Mifepristone + NSAIDs ❓

Theoretically NSAIDs might reduce the efficacy of mifepristone, and combined use is often not recommended. However, evidence from two studies with naproxen and diclofenac suggests no reduction in mifepristone efficacy.

Because of theoretical concerns of antagonistic effects, NSAID analgesics have been avoided in protocols for medical abortion. However, the limited available evidence suggests that this might not be necessary.

Mirtazapine

Mirtazapine + Phenobarbital ⚠

Phenytoin decreases the AUC and maximum plasma levels of mirtazapine by 47% and 33%, respectively. Phenobarbital (and therefore primidone) would be expected to interact similarly.

The mirtazapine dose may need to be increased in the presence of phenobarbital. Monitor concurrent use to ensure mirtazapine is effective.

Mirtazapine + Phenytoin ⚠

Mirtazapine does not appear to affect the pharmacokinetics of phenytoin. Phenytoin decreases the AUC and maximum plasma levels of mirtazapine by 47% and 33%, respectively. Fosphenytoin, a prodrug of phenytoin, may interact similarly.

The mirtazapine dose may need to be increased in the presence of phenytoin. Monitor concurrent use to ensure mirtazapine is effective.

Mirtazapine + Protease inhibitors ⚠

The protease inhibitors are predicted to inhibit the metabolism of mirtazapine by CYP3A4. Other CYP3A4 inhibitors (such as ketoconazole) have been shown to have this effect.

The manufacturers advise caution on concurrent use. Monitor for adverse effects (e.g. oedema, sedation).

Mirtazapine + Rifampicin (Rifampin) ⚠

Rifampicin is predicted to lower mirtazapine levels. Other enzyme inducers (e.g. phenytoin) have been shown to have this effect.

The mirtazapine dose may need to be increased during concurrent use. Monitor to ensure that mirtazapine is effective.

Mirtazapine + SSRIs ❓

There are a couple of isolated cases of possible serotonin syndrome, page 392, when mirtazapine was used with fluoxetine and fluvoxamine, and there is a report of hypomania associated with combined use with sertraline. Restless legs syndrome occurred with fluoxetine and mirtazapine. Fluvoxamine markedly increased plasma levels of mirtazapine in two cases.

Caution is warranted on concurrent use. Monitor for adverse effects (e.g. oedema, sedation) and be aware that CNS excitation may occur. Extra caution might be appropriate with fluvoxamine, since the limited evidence suggests that this might markedly raise mirtazapine levels. However, this needs confirming.

Mirtazapine + Warfarin and other oral anticoagulants ⚠

Mirtazapine may cause small but clinically insignificant increases in INR in patients taking warfarin.

No action needed.

M

Moclobemide

Moclobemide + Nasal decongestants ⊗

Limited evidence suggests that blood pressure elevations may occur when patients taking moclobemide are given nasal decongestants with indirect sympathomimetic actions, such as ephedrine. However, these rises in blood pressure do not seem to be as large as those seen with the non-selective MAOIs. Ephedrine has been successfully and uneventfully used in the presence of moclobemide (omitted on the day of surgery) during anaesthesia to control hypotension.

The manufacturers of moclobemide advise avoiding drugs such as ephedrine, pseudoephedrine and phenylpropanolamine.

Moclobemide + Opioids ⊗

One report suggests that on the basis of *animal* studies the combination of moclobemide and pethidine (meperidine) should be avoided or used with caution. A report of suspected serotonin syndrome in a patient given pethidine (meperidine) in addition to her usual treatment with moclobemide, nortriptyline and lithium, adds some weight to this suggestion. Similar predictions have been made for tramadol, and serotonin syndrome, page 392, has been seen in a patient given tramadol with moclobemide and clomipramine.

Concurrent use should be avoided or undertaken with great caution.

Moclobemide + SSRIs ⊗

Some studies suggest that moclobemide may not interact with the SSRIs, but there have been case reports of serotonin syndrome, page 392, in patients taking the combination.

Concurrent use is contraindicated. Because the effects of moclobemide are readily reversible, only one day need elapse between stopping moclobemide and starting an SSRI. However, if stopping an SSRI and starting moclobemide the same intervals as for the irreversible MAOIs are required. The manufacturers say that any type of MAOI should not be added until sertraline has been stopped for 14 days, or citalopram, escitalopram, fluvoxamine or paroxetine have been stopped for 7 days, (14 days in the US). The manufacturers of fluoxetine recommend that at least 5 weeks should elapse between stopping the fluoxetine and starting the MAOI. A longer interval is suggested if long-term or high-dose fluoxetine has been used.

Moclobemide + Trazodone ⊗

A number of studies suggest that no interaction, or only a moderate non-significant rise in *tricyclic antidepressant* levels occurs when they are given with moclobemide. However, several case reports describe serotonin syndrome, page 392, in patients receiving the combination. It seems likely that trazodone will also interact in this way.

Concurrent use is not advised. Moclobemide has a short duration of action so no treatment free period is required before starting trazodone. However, some

M

recommend waiting 24 hours. Moclobemide should not be started until at least one week after trazodone has been stopped.

Moclobemide + Tricyclics ⊗

A number of studies suggest that no interaction, or only a moderate non-significant rise in tricyclic antidepressant levels occurs when they are given with moclobemide. However, several case reports describe serotonin syndrome, page 392, in patients receiving the combination.

Concurrent use should be avoided. Moclobemide has a short duration of action so no treatment free period is required before starting a tricyclic antidepressant. However, some recommend waiting 24 hours. Moclobemide should not be started until at least one week after a tricyclic antidepressant has been stopped.

Moclobemide + Triptans ⚠

Moclobemide markedly inhibits the metabolism of rizatriptan, modestly inhibits the metabolism of zolmitriptan and approximately doubles the bioavailability of sumatriptan. Note that there is a potential risk of serotonin syndrome, page 392, if triptans are given with moclobemide.

The manufacturers contraindicate the use of moclobemide with rizatriptan or sumatriptan. In the UK, a maximum intake of 5 mg of zolmitriptan in 24 hours is recommended by the manufacturers, whereas in the US the combination is contraindicated.

Moclobemide + Venlafaxine ⊗

The concurrent use of moclobemide and venlafaxine has led to the potentially fatal serotonin syndrome, page 392.

The manufacturers of venlafaxine recommend that one week should elapse between stopping the venlafaxine and starting the MAOI, and 2 weeks between stopping an MAOI and starting venlafaxine.

Modafinil

Modafinil + Phenytoin ⚠

There is some *in vitro* evidence to indicate that modafinil may possibly inhibit the metabolism of phenytoin. Fosphenytoin, a prodrug of phenytoin, may interact similarly.

It may be prudent to monitor the effects of phenytoin in the presence of modafinil, taking levels if any evidence of toxicity occurs (e.g. blurred vision, nystagmus, ataxia or drowsiness).

M

Montelukast

Montelukast + Phenobarbital ⚠

Phenobarbital reduces the AUC and maximum serum levels of montelukast by 38% and 20%, respectively. However, there is so far no clinical evidence that the montelukast dosage needs adjustment. Note that primidone is metabolised to phenobarbital and therefore may interact similarly.

> The manufacturers caution concurrent use, especially in children. Monitor for a reduction in montelukast efficacy.

Montelukast + Phenytoin ⚠

Phenytoin (and therefore possibly fosphenytoin) is predicted to reduce montelukast levels.

> The manufacturers caution concurrent use, especially in children. Monitor for a reduction in montelukast efficacy.

Montelukast + Rifampicin (Rifampin) ⚠

Rifampicin is predicted to reduce montelukast levels.

> The manufacturers caution concurrent use, especially in children. Monitor for a reduction in montelukast efficacy.

Moxonidine

Moxonidine + Tricyclics ✖

Tricyclic antidepressants may antagonise the blood pressure lowering effects of clonidine, page 193. As moxonidine is related to clonidine it is expected to interact similarly. Tricyclics can also cause postural hypotension, and can cause sedation, both of which could potentially be additive with the effects of moxonidine.

> The manufacturers of moxonidine advise avoiding tricyclic antidepressants, because of the lack of clinical experience of combined use. If the combination is used, it would be prudent to carefully monitor blood pressure and sedation.

M

Mycophenolate

Mycophenolate + Rifampicin (Rifampin) ⚠

Rifampicin reduces the levels of mycophenolic acid (the active metabolite of mycophenolate) and increases the levels of the metabolite associated with mycophenolate adverse effects.

> Mycophenolate should be monitored for efficacy and adverse effects if rifampicin is given and the dose adjusted as required, both on starting and stopping rifampicin.

Mycophenolate + Sevelamer ⚠

Sevelamer reduces the AUC of mycophenolate by 25%.

> The clinical significance of this interaction is unclear, but it would seem prudent to monitor mycophenolate levels in any patient given sevelamer.

Mycophenolate + Vaccines ✖

The body's immune response is suppressed by mycophenolate. The antibody response to vaccines may be reduced. The use of live attenuated vaccines may result in generalised infection.

> For many inactivated vaccines even the reduced response seen is considered clinically useful, and in the case of renal transplant patients influenza vaccination is actively recommended. If a vaccine is given, it may be prudent to monitor the response, so that alternative prophylactic measures can be considered where the response is inadequate. Note that even where effective antibody titres are produced, these may not persist as long as in healthy subjects, and more frequent booster doses may be required. The use of live vaccines is generally considered to be contraindicated.

M

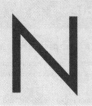

Nasal decongestants

Nasal decongestants + **Sibutramine**

There do not appear to be any studies on the use of sibutramine with decongestants, cough and cold medications, but the manufacturers predict that a rise in blood pressure or heart rate could occur. Ephedrine, phenylpropanolamine, pseudoephedrine, and xylometazoline (all indirect-acting sympathomimetics) have been specifically named.

Avoid concurrent use where possible. If both drugs are given monitor the outcome closely.

Nasal decongestants + **Theophylline**

There is some information suggesting an increased frequency of adverse effects when ephedrine is used with theophylline.

Note that ephedrine is an ingredient of a number of cough and cold remedies. It may be prudent to use an alternative.

Neomycin

Neomycin + **Penicillins**

The serum levels of oral phenoxymethylpenicillin can be halved by neomycin.

The clinical significance of this interaction is unclear. Monitor concurrent use to ensure phenoxymethylpenicillin is effective.

Neomycin + Vitamin A ❓

Neomycin can markedly reduce the absorption of vitamin A (retinol). The extent to which chronic treatment with neomycin would impair the treatment of vitamin A deficiency has not been determined.

> The general importance of this interaction is unknown, but bear it in mind in case of an unexpected response to treatment.

Neomycin + Warfarin and other oral anticoagulants ✅

Normally no interaction occurs, but in rare cases neomycin can cause a malabsorption syndrome, which may reduce vitamin K absorption and lead to over-anticoagulation.

> This interaction seems rare, but bear it in mind in case of an excessive response to anticoagulant treatment.

Nicorandil

Nicorandil + Phosphodiesterase type-5 inhibitors ❌

The manufacturers of sildenafil contraindicate the concurrent use of sildenafil and *nitrates* because potentially serious hypotension can occur, and myocardial infarction may possibly be precipitated. A number of fatalities have occurred as a result of this interaction with nitrates. Tadalafil and vardenafil interact similarly. Nicorandil is expected to interact in the same way as the nitrates.

> The concurrent use of these phosphodiesterase inhibitors and nicorandil is contraindicated. Sildenafil should not be used within 24 hours of a nitrate, and some evidence suggests this is also a suitable separation for vardenafil. Nitrates should not be given for at least 48 hours after the last dose of tadalafil. Similar cautions would seem to apply to nicorandil.

Nicotinic acid (Niacin)

Nicotinic acid (Niacin) + Statins ⚠️

The combination of a statin and nicotinic acid has been implicated in cases of rhabdomyolysis.

> If the decision is made to use nicotinic acid with a statin the outcome should be very well monitored. All patients should be warned to report promptly any unexplained muscle aches, tenderness, cramps, stiffness or weakness. The manufacturers of simvastatin say that the dose should not exceed 10 mg daily in patients taking nicotinic acid in doses of at least 1 g daily.

Nitrates

Nitrates + **Phosphodiesterase type-5 inhibitors** ✕

The manufacturers of sildenafil contraindicate the concurrent use of sildenafil and organic nitrates (e.g. glyceryl trinitrate (nitroglycerin), isosorbide dinitrate, isosorbide mononitrate) because potentially serious hypotension can occur, and myocardial infarction may possibly be precipitated. A number of fatalities have occurred as a result of this interaction. Tadalafil and vardenafil interact similarly.

> The concurrent use of these phosphodiesterase inhibitors and all organic nitrates is contraindicated. Sildenafil should not be used within 24 hours of a nitrate, and some evidence suggests this is also a suitable separation for vardenafil. Nitrates should not be given for at least 48 hours after the last dose of tadalafil.

NNRTIs

The NNRTIs are extensively metabolised by cytochrome P450, particularly by CYP3A4. They are also inducers (nevirapine, efavirenz) or inhibitors (delavirdine) of CYP3A4. The NNRTIs therefore have the potential to interact with drugs metabolised by CYP3A4, and are also affected by CYP3A4 inhibitors and inducers. Delavirdine and efavirenz may also inhibit some other cytochrome P450 isoenzymes.

NNRTIs + **Opioids** ⚠

Methadone plasma levels can be markedly reduced by efavirenz or nevirapine, and methadone withdrawal symptoms have been seen.

> If efavirenz or nevirapine are added to established treatment with methadone, be alert for evidence of opiate withdrawal, and raise the methadone dose accordingly. Some patients may require an increase in the methadone dose frequency to twice daily. In patients who subsequently discontinue the NNRTI, the methadone dose should be gradually reduced.

NNRTIs + **Phenobarbital** ⚠

The concurrent use of *carbamazepine* and efavirenz leads to a modest reduction in the plasma levels of both drugs; similar effects are predicted to occur with phenobarbital (and therefore primidone) .

> The manufacturers say that when efavirenz is given with phenobarbital, there is a potential for reduction or increase in the plasma levels of each drug: they therefore recommend periodic monitoring of plasma levels.

NNRTIs + **Phenytoin** ⚠️

The concurrent use of *carbamazepine* and efavirenz leads to a modest reduction in the plasma levels of both drugs; similar effects are predicted to occur with phenytoin (and therefore possibly fosphenytoin).

> The manufacturers say that when efavirenz is given with phenytoin, there is a potential for reduction or increase in the plasma levels of each drug: they therefore recommend periodic monitoring of plasma levels.

NNRTIs + **Phosphodiesterase type-5 inhibitors** ⚠️

Efavirenz and nevirapine are predicted to reduce the levels of phosphodiesterase type-5 inhibitors, because other inducers of CYP3A4 have been shown to do so. For example, sildenafil levels are reduced by 70% by *bosentan* and tadalafil levels are reduced by 88% by *rifampicin*. Vardenafil is also metabolised by CYP3A4, and therefore its levels may possibly be lowered by efavirenz and nevirapine.

> If these phosphodiesterase type-5 inhibitors are not effective in patients taking efavirenz or nevirapine, it would seem sensible to try a higher dose with close monitoring.

NNRTIs + **Proton pump inhibitors** ✖️

Antacids roughly halve the AUC of delavirdine, and proton pump inhibitors are predicted to interact similarly. This is because delavirdine is poorly soluble at pHs greater than 3.

> Long-term concurrent use is not recommended.

NNRTIs + **Rifabutin**

Delavirdine ✖️

Rifabutin causes a 5-fold increase in delavirdine clearance, and an 84% fall in the steady-state plasma levels.

> The US Center for Disease Control and Prevention recommends that rifabutin should not be used with delavirdine.

Efavirenz ⚠️

Rifabutin does not affect efavirenz levels, but efavirenz may decrease rifabutin levels.

> The US Center for Disease Control and Prevention states that the combination is probably clinically useful, and they suggest increasing the dose of rifabutin to 450 mg or 600 mg daily, or 600 mg two to three times weekly. Monitor the outcome of concurrent use carefully.

N

NNRTIs + Rifampicin (Rifampin)

Delavirdine ✗

Rifampicin causes a 27-fold increase in clearance of delavirdine, and the steady-state plasma levels become almost undetectable.

> The US Center for Disease Control and Prevention recommends that rifampicin should not be used with delavirdine.

Efavirenz ⚠

Rifampicin reduces the AUC of efavirenz by about 25%.

> The manufacturers advise that the dose of efavirenz should be raised to 800 mg daily. Monitor well for efavirenz efficacy and adverse effects.

Nevirapine ⚠

A clinical study showed that the AUC of nevirapine was reduced by 31% in patients given rifampicin. Other information suggests that rifampicin reduces the AUC of nevirapine by 58%.

> In the UK the combination is not advised. The US Center for Disease Control and Prevention recommends *rifabutin*, and says that rifampicin should be used only if clearly indicated and with close monitoring.

NNRTIs + SSRIs ⚠

A case of serotonin syndrome, page 392, occurred in a woman taking fluoxetine when efavirenz was added; this resolved when the dose of fluoxetine was halved. Efavirenz decreases sertraline levels, and nevirapine decreases fluoxetine levels, whereas fluvoxamine increases nevirapine levels.

> Monitor for fluoxetine efficacy if nevirapine is given, and sertraline efficacy if efavirenz is given; adjust the SSRI dose as required. Monitor for signs of nevirapine adverse effects in patients also taking fluvoxamine. Bear the case of serotonin syndrome in mind if efavirenz and fluoxetine are both given.

NNRTIs + Statins

Delavirdine ⚠

Delavirdine is expected to raise the levels of atorvastatin, simvastatin and lovastatin. This expectation is supported by a case of rhabdomyolysis, which developed in a patient taking atorvastatin and delavirdine.

> One of the manufacturers of simvastatin contraindicates delavirdine, and the US manufacturer of delavirdine advises against the use of either simvastatin or lovastatin. Patients should be made aware of the risks of myopathy and rhabdomyolysis, and asked to promptly report muscle pain, tenderness or weakness, especially if accompanied by malaise, fever or dark urine.

Efavirenz ⚠

Efavirenz (and possibly nevirapine) lowers the levels of atorvastatin, simvastatin, and pravastatin.

It would seem prudent to monitor the lipid profile of patients taking efavirenz and any of these statins, although bear in mind that NNRTIs are often used with protease inhibitors, page 376, which dramatically *increase* the levels of some statins.

NNRTIs + Tacrolimus ❓

A single case reports a decrease in the metabolism of tacrolimus by efavirenz.

Although this is only an isolated case it is in line with the way both drugs are known to interact. It would seem prudent to closely monitor tacrolimus levels in any patient given efavirenz.

NNRTIs + Warfarin and other oral anticoagulants ⚠

Three cases suggest that warfarin requirements are approximately doubled by nevirapine.

Monitor the effect of concurrent use on the anticoagulant response and adjust the dose as necessary.

NRTIs

NRTIs are prodrugs, which need to be activated by phosphorylation within cells. Drugs may therefore interact with NRTIs by increasing or decreasing intracellular activation. NRTIs are water soluble, and are mainly eliminated by the kidneys (didanosine, lamivudine, stavudine, and zalcitabine) or undergo hepatic glucuronidation (abacavir, zidovudine). The few important interactions with these drugs primarily involve altered renal clearance. For zidovudine (and possibly abacavir) some interactions occur via altered glucuronidation, but the clinical relevance of these are less clear. Cytochrome P450-mediated interactions are not important for this class of drugs. Didanosine chewable tablets are formulated with antacid buffers that are intended to facilitate didanosine absorption by minimising acid-induced hydrolysis in the stomach. These preparations can therefore alter the absorption of other drugs that are affected by antacids (e.g. azole antifungals, quinolone antibacterials, tetracyclines). This interaction may be minimised by separating administration by at least 2 hours. Alternatively, the enteric-coated preparation of didanosine (gastro-resistant capsules) may be used.

NRTIs + Opioids ❓

Zidovudine had no effect on methadone levels in one study, but there is one report of a patient requiring a modest increase in his methadone dose after starting zidovudine. Similarly, small changes in the pharmacokinetics of abacavir and methadone may occur on concurrent use, and there is a report of 2 patients requiring increases in their methadone doses. Methadone can increase zidovudine serum levels, and reduce levels of didanosine from the tablet formulation, but not the enteric-coated capsule preparation. Methadone may cause small decreases in stavudine levels.

The clinical relevance of these minor changes is unclear. It may be prudent to monitor methadone dose requirements until more is known.

NRTIs + Pentamidine ❌

Additive pancreatic toxicity has occurred with the concurrent use of zalcitabine and intravenous pentamidine, and a similar interaction is expected with didanosine or stavudine. Didanosine, stavudine and zalcitabine alone have all been associated with fatal pancreatitis.

The manufacturers of zalcitabine recommend that if pentamidine is needed, treatment with zalcitabine should be interrupted. A similar recommendation has been made for didanosine, although the manufacturers suggest that close monitoring is adequate. Careful monitoring is recommended if pentamidine is given with stavudine.

NRTIs + Phenobarbital ⚠

The UK manufacturer of abacavir says that potent enzyme inducers such as phenobarbital (and therefore probably primidone) may slightly decrease abacavir concentrations.

The clinical significance of this prediction is unclear but it may be prudent to monitor to ensure abacavir is effective.

NRTIs + Phenytoin ⚠

Phenytoin is predicted to decrease abacavir levels. Zidovudine may alter the pharmacokinetics of phenytoin, although this may be due to HIV infection itself. Fosphenytoin, a prodrug of phenytoin, may interact similarly.

The clinical significance of these interactions is unclear. However, it may be prudent to monitor the efficacy of abacavir. Be aware that larger phenytoin doses may be needed in the presence of zidovudine.

NRTIs + Probenecid ⚠

Probenecid reduces the clearance of zalcitabine and zidovudine, increasing their serum levels.

The combination of zalcitabine and probenecid is well tolerated, but the incidence of adverse effects is reported to be very much increased when probenecid is taken with zidovudine. Concurrent use need not be avoided, but monitor carefully for zidovudine toxicity.

NRTIs + Rifabutin ⚠

Rifabutin may increase the clearance of zidovudine by up to 50%.

> The clinical implications of this interaction are unknown. Be alert for any evidence of a reduced response to zidovudine if rifabutin is given. Didanosine, stavudine and zalcitabine are not expected to interact with rifabutin.

NRTIs + Rifampicin (Rifampin) ⚠

Several studies suggest that rifampicin more than doubles the clearance of zidovudine. In some subjects increased haematological toxicity was also seen. Rifampicin is predicted to interact similarly with abacavir.

> Be alert for any evidence of a reduced response to these antivirals and monitor for haematological toxicity.

NRTIs + Valproate ⚠

Sodium valproate increases the AUC of zidovudine by 80%. In one case sodium valproate increased serum zidovudine levels by up to 3-fold, and increased the CSF levels of zidovudine by 74%.

> It would seem prudent to monitor for zidovudine adverse effects and possible toxicity. Other NRTIs do not undergo significant glucuronidation and are therefore not expected to interact in this way with sodium valproate.

NSAIDs

NSAIDs + NSAIDs ✖

The combined use of two or more NSAIDs increases the risk of gastrointestinal damage.

> As there is no clear clinical rationale for the combined use of different NSAIDs, such use should be avoided.

NSAIDs + Opioids

NSAIDs, general ✔

On the whole the concurrent use of NSAIDs and opioids is successful and without incident. The following specifically studied pairs have not been found to interact adversely: alfentanil with parecoxib, codeine with diclofenac, dextropropoxyphene (propoxyphene) with meclofenamate, dextropropoxyphene (propoxyphene) with sulindac, fentanyl with parecoxib, methadone with intramuscular diclofenac, and morphine with ketoprofen. There seems no reason to assume other NSAIDs and opioids will interact. However, see the specific instances discussed below.

> No action needed.

Diclofenac ❓

An isolated report describes grand mal seizures in a patient given diclofenac and pentazocine. Diclofenac did not alter morphine pharmacokinetics in one study. However, in another, diclofenac slightly increased respiratory depression despite a reduction in morphine use, possibly because of persistent levels of an active metabolite of morphine.

> These interactions are not established and they seem unlikely to be of general significance, but be alert to the possibility of increased sedation, or, with pentazocine, use with caution in patients who are known to be seizure-prone.

Ketorolac ❓

A single case report describes marked respiratory depression in a man taking buprenorphine with ketorolac.

> This seems unlikely to be of general significance but be alert to the possibility of increased sedation.

NSAIDs + Paracetamol (Acetaminophen) ✅

On the whole the concurrent use of NSAIDs with paracetamol is beneficial and without serious adverse effects. However, one epidemiological study found that paracetamol alone, and particularly when combined with NSAIDs, was associated with an increased risk of gastrointestinal bleeding, but other studies have not found such an effect. Diflunisal raises paracetamol levels by 50% but does not alter the total bioavailability.

> The interaction with diflunisal has not been shown to be clinically significant but the manufacturers advise caution because of the risks of increased paracetamol levels. There is no evidence to suggest that the concurrent use of paracetamol and any NSAID should be avoided.

NSAIDs + Penicillamine ❓

Indometacin has been found to increase the peak levels of penicillamine by about 22%. The manufacturers warn that the concurrent use of NSAIDs and penicillamine may increase the risk of nephrotoxicity.

> The US manufacturer specifically recommends avoiding oxyphenbutazone or phenylbutazone because these drugs are also associated with serious haematological and renal effects. There seems to be no reason to avoid other NSAIDS and penicillamine, but if problems occur bear the possibility of a drug interaction in mind.

NSAIDs + Pentoxifylline ❌

The manufacturers of ketorolac say that there is an increased risk of bleeding events if pentoxifylline is given concurrently.

> The manufacturers say that concurrent use should be avoided.

NSAIDs + Phenytoin ⊗

Serum phenytoin levels can be markedly increased by azapropazone, and toxicity can develop rapidly. A similar interaction has been seen with phenylbutazone, and it seems likely that oxyphenbutazone will interact similarly. Fosphenytoin, a prodrug of phenytoin, may interact similarly with these NSAIDs.

It has been suggested that the concurrent use of phenytoin and these NSAIDs should be avoided.

NSAIDs + Probenecid ❓

Probenecid reduces the loss of dexketoprofen, diflunisal, ketoprofen, ketorolac, indometacin, meclofenamate, naproxen, tenoxicam and tiaprofenic acid from the body, and raises their serum levels. Increased clinical effects have been seen for indometacin, but indometacin toxicity has also occurred.

Increased levels do occur, which could reasonably be expected to result in increased beneficial and adverse effects. However, the clinical outcome of this interaction is uncertain and so action (e.g. dose adjustments) should be based on the response of the patient. Note that probenecid is specifically contraindicated by the manufacturers of ketorolac.

NSAIDs + Quinolones ⚠

Convulsions have been seen in patients given fenbufen with enoxacin, and several NSAIDs with ofloxacin or ciprofloxacin. The CSM in the UK warns that this interaction could occur with any NSAID/quinolone combination.

Convulsions are rare, so in the majority of patients concurrent use should be without problem. Epileptics, or those predisposed to convulsions, seem to be at greater risk, so avoid concurrent use or monitor very closely.

NSAIDs + Rifampicin (Rifampin) ⚠

The plasma levels of celecoxib, diclofenac, and etoricoxib are reduced by rifampicin.

The clinical relevance of these interactions is unclear, but it seems likely that the efficacy of these NSAIDs will be reduced by rifampicin. Combined use should be well monitored, and the NSAID dosage increased if necessary.

NSAIDs + SSRIs ❓

The SSRIs may increase the risk of upper gastrointestinal bleeding and the risk appears to be further increased by the concurrent use of NSAIDs.

The manufacturers of the SSRIs warn that patients should be cautioned about the concurrent use of NSAIDs. Alternatives such as paracetamol (acetaminophen) or less gastrotoxic NSAIDs such as ibuprofen may be considered, but if the combination of an SSRI and NSAID cannot be avoided, prescribing of gastro-protective drugs such as proton pump inhibitors, or H_2-receptor antagonists should be considered, especially in elderly patients or those with a history of gastrointestinal bleeding.

NSAIDs + Tacrolimus ⚠

The UK manufacturers of tacrolimus suggest that all NSAIDs may have additive nephrotoxic effects with tacrolimus. Cases of renal failure have been reported in patients receiving the combination.

Tacrolimus levels and/or effects (e.g. on renal function) should be monitored as a matter of routine, but it may be prudent to increase monitoring if NSAIDs are started.

NSAIDs + Ticlopidine ❓

The risk of faecal blood loss, gastrointestinal haemorrhage and other bleeding is increased by concurrent use of *clopidogrel* and NSAIDs. Ticlopidine is expected to interact similarly.

The manufacturers advise caution if NSAIDs and ticlopidine are given together. Consider giving additional gastrointestinal prophylaxis such as a proton pump inhibitor in patients at risk of gastrointestinal ulceration and bleeding.

NSAIDs + Vancomycin ⚠

Indometacin reduces the renal clearance of vancomycin in premature neonates. This interaction appears not to have been studied in adults.

The effect in adults is unclear, but in neonates be prepared to reduce the dose of vancomycin in the presence of indometacin.

NSAIDs + Warfarin and other oral anticoagulants

Azapropazone, Ketorolac, Oxyphenbutazone, Phenylbutazone ✗

The anticoagulant effects of warfarin are markedly increased by azapropazone, ketorolac, oxyphenbutazone and phenylbutazone.

Concurrent use is contraindicated.

Coxibs ❓

There is some evidence to suggest that celecoxib, parecoxib and rofecoxib do not normally interact with warfarin. However, raised INRs accompanied by bleeding, particularly in the elderly, have been attributed to the use of warfarin and celecoxib or rofecoxib, and fluindione with rofecoxib. Etoricoxib causes a small increase in INR when it is taken with warfarin.

Monitor the anticoagulant effect if these NSAIDs are added to or withdrawn from the treatment of patients taking anticoagulants.

Other NSAIDs ⚠

Case reports suggest that most NSAIDs can occasionally enhance the effects of warfarin and other coumarins (acenocoumarol, phenprocoumon), resulting in increased anticoagulant effects and sometimes severe bleeding events.

Monitor the anticoagulant effect if NSAIDs are added to or withdrawn from the treatment of patients taking anticoagulants. Note that since NSAIDs reduce platelet aggregation and cause gastrointestinal irritation they can prolong and worsen any bleeding events.

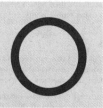

Opioids

Opioids with mixed agonist/antagonist properties (e.g. buprenorphine, butorphanol, nalbuphine, pentazocine) may precipitate opioid withdrawal symptoms in patients taking pure opioid agonists such as fentanyl, methadone, morphine and tramadol.

Opioids + Phenobarbital

Fentanyl, Methadone or Pethidine (Meperidine) ⚠

Phenobarbital and primidone appear to increase fentanyl and methadone requirements. Methadone withdrawal reactions have been seen. The analgesic effects of pethidine can be reduced by barbiturates.

Monitor concurrent use to ensure the opioid effects are adequate.

Opioids, general ⚠

The concurrent use of opioids (including weak opioids such as codeine) and barbiturates appears to increase sedation and respiratory depression. Although phenobarbital decreased the analgesic effects of pethidine (meperidine) in one study increased sedation has been reported with the combination.

Concurrent use need not be avoided, but be aware of the potential for respiratory depression, especially in patients with a restricted respiratory capacity.

Opioids + Phenytoin ⚠

Phenytoin appears to increase fentanyl and methadone requirements. Methadone withdrawal reactions have been seen. Fosphenytoin, a prodrug of phenytoin, may interact similarly.

Monitor concurrent use to ensure the opioid effects are adequate.

Opioids + Pregabalin ❓

The manufacturer of pregabalin notes that there was no clinically relevant pharmacokinetic interaction between pregabalin and oxycodone, and that there was no clinically important effect on respiration. However, pregabalin appeared to cause an additive impairment in cognitive and gross motor function when given with oxycodone. It seems possible that all opioids may have this effect.

Caution is warranted during the combined use of pregabalin and any opioid.

Opioids + Protease inhibitors

Alfentanil and Fentanyl ⚠

Ritonavir markedly increases the levels of fentanyl, and markedly increases alfentanil-induced miosis. Other protease inhibitors may also be expected to interact similarly but there seems little documented about these effects in practice. Care should also be taken if ritonavir is used with other protease inhibitors as a pharmacokinetic enhancer.

Concurrent use should be monitored. Dose reductions of fentanyl (given by any route) or alfentanil may be required, particularly with long-term use.

Buprenorphine ⚠

Atazanavir with ritonavir can increase the levels of buprenorphine and increase its adverse effects such as sedation. Other protease inhibitors may also be expected to interact similarly but there seems little documented about these effects in practice.

The manufacturers recommend avoiding concurrent use as the magnitude of the interaction is unknown. However if concurrent use is needed in patients taking protease inhibitors, the initial dose of buprenorphine should be halved.

Dextropropoxyphene (Propoxyphene) ✖

Ritonavir is predicted to increase the effects of dextropropoxyphene. Other protease inhibitors may also be expected to interact similarly but there seems little documented about these effects in practice.

The UK manufacturer of ritonavir contraindicates its use with dextropropoxyphene as extremely raised dextropropoxyphene levels may occur, which would increase the risk of serious adverse events (e.g. respiratory depression). However, the US manufacturer only suggests that a dose decrease may be needed.

Methadone ⚠

Methadone serum levels can be reduced by amprenavir, nelfinavir, lopinavir/ritonavir, ritonavir/saquinavir, tipranavir/ritonavir and possibly ritonavir. Not all patients appear to be affected. Amprenavir levels may be reduced by methadone.

An increased methadone dosage may be needed in some patients to prevent opiate withdrawal. Monitor amprenavir to ensure it remains effective. It has been suggested that alternative antiretrovirals should be considered.

Morphine ⚠

Ritonavir is predicted to decrease the levels of morphine.

> The clinical significance of this prediction is unclear however it would be prudent to monitor concurrent use to ensure morphine is effective and pain control is adequate.

Pethidine (Meperidine) ✖

Ritonavir decreased pethidine levels but increased norpethidine levels, which may possibly increase toxicity on long-term use.

> The manufacturers of pethidine oral preparations and injection contraindicate or advise against its use with ritonavir because of the risk of norpethidine toxicity. Long-term use of pethidine with other protease inhibitors that are given with low-dose ritonavir is also not recommended.

Other opioids ❓

Ritonavir is predicted to increase the effects of dihydrocodeine, oxycodone, and tramadol. However, there is no clinical evidence that this occurs. Ritonavir may also *decrease* the effects of codeine by inhibiting its metabolism to an active metabolite.

> Caution and careful monitoring of effects is warranted with dihydrocodeine, oxycodone, and tramadol as high levels may lead to CNS depression. Smaller initial doses may be appropriate. In contrast, codeine may be less effective than expected. Low-dose ritonavir would be expected to have a less potent effect on the metabolism of these opioids and dose adjustments would not generally be required.

Opioids + **Quinidine** ⚠

The analgesic effects of codeine, and hydrocodone appear to be reduced or abolished by quinidine in most patients. Quinidine appears to increase the oral absorption and effects of fentanyl, methadone, and morphine.

> The interaction with codeine, and hydrocodone is possible in the majority of patients. Consider the use of an alternative analgesic. Dihydrocodeine, oxycodone and tramadol do not appear to be affected. Monitor for increased opioid effects after the oral administration of fentanyl, methadone, and morphine. Note that quinidine and high-dose methadone may prolong the QT interval, see drugs that prolong the QT interval, page 237.

Opioids + **Quinolones** ⚠

It has been suggested that opioids decrease oral ciprofloxacin levels, but good evidence for this appears to be lacking.

> The manufacturers of ciprofloxacin state that the use of ciprofloxacin tablets is not recommended with opiate premedicants due to the risks of inadequate ciprofloxacin levels. Note that both high-dose methadone and some quinolones (gatifloxacin, levofloxacin, moxifloxacin and in particular sparfloxacin) may prolong the QT interval, see drugs that prolong the QT interval, page 237.

Opioids + **Rifampicin (Rifampin)** ⚠

Serum methadone levels can be markedly reduced by rifampicin, and withdrawal symptoms have occurred in some patients. Similarly, rifampicin markedly increases the metabolism of alfentanil, codeine, fentanyl and morphine, and reduces their effects.

> Monitor concurrent use for reduced opioid effects and adjust the dose accordingly. Note that rifabutin only appears to interact in a small number of patients, and to a lesser extent, so it may be a suitable alternative.

Opioids + **Sibutramine** ✖

The concurrent use of serotonergic drugs and sibutramine may theoretically lead to the potentially fatal serotonin syndrome, page 392.

> The manufacturers of sibutramine state that it should not be taken with any serotonergic drugs including fentanyl, pentazocine and pethidine (meperidine).

Opioids + **SSRIs**

Tramadol ⚠

Several case reports describe the development of serotonin syndrome, page 392, in patients taking fluoxetine, paroxetine or sertraline with tramadol. Another patient developed hallucinations when taking tramadol with paroxetine.

> There would seem to be little reason for totally avoiding the concurrent use of the SSRIs and tramadol but it would clearly be prudent to use the combination cautiously and monitor the outcome closely. Tramadol should be used with caution with SSRIs because of the possible increased risk of seizures.

Other opioids ❓

In isolated cases the concurrent use of SSRIs and opioids (including fentanyl, hydromorphone, oxycodone, pentazocine, pethidine (meperidine), and possibly morphine) has resulted in the serotonin syndrome. Methadone levels are modestly increased by fluvoxamine, paroxetine and sertraline, and possibly fluoxetine.

> Serotonin syndrome, page 392, seems to be a rare occurrence, but the possibility should be borne in mind if an SSRI is given with one of these opioids. Be aware that the use of fluvoxamine, paroxetine, sertraline or fluoxetine may alter the response to methadone. Monitor the outcome of concurrent use for methadone adverse effects.

Opioids + **Tricyclics**

Opioids, general ⚠

The incidence of myoclonus (muscle twitching or spasm) in patients on high doses of morphine appeared to be increased by tricyclic antidepressants in one study. Some studies suggest that the concurrent use of opioids and tricyclics may result in raised drug levels (amitriptyline and clomipramine increased the AUC of morphine, dextropropoxyphene (propoxyphene) raised amitriptyline and doxepin levels, and methadone raised desipramine levels). There is some evidence that suggests that combined use of opioids and tricyclics makes patients drowsier, clumsier and therefore more accident-prone, and may increase the risk of respiratory depression.

> Serious adverse interactions seem rare. An increase in opioid levels could be beneficial, but be aware that increased adverse effects are a possibility. Be alert for any evidence of increased CNS depression and increased tricyclic antidepressant adverse effects. Warn patients that sedation can occur. Respiratory depression is more likely to be of significance in those who already have respiratory impairment. Note that some tricyclics and high-dose methadone may prolong the QT interval, see drugs that prolong the QT interval, page 237.

Tramadol ⚠

The CSM in the UK recommends caution if tramadol is used with a tricyclic antidepressant as both drugs may reduce the seizure threshold. There have been reports of seizures on concurrent use.

> Consider an alternative analgesic or antidepressant if possible or use with caution.

Opioids + Triptans ⚠

Sumatriptan given by injection appears not to interact with butorphanol nasal spray, but if both drugs are given by nasal spray a significant interaction may occur, resulting in a reduction in butorphanol levels.

> When butorphanol was given 30 minutes after sumatriptan no significant pharmacokinetic interaction was noted. It would therefore seem wise to separate administration to ensure the full effects of butorphanol are achieved.

Opioids + Warfarin and other oral anticoagulants ⚠

Tramadol has been reported to increase the anticoagulant effects of warfarin and phenprocoumon in a few patients. Similarly, several patients taking warfarin have shown a marked increase in prothrombin times and/or bleeding when given co-proxamol (which contains dextropropoxyphene (propoxyphene)), but the interaction seems to be uncommon.

> It would be prudent to consider monitoring prothrombin times in any patient taking anticoagulants when tramadol is first added, being alert for the need to reduce the anticoagulant dosage.

Orlistat

Orlistat + Vitamins ⚠

Orlistat decreases the absorption of supplemental beta-carotene and vitamin E. There is some evidence to suggest that some patients may have low vitamin D levels while taking orlistat, even if they are also taking multivitamins.

It is recommended that multivitamin preparations should be taken at least 2 hours after orlistat, or at bedtime. The US manufacturers suggest that patients taking orlistat should be advised to take multivitamins, because of the possibility of reduced vitamin levels. Note that it has been suggested that monitoring of vitamin D may be required, even if multivitamins are given.

Orlistat + Warfarin and other oral anticoagulants ⚠

Several cases of increased INR have been reported in patients taking either warfarin or acenocoumarol after also taking orlistat. In contrast, a study in healthy subjects found no interaction. The manufacturers suggest that an interaction between orlistat and anticoagulants is possible.

Close monitoring is recommended for the first 4 weeks of concurrent use. As changes in diet are known to affect anticoagulant levels this seems prudent.

Oxcarbazepine

Oxcarbazepine is a derivative of carbamazepine, but has a lesser effect on CYP3A4. Oxcarbazepine can also act as an inhibitor of CYP2C19.

Oxcarbazepine + Phenytoin ❓

High doses of oxcarbazepine increase phenytoin levels, and a reduction in the phenytoin dose may be required. Elevations in phenytoin levels of up to 40% have been seen in retrospective studies. Fosphenytoin, a prodrug of phenytoin, may interact similarly.

Bear this interaction in mind on concurrent use, and with high oxcarbazepine doses consider monitoring phenytoin levels. Indicators of phenytoin toxicity include blurred vision, nystagmus, ataxia or drowsiness.

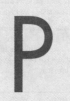

Paracetamol (Acetaminophen)

Paracetamol (Acetaminophen) + **Rifampicin (Rifampin)** [?]

Rifampicin induces the glucuronidation of paracetamol and increases its clearance, but does not increase the formation of hepatotoxic metabolites of paracetamol.

The clinical importance of these findings awaits further study, but they suggest that rifampicin may reduce the efficacy of paracetamol.

Paracetamol (Acetaminophen) + **Warfarin and other oral anticoagulants** [?]

An equal number of randomised studies have found a modest increase in the anticoagulant effect (e.g. an increase in INR of 1) of coumarins as have reported no effect. There are isolated case reports of an increase in anticoagulant effects in patients taking warfarin or acenocoumarol and paracetamol.

On the basis of the available data, it is not possible to firmly recommend increased monitoring, or dismiss its advisability. Further study is clearly needed. Paracetamol is still considered to be safer than aspirin or NSAIDs as an analgesic in the presence of an anticoagulant because it does not affect platelets or cause gastric bleeding.

Penicillins

Penicillins + **Probenecid** [?]

Probenecid reduces the excretion of the penicillins, and usually raises their levels.

Concurrent use can be beneficial, but consider any detrimental effect that elevated penicillin levels may have in individual patients.

Penicillins + **Warfarin and other oral anticoagulants** ⚠

The effects of the oral anticoagulants are not normally altered by the penicillins but isolated cases of increased prothrombin times and/or bleeding have been seen in patients given amoxicillin, ampicillin/flucloxacillin, benzylpenicillin, co-amoxiclav, or talampicillin. Carbenicillin, in the absence of an anticoagulant, can prolong prothrombin times. In contrast, a handful of cases of reduced warfarin effects have been seen with dicloxacillin, nafcillin, and possibly amoxicillin.

Even though the general picture is of no interaction some individual physicians say that they have seen changes with otherwise normally non-interacting penicillins. It has been said that experience in anticoagulant clinics suggests that the INR can be altered by courses of broad-spectrum antibacterials such as ampicillin, even though studies do not demonstrate an interaction. For this reason consider monitoring concurrent use so that the very occasional and unpredictable cases (increases or decreases in the anticoagulant effects) can be identified and handled accordingly. Any significant changes appear to occur after 4 days of concurrent use.

P

Pentoxifylline

Pentoxifylline + **Quinolones** ⚠

Evidence from one study suggests that ciprofloxacin increases the peak serum levels of pentoxifylline by 60%, and may increase the incidence of adverse effects. In some clinical studies ciprofloxacin has been used to boost the levels of pentoxifylline.

It has been suggested that the dosage of pentoxifylline should be halved if ciprofloxacin is also given, which may be a sensible precaution. Alternatively, it may be sufficient to recommend a reduction in pentoxifylline dose only in those who experience adverse effects (e.g. nausea, headache). Note that other quinolones may also interact, see quinolones, page 382.

Pentoxifylline + **Theophylline** ⚠

Pentoxifylline can raise serum theophylline serum levels by about 30%.

Patients should be well monitored for theophylline adverse effects (headache, nausea, palpitations) while taking both drugs and it may be necessary to decrease the theophylline dose in some cases.

Pentoxifylline + **Warfarin and other oral anticoagulants** ❓

The anticoagulant effects of phenprocoumon were not significantly altered by pentoxifylline in one study, but serious bleeding has been seen with pentoxifylline, both alone and in the presence of acenocoumarol. Other oral anticoagulants would be expected to interact similarly.

> It may be prudent to monitor concurrent use for any increase in bleeding events. Some have suggested the combination should be avoided.

Phenobarbital

Studies in man and *animals* clearly show that the barbiturates are potent liver enzyme inducers. The most commonly used barbiturate is phenobarbital, which is known to induce CYP3A4, amongst other isoenzymes. Most of the interaction information concerns phenobarbital, but all barbiturates would be expected to share its interactions to a greater or lesser extent. Note that primidone is metabolised to phenobarbital, and so would therefore also be expected to share many of its interactions.

Phenobarbital + Phenytoin ⚠

The concurrent use of phenytoin and phenobarbital is normally uneventful. However, changes in phenytoin levels (often decreases but sometimes increases) can occur if phenobarbital is added, but seizure control is not usually affected by this pharmacokinetic interaction. Phenytoin toxicity following barbiturate withdrawal has been seen. Increased phenobarbital levels and possibly toxicity may occur as a result of the addition of phenytoin to phenobarbital. Similar interaction may occur with primidone and fosphenytoin.

> Given the unpredictable outcome of concurrent use it would seem prudent to monitor levels if one drug is added to the other or if a dose is changed. Indicators of phenobarbital toxicity include drowsiness, ataxia or dysarthria.

Phenobarbital + Phosphodiesterase type-5 inhibitors ❓

Phenobarbital and therefore probably primidone are expected to reduce the levels of phosphodiesterase type-5 inhibitors, because other inducers of CYP3A4 have been shown to do so. For example, sildenafil levels are reduced by 70% by *bosentan* and tadalafil levels are reduced by 88% by *rifampicin*. Vardenafil is also metabolised by CYP3A4, and therefore its levels may possibly be lowered by phenobarbital and primidone.

> If these phosphodiesterase type-5 inhibitors are not effective in patients taking phenobarbital or primidone, it would seem sensible to try a higher dose with close monitoring.

Phenobarbital + Praziquantel ⚠

Phenobarbital (and therefore probably primidone) markedly reduces the serum levels of praziquantel, but whether this results in neurocysticercosis treatment failures is unclear.

When treating systemic worm infections such as neurocysticercosis some authors advise increasing the praziquantel dosage from 25 to 50 mg/kg if phenobarbital is being used. Note that the manufacturers current recommended dose for praziquantel for neurocysticercosis is 50 mg/kg daily in 3 divided doses. The interaction with antiepileptics is of no importance when praziquantel is used for intestinal worm infections (where its action is a local effect on the worms in the gut).

P

Phenobarbital + Propafenone ⚠

Phenobarbital reduces the peak levels of propafenone by 26 to 87%. Primidone is metabolised to phenobarbital and may therefore interact similarly.

The clinical importance of this interaction awaits assessment but check that propafenone remains effective if phenobarbital is added, and that toxicity does not occur if it is stopped.

Phenobarbital + Protease inhibitors ⚠

It is likely that phenobarbital and other barbiturates will increase the metabolism of the protease inhibitors, thereby reducing their levels and possibly resulting in antiretroviral therapy failure. However, one case suggested that this may not have occurred when primidone was given with ritonavir/saquinavir, although this should be viewed with caution.

The combination of protease inhibitors and barbiturates should be used with caution. Monitor for antiviral efficacy.

Phenobarbital + Pyridoxine ❓

Daily doses of pyridoxine 200 mg can cause reductions of 40 to 50% in phenobarbital levels in some patients. Primidone is metabolised to phenobarbital and may therefore be affected similarly, although this does not appear to have been studied.

Concurrent use should be monitored if large doses of pyridoxine are used, being alert for the need to increase the phenobarbital dosage. It seems unlikely that small doses (as in multivitamin preparations) will interact to any great extent.

Phenobarbital + Quinidine ⚠

Quinidine levels can be reduced by the concurrent use of phenobarbital or primidone. Loss of arrhythmia control is possible if the quinidine dosage is not increased.

Concurrent use need not be avoided, but be alert for the need to increase the quinidine dosage. If phenobarbital or primidone are withdrawn the quinidine dosage may need to be reduced to avoid quinidine toxicity. Quinidine serum levels should be monitored if possible.

Phenobarbital + Rifampicin (Rifampin) ⚠️

Phenobarbital possibly modestly increases the clearance of rifampicin (up to a 40% reduction in rifampicin levels in one study). The effect of rifampicin on phenobarbital levels is unknown, but note that rifampicin markedly increases the clearance of hexobarbital. Primidone is metabolised to phenobarbital and may therefore interact similarly with rifampicin.

> The outcome of concurrent use is unclear. Concurrent use need not be avoided, but be alert for a reduced response to both drugs.

Phenobarbital + Rimonabant ❓

The manufacturers predict that potent inducers of CYP3A4 such as phenobarbital (and therefore probably primidone) may lower the serum levels of rimonabant. This is based on the fact that potent *inhibitors* of CYP3A4 *increase* rimonabant levels (see under azoles, page 122).

> Caution is recommended with concurrent use of phenobarbital. Patients should be monitored to ensure rimonabant remains effective.

Phenobarbital + Sirolimus ⚠️

The manufacturers of sirolimus predict that phenobarbital (and therefore probably primidone) may lower its serum levels, probably because rifampicin (rifampin), another CYP3A4 inducer, has been shown to do so.

> The extent of any change in sirolimus levels is uncertain, but it would seem prudent to increase the frequency of monitoring of sirolimus levels during concurrent use.

Phenobarbital + Solifenacin ⚠️

Ketoconazole increases solifenacin levels 2- to 3-fold by *inhibiting* CYP3A4. The manufacturers predict that potent CYP3A4 *inducers* (e.g. phenobarbital, and therefore probably primidone) will decrease solifenacin levels.

> Be alert for a reduction in the efficacy of solifenacin in patients taking phenobarbital.

Phenobarbital + SSRIs ❓

In one study in 6 subjects phenobarbital caused reductions of 10 to 86% in the AUC of paroxetine, but the mean values were unaltered. One subject showed a 56% *increase* in their AUC. Primidone is metabolised to phenobarbital and may therefore interact similarly with rifampicin.

> Although there seems to be little correlation between plasma paroxetine levels and its efficacy, be alert for the need to increase its dosage if phenobarbital is given. Note that SSRIs can decrease the seizure threshold.

Phenobarbital + Tacrolimus ⚠

Phenobarbital (and therefore probably primidone) is predicted to reduce tacrolimus levels. This effect has been seen with other CYP3A4 inducers, such as phenytoin.

No interaction is established, but based on the known metabolism of these drugs it would be prudent to monitor tacrolimus levels in a patient given phenobarbital or primidone.

Phenobarbital + Tetracyclines ⚠

The serum levels of doxycycline are reduced and may fall below the accepted minimum inhibitory concentration in patients receiving long-term treatment with barbiturates.

It has been suggested that the doxycycline dosage could be doubled. Alternatively, tetracycline, oxytetracycline, and chlortetracycline appear not to interact and may therefore be suitable alternatives.

Phenobarbital + Theophylline ⚠

Theophylline serum levels can be reduced by phenobarbital or pentobarbital (clearance increased by roughly one-third). A single report describes a similar interaction with secobarbital, and an interaction would be expected to occur with other barbiturates. Limited evidence suggests that the barbiturates may have a greater effect in children, and if given in high dose.

It would be prudent to monitor theophylline levels if a barbiturate is added to or withdrawn from theophylline treatment.

Phenobarbital + Tiagabine ⚠

The plasma concentration of tiagabine may be reduced by 1.5- to 3-fold by both phenobarbital and primidone.

The manufacturers recommend that tiagabine 30 to 45 mg (in divided doses) should be given to patients taking enzyme-inducing antiepileptics.

Phenobarbital + Tibolone ❓

The manufacturers warn that phenobarbital or primidone may increase the metabolism of tibolone and thereby reduce its effects.

The clinical significance of this warning is unclear. There appear to be no reports of an interaction in practice.

Phenobarbital + Topiramate ❓

Phenobarbital and primidone can reduce the serum levels of topiramate by about 30%.

When topiramate is added to phenobarbital or primidone therapy, its dose should

P

be titrated to effect. If phenobarbital or primidone are added or withdrawn be aware that the dose of topiramate may be need adjustment.

Phenobarbital + Toremifene ⚠

Phenobarbital can reduce the serum levels of toremifene. Primidone is metabolised to phenobarbital and may therefore interact similarly.

The manufacturers of toremifene suggest that its dosage may need to be doubled in the presence of phenobarbital.

Phenobarbital + Tricyclics ⚠

Barbiturates reduce the levels of the tricyclic antidepressants, which has been associated with the re-emergence of depression. Although not all combinations have been studied, they would all be expected to interact similarly.

Monitor the outcome of concurrent use anticipating reduced tricyclic antidepressant effects. Consider an alternative to the barbiturate, or raise the tricyclic dose if problems occur. Note that tricyclics lower the seizure threshold.

Phenobarbital + Vaccines ⚠

Influenza vaccine can cause a transient moderate (30%) rise in serum phenobarbital levels. Primidone is metabolised to phenobarbital and may therefore interact similarly.

Warn the patient to monitor for indicators of phenobarbital toxicity (drowsiness, ataxia or dysarthria), and take levels if necessary. Levels may still be moderately raised after 28 days. However, most patients seem unlikely to require dosage adjustments.

Phenobarbital + Valproate ⚠

Serum phenobarbital levels can be increased by sodium valproate. Small reductions in sodium valproate levels have also been reported. Valproate has been reported to cause increases, decreases, and no change in serum primidone levels. Primidone-derived phenobarbital levels appear to be increased by valproate. Combined use of phenobarbital and valproate may cause an increase in serum liver enzymes.

Use of this combination may result in excessive sedation and lethargy. To control this interaction the dosage of phenobarbital has been reduced by about 30 to 50%, without loss of seizure control. Indicators of phenobarbital toxicity include drowsiness, ataxia or dysarthria. Monitor levels as necessary. Valproate has been associated with serious hepatotoxicity, especially in children aged less than 3 years, and this has been more common in those receiving other antiepileptics. Valproate monotherapy is to be preferred in this group.

Phenobarbital + Vigabatrin ❓

Vigabatrin causes a trivial decrease in phenobarbital and primidone levels. There is some evidence that phenobarbital may reduce the efficacy of vigabatrin in infantile spasms.

The clinical significance of this potential interaction is unclear.

Phenobarbital + Vitamin D ❓

The long-term use of phenobarbital can disturb vitamin D and calcium metabolism, which may result in osteomalacia. There are a few reports of patients taking vitamin D supplements as replacement therapy who responded poorly while taking phenobarbital or primidone.

Monitor the outcome of concurrent use. Larger doses of vitamin D may be needed.

Phenobarbital + Warfarin and other oral anticoagulants ⚠

The effects of a large number of oral anticoagulants (acenocoumarol, dicoumarol, ethyl biscoumacetate, phenprocoumon and warfarin) are reduced by the barbiturates.

Reduced anticoagulant effects may occur within 2 to 4 days (maximum effect after about 3 weeks). Monitor the INR closely until stable and be aware that dose increases of 30 to 60% are likely to be needed. Also monitor if the barbiturate is stopped (note that the interaction may persist for up to 6 weeks after concurrent use is stopped). The benzodiazepines do not usually interact with anticoagulants, and may therefore be a suitable alternative in some circumstances.

Phenobarbital + Zonisamide ❓

Phenobarbital (and therefore probably primidone) can cause a small to moderate reduction in the serum levels of zonisamide, but zonisamide appears not to affect phenobarbital or primidone levels.

The clinical importance of this interaction is unknown, but bear the possibility of reduced zonisamide levels in mind.

Phenytoin

Phenytoin is extensively metabolised by hydroxylation, principally by CYP2C9, although CYP2C19 also plays a role. These isoenzymes show genetic polymorphism, and CYP2C19 may assume a greater role in individuals who have a poor metaboliser phenotype of CYP2C9. The concurrent use of inhibitors of CYP2C9, and sometimes also CYP2C19, can lead to phenytoin toxicity. In addition, phenytoin metabolism is saturable (it shows nonlinear pharmacokinetics), therefore, small changes in metabolism or phenytoin dose can result in marked changes in plasma levels. Fosphenytoin is a prodrug of phenytoin, which is rapidly and completely hydrolysed to phenytoin in the body. It is predicted to interact with other drugs in the same way as phenytoin. No drugs are known to interfere with the conversion of fosphenytoin to phenytoin.

Phenytoin + **Phosphodiesterase type-5 inhibitors** ⚠

Phenytoin is predicted to reduce the levels of phosphodiesterase type-5 inhibitors, because other inducers of CYP3A4 have been shown to do so. For example, sildenafil levels are reduced by 70% by *bosentan* and tadalafil levels are reduced by 88% by *rifampicin*. Vardenafil is also metabolised by CYP3A4, and therefore its levels may possibly be lowered by phenytoin.

> If these phosphodiesterase type-5 inhibitors are not effective in patients taking phenytoin, it would seem sensible to try a higher dose with close monitoring. Note that fosphenytoin, a prodrug of phenytoin, may interact similarly.

Phenytoin + **Praziquantel** ⚠

Phenytoin markedly reduces the serum levels of praziquantel, but whether this results in neurocysticercosis treatment failures is unclear. Fosphenytoin, a prodrug of phenytoin, may interact similarly.

> When treating systemic worm infections such as neurocysticercosis some authors advise increasing the praziquantel dosage from 25 to 50 mg/kg if phenytoin is being used, but in one case this dose was not effective. Note that the manufacturers current recommended dose for praziquantel for neurocysticercosis is 50 mg/kg daily in 3 divided doses. The interaction with anticonvulsants is of no importance when praziquantel is used for intestinal worm infections (where its action is a local effect on the worms in the gut).

Phenytoin + **Protease inhibitors** ⚠

Nelfinavir, fosamprenavir/ritonavir, and lopinavir/ritonavir modestly reduced phenytoin levels in pharmacokinetic studies. In case reports, ritonavir has decreased, increased or not altered phenytoin levels. Phenytoin decreased lopinavir levels, and possibly also indinavir and ritonavir levels, had only had a minor effect on the levels of amprenavir (given as fosamprenavir/ritonavir), but did not alter nelfinavir levels. Phenytoin is predicted to decrease darunavir and saquinavir levels.

> Phenytoin should be used with caution in combination with any protease inhibitor, with close monitoring of antiviral efficacy and phenytoin levels. Consider using an alternative antiepileptic where possible. Note that fosphenytoin, a prodrug of phenytoin, may interact similarly.

Phenytoin + **Proton pump inhibitors** ❓

A study found that omeprazole 20 mg daily did not affect phenytoin levels, whereas earlier studies suggested that phenytoin levels might be modestly raised by omeprazole 40 mg daily. A study with esomeprazole also suggests that it may cause a minor rise in phenytoin levels. Lansoprazole does not normally interact with phenytoin, but an isolated case report of toxicity is tentatively attributed to an interaction. Fosphenytoin, a prodrug of phenytoin, may interact similarly with these proton pump inhibitors.

> This interaction is unlikely to be generally significant, but bear it in mind in case of an unexpected response to treatment. Indicators of phenytoin toxicity include blurred vision, nystagmus, ataxia or drowsiness. However, note that the manufacturers of esomeprazole recommend monitoring phenytoin levels.

P

Phenytoin + Pyridoxine ❓

Daily doses of pyridoxine 80 to 400 mg can cause reductions of about 35% in phenytoin levels in some patients. The effect on fosphenytoin, a prodrug of phenytoin, does not appear to have been studied, but it may be prudent to assume it may interact similarly.

> Concurrent use should be monitored if large doses of pyridoxine are used, being alert for the need to increase the phenytoin dosage. It seems unlikely that small doses (as in multivitamin preparations) will interact to any great extent.

Phenytoin + Quinidine ⚠

Quinidine levels can be reduced by phenytoin. Loss of arrhythmia control is possible if the quinidine dosage is not increased. Fosphenytoin, a prodrug of phenytoin, may interact similarly.

> Concurrent use need not be avoided, but be alert for the need to increase the quinidine dosage. If phenytoin is withdrawn the quinidine dosage may need to be reduced to avoid quinidine toxicity. Quinidine serum levels should be monitored if possible.

Phenytoin + Quinolones ⚠

Studies suggest that ciprofloxacin, clinafloxacin, and enoxacin do not usually have a clinically significant effect on phenytoin levels. However, case reports describe both a rise and a fall in phenytoin levels in patients given ciprofloxacin. Fosphenytoin, a prodrug of phenytoin, may interact similarly.

> The clinical importance of these changes in levels is unknown, but bear them in mind in case of an unexpected response to treatment. It has been suggested that it may be prudent to monitor phenytoin levels in those given ciprofloxacin. Quinolones alone very occasionally cause convulsions, therefore they should be used with caution in patients with epilepsy.

Phenytoin + Rifampicin (Rifampin) ⚠

Serum phenytoin levels can be markedly reduced by rifampicin (clearance doubled in one study). If rifampicin is given with isoniazid, phenytoin levels may fall in patients who are fast acetylators of isoniazid, but may occasionally rise in those who are slow acetylators. Fosphenytoin, a prodrug of phenytoin, may interact similarly.

> It is unlikely that the acetylator status of the patient will be known. Therefore monitor phenytoin levels and adjust the dose accordingly.

Phenytoin + Rimonabant ❓

The manufacturers predict that potent inducers of CYP3A4 such as phenytoin (and therefore possibly fosphenytoin) may lower the serum levels of rimonabant. This is based on the fact that potent *inhibitors* of CYP3A4 *increase* rimonabant levels (see under azoles, page 122).

> Caution is recommended with concurrent use of phenytoin. Patients should be monitored to ensure rimonabant remains effective.

Phenytoin + Sirolimus ❓

The manufacturers predict that phenytoin (and therefore possibly fosphenytoin) may lower the serum levels of sirolimus, probably because rifampicin (rifampin), another CYP3A4 inducer, has been shown to do so. This prediction seems to be confirmed by 2 patients who needed an increase in their sirolimus doses when they were given phenytoin.

> The extent of any change in sirolimus levels is uncertain, but it would seem prudent to increase the frequency of monitoring sirolimus levels, both during concurrent use and also if phenytoin is withdrawn.

Phenytoin + Solifenacin ⚠

Ketoconazole increases solifenacin levels 2- to 3-fold by *inhibiting* CYP3A4. The manufacturers predict that potent CYP3A4 *inducers* (e.g. phenytoin, and therefore probably fosphenytoin) will decrease solifenacin levels.

> Be alert for a reduction in the efficacy of solifenacin in patients taking phenytoin.

Phenytoin + SSRIs ⚠

Phenytoin serum levels can be increased by fluoxetine in some patients and toxicity may occur. There are also isolated reports of phenytoin toxicity when fluvoxamine was also taken. Phenytoin and sertraline do not normally interact, but 2 patients have shown increased serum phenytoin levels while taking sertraline. Fosphenytoin, a prodrug of phenytoin, may interact similarly with these SSRIs.

> Monitor patients for signs of phenytoin toxicity, such as blurred vision, nystagmus, ataxia or drowsiness. Consider monitoring phenytoin levels and adjust the dose accordingly. Note that SSRIs should be avoided in unstable epilepsy and used with care in other epileptics.

Phenytoin + Sulfinpyrazone ⚠

Some limited evidence indicates that phenytoin levels may be markedly increased by sulfinpyrazone. Fosphenytoin, a prodrug of phenytoin, may interact similarly.

> Warn the patient to monitor for indicators of phenytoin toxicity (blurred vision, nystagmus, ataxia or drowsiness). It would seem advisable to monitor phenytoin levels.

Phenytoin + **Sulfonamides** ⚠

Phenytoin serum levels can be raised by co-trimoxazole (which contains sulfamethoxazole), sulfamethizole, sulfamethoxazole, and sulfadiazine. Phenytoin toxicity may develop in some cases. Fosphenytoin, a prodrug of phenytoin, may interact similarly.

> The risk of toxicity is small and is most likely in those with serum phenytoin levels at the top end of the range. Monitor phenytoin levels and adjust the dose accordingly. Indicators of phenytoin toxicity include blurred vision, nystagmus, ataxia or drowsiness.

Phenytoin + **Tacrolimus** ❓

An isolated report describes an increase in serum phenytoin levels attributed to the use of tacrolimus. Phenytoin decreased tacrolimus levels in one case, and has been used to reduce tacrolimus levels after an overdose. Fosphenytoin, a prodrug of phenytoin, may interact similarly

> No interaction is established, but based on the known metabolism of these drugs it would be prudent to monitor tacrolimus levels in a patient given phenytoin. Similarly, based on the single case of phenytoin toxicity, it may also be advisable to monitor phenytoin levels.

Phenytoin + **Tetracyclines** ⚠

The serum levels of doxycycline are reduced and may fall below the accepted minimum inhibitory concentration in patients receiving long-term treatment with phenytoin. Fosphenytoin, a prodrug of phenytoin, may interact similarly.

> It has been suggested that the doxycycline dosage could be doubled to counteract this interaction. Tetracycline, oxytetracycline and chlortetracycline appear not to interact and may therefore be suitable alternatives.

Phenytoin + **Theophylline** ⚠

The serum levels of theophylline can be markedly reduced by phenytoin and dosage increases may be needed to maintain therapeutic theophylline levels. Fosphenytoin, a prodrug of phenytoin, may interact similarly. Some limited evidence suggests that theophylline may also reduce phenytoin levels.

> Ideally theophylline levels should be measured to confirm that they remain within the therapeutic range. Dosage increases of theophylline of up to 50% or more may be required. The effect of theophylline on phenytoin is not established. It may be prudent to monitor phenytoin levels as well. Separating the oral dosage by 1 to 2 hours appears to minimise the effects of theophylline on phenytoin.

Phenytoin + **Tiagabine** ⚠

The plasma concentrations of tiagabine may be reduced by 1.5 to 3-fold by phenytoin. Fosphenytoin, a prodrug of phenytoin, may interact similarly

> The manufacturers recommend that tiagabine 30 to 45 mg (in divided doses) should be given to patients taking enzyme-inducing antiepileptics.

P

Phenytoin + Tibolone ❓

The manufacturers warn that phenytoin (and therefore possibly fosphenytoin) may increase the metabolism of tibolone and thereby reduce its effects.

The clinical significance of this warning is unclear. There appear to be no reports of an interaction in practice.

Phenytoin + Ticlopidine ⚠

There are a number of case reports of patients taking phenytoin who developed toxicity when ticlopidine was added. Ticlopidine appears to inhibit phenytoin metabolism. Fosphenytoin, a prodrug of phenytoin, may interact similarly.

It would be prudent to monitor serum phenytoin levels if ticlopidine is added. Warn the patient to monitor for indicators of phenytoin toxicity (blurred vision, nystagmus, ataxia or drowsiness).

Phenytoin + Topiramate ⚠

Phenytoin increases the clearance of topiramate 2- to 3-fold, which appears to result in topiramate levels that are up to 50% lower. Topiramate slightly increases the phenytoin AUC (raised about 25%) but this is said not to be clinically significant. Fosphenytoin, a prodrug of phenytoin, may interact similarly.

Topiramate dose adjustments may be required if phenytoin is added or discontinued. Be aware that a few patients may have increased phenytoin levels, particularly at high topiramate doses. Warn the patient to monitor for indicators of phenytoin toxicity (blurred vision, nystagmus, ataxia or drowsiness). Consider monitoring phenytoin levels.

Phenytoin + Toremifene ⚠

Phenytoin can reduce the serum levels of toremifene. Fosphenytoin, a prodrug of phenytoin, may interact similarly.

The manufacturers of toremifene suggest that the dosage may need to be doubled in the presence of phenytoin.

Phenytoin + Tricyclics ❓

Some very limited evidence suggests that imipramine can raise serum phenytoin levels. Phenytoin possibly reduces serum desipramine levels. Fosphenytoin, a prodrug of phenytoin, may interact similarly.

Care should be taken if deciding to use this combination in epileptic patients. If concurrent use is undertaken the effects should be very well monitored. Note that the tricyclics lower the convulsive threshold.

Phenytoin + **Trimethoprim** ⚠

Phenytoin serum levels can be raised by co-trimoxazole (which contains trimethoprim). Trimethoprim can increase decrease the clearance of phenytoin by 30% and prolong its half-life. Phenytoin toxicity may develop in some cases. Fosphenytoin, a prodrug of phenytoin, may interact similarly.

> The risk of toxicity is small and is most likely in those with serum phenytoin levels at the top end of the range. Monitor phenytoin levels and adjust the dose accordingly. Indicators of phenytoin toxicity include blurred vision, nystagmus, ataxia or drowsiness.

P

Phenytoin + **Vaccines** ✓

Influenza vaccine is reported to increase, decrease or to have no effect on the serum levels of phenytoin. Fosphenytoin, a prodrug of phenytoin, may interact similarly. The efficacy of the vaccine is unaffected.

> Phenytoin levels appear to return to normal after about 14 days. Warn the patient to monitor for indicators of phenytoin toxicity (blurred vision, nystagmus, ataxia or drowsiness). However, be aware that any alteration in levels may take a couple of weeks to develop and usually resolves spontaneously.

Phenytoin + **Valproate** ⚠

Concurrent use is usually uneventful. Initially total serum phenytoin levels may fall by 20 to 50% but this is offset by a rise in the levels of free (and active) phenytoin, which may very occasionally cause some toxicity. After continued use the total serum phenytoin levels rise once again. Phenytoin also reduces valproate levels. Fosphenytoin, a prodrug of phenytoin, may interact similarly.

> Monitor phenytoin and adjust the dose accordingly. When monitoring concurrent use it is important to understand fully the implications of changes in 'total', and 'free' or 'unbound' serum phenytoin levels. Where monitoring of free phenytoin levels is not available, various nomograms have been designed for predicting unbound phenytoin levels during the use of sodium valproate. Consider monitoring valproate levels for an indication of toxicity if phenytoin is stopped.

Phenytoin + **Vigabatrin** ❓

Vigabatrin causes a small to moderate 20 to 30% fall in serum phenytoin levels. Fosphenytoin, a prodrug of phenytoin, may interact similarly

> Occasional patients may require a small adjustment in dose. Note that this interaction can take several weeks to develop.

Phenytoin + **Vitamin D** ⚠

The long-term use of phenytoin can disturb vitamin D and calcium metabolism, which may result in osteomalacia. There are a few reports of patients taking vitamin D supplements for replacement therapy who responded poorly while taking phenytoin. Fosphenytoin, a prodrug of phenytoin, may interact similarly.

Monitor the outcome of concurrent use. Larger doses of vitamin D may be needed.

Phenytoin + **Warfarin and other oral anticoagulants** ❓

Phenytoin would be expected to reduce the anticoagulant effects of the coumarins and this has been seen with warfarin. However, cases where the effects of warfarin were *increased* have been reported, and one study showed the effects of phenprocoumon were generally unaltered by phenytoin. A single case of severe bleeding has been described in a patient taking acenocoumarol, paroxetine and phenytoin. Fosphenytoin, a prodrug of phenytoin, may interact similarly. Limited evidence suggests that phenytoin levels may rise in patients taking phenprocoumon or warfarin.

None of these interactions have been extensively studied nor are they well established. Warn patients to monitor for indicators of phenytoin toxicity (blurred vision, nystagmus, ataxia or drowsiness) and to report any increased bruising or bleeding. Consider monitoring phenytoin levels and anticoagulant control if acenocoumarol, phenprocoumon or warfarin is given with phenytoin.

Phenytoin + **Zonisamide** ❓

Phenytoin can cause a small to moderate reduction in the serum levels of zonisamide. Zonisamide appears not to affect phenytoin levels in most studies, although two studies suggest a modest rise of about 20% may occur. Fosphenytoin, a prodrug of phenytoin, may interact similarly

The general importance of this interaction is unknown although a serious interaction is unlikely. Consider the importance of a possible reduction in zonisamide levels. Bear the potential for a modest increase in phenytoin levels in mind should a patient taking zonisamide develop signs of phenytoin toxicity (blurred vision, nystagmus, ataxia or drowsiness).

Phosphodiesterase type-5 inhibitors

Phosphodiesterase type-5 inhibitors + **Procainamide** ❌

Vardenafil causes a slight prolongation of the QT interval. The manufacturers therefore contraindicate class Ia antiarrhythmics such as procainamide. Consider also drugs that prolong the QT interval, page 237.

Avoid concurrent use.

Phosphodiesterase type-5 inhibitors + **Protease inhibitors**

Ritonavir with Sildenafil ❌

Ritonavir can cause marked rises in serum sildenafil levels. A fatal heart attack occurred in a man taking ritonavir and saquinavir when he also took sildenafil.

> If the decision is taken to use sildenafil in a patient taking ritonavir, the dose of sildenafil should not exceed 25 mg in a 48-hour period, but note that the fatality described above occurred despite the use of this dose. There appears to be no direct information about ritonavir used as a pharmacokinetic enhancer, but given the magnitude of the effect with ritonavir 400 mg (11-fold rise), it would seem prudent to take a cautious approach, and follow the advice for high-dose ritonavir. Use of ritonavir with sildenafil used for the management of pulmonary hypertension is contraindicated.

P

Other protease inhibitors ⚠

Indinavir and saquinavir can cause marked rises in serum sildenafil levels; ritonavir raises tadalafil levels; and ritonavir and indinavir raise vardenafil levels. It seems likely that all protease inhibitors will interact with these phosphodiesterase inhibitors.

> In general, it is recommended that a low sildenafil starting dose of 25 mg should be considered for erectile dysfunction, and 20 mg twice daily for pulmonary hypertension in those taking protease inhibitors (but see ritonavir, above). For indinavir a starting dose of 12.5 mg may be more appropriate for erectile dysfunction, and the maximum dosage frequency should be reduced to once or twice weekly. The US manufacturer advises that the dose of tadalafil should not exceed 10 mg every 72 hours in patients taking ritonavir. Similar precautions would seem prudent with other protease inhibitors. Due to the large rises in vardenafil levels, the UK manufacturer contraindicates its use with protease inhibitors that are potent CYP3A4 (they name ritonavir and indinavir). In contrast, the US prescribing information recommends dose restrictions as follows: the dose of vardenafil should not exceed 2.5 mg in 24 hours when used with atazanavir, indinavir, or saquinavir, and should not exceed 2.5 mg in 72 hours when used with ritonavir. Similar precautions would seem prudent with other protease inhibitors.

Phosphodiesterase type-5 inhibitors + **Quinidine** ❌

Vardenafil causes a slight prolongation of the QT interval. The manufacturers therefore contraindicate class Ia antiarrhythmics such as quinidine. Consider also drugs that prolong the QT interval, page 237.

> Avoid concurrent use.

Phosphodiesterase type-5 inhibitors + **Rifabutin** ⚠

Rifabutin is predicted to reduce the levels of phosphodiesterase type-5 inhibitors, because other inducers of CYP3A4 have been shown to do so. For example, sildenafil levels are reduced by 70% by *bosentan* and tadalafil levels are reduced by 88% by *rifampicin*. Vardenafil is also metabolised by CYP3A4, and therefore its levels may possibly be lowered by rifabutin.

> If these phosphodiesterase type-5 inhibitors are not effective in patients taking rifabutin, it would seem sensible to try a higher dose with close monitoring.

Phosphodiesterase type-5 inhibitors + **Rifampicin (Rifampin)** ❓

Tadalafil levels are reduced by 88% by rifampicin, by inhibiting CYP3A4. Rifampicin is predicted to reduce the levels of other phosphodiesterase type-5 inhibitors, which are also metabolised by CYP3A4.

> If these phosphodiesterase type-5 inhibitors are not effective in patients taking rifampicin, it would seem sensible to try a higher dose with close monitoring.

Praziquantel

Praziquantel + **Rifampicin (Rifampin)** ❌

Plasma levels of praziquantel are markedly reduced by rifampicin pretreatment, to undetectable levels in over half of the subjects in one study.

> It is predicted that rifampicin will reduce the efficacy of praziquantel, and therefore the combination should be avoided.

Probenecid

Probenecid + **Pyrazinamide** ❌

The interactions of probenecid and pyrazinamide and their effects on the excretion of uric acid are complex. The overall effect is that if probenecid were to be used to treat the hyperuricaemia caused by pyrazinamide, the normal uricosuric effects of probenecid would be diminished and larger doses would be required.

> Note that hyperuricaemia is a contraindication to pyrazinamide use and it should be stopped if gouty arthritis occurs.

Probenecid + **Quinolones** ✅

Probenecid increases the serum levels and/or decreases the urinary excretion of cinoxacin, ciprofloxacin, clinafloxacin, enoxacin, fleroxacin, levofloxacin, nalidixic acid and norfloxacin.

> This is unlikely to be of clinical significance unless other drugs that affect renal

clearance are taken concurrently. Grepafloxacin, moxifloxacin, sparfloxacin, and probably ofloxacin, appear not to interact with probenecid.

Procainamide

Procainamide + Trimethoprim ⚠

Trimethoprim causes a marked increase in the plasma levels of procainamide and its active metabolite, N-acetylprocainamide.

The need to reduce the procainamide dosage should be anticipated if trimethoprim is given to patients already controlled on procainamide.

Proguanil

Proguanil + Warfarin and other oral anticoagulants ❓

An isolated report describes bleeding in a patient taking warfarin after she took proguanil for about 5 weeks.

Any interaction seems rare, but bear it in mind in case of an excessive response to warfarin.

Propafenone

Propafenone + Quinidine ⚠

Quinidine doubles the plasma levels of propafenone and halves the levels of its active metabolite, but the antiarrhythmic effects appear to be unaffected.

Anticipate the need to reduce the propafenone dosage (possibly by half) if the combination is used. Monitor well.

Propafenone + Rifampicin (Rifampin) ⚠

When given orally, propafenone serum levels can be markedly reduced by rifampicin (bioavailability reduced by at least half). This has resulted in the re-emergence of arrhythmias in some cases. Limited evidence suggests that intravenous propafenone is not affected.

The dosage of oral propafenone will probably need increasing if rifampicin is given. Alternatively, if possible, it has been advised that another antibacterial be used because of the probable difficulty in adjusting the propafenone dosage.

Propafenone + SSRIs ⚠

Fluoxetine markedly inhibits the metabolism (5-hydroxylation) of propafenone, and paroxetine would also be expected to behave similarly, but the clinical consequences of this are unknown. Fluvoxamine would be expected to inhibit the metabolism of propafenone by *N*-dealkylation, but in most patients this is only expected to have a small effect.

Until more is known, it would be prudent to use caution when giving fluoxetine or paroxetine with propafenone. Sertraline, citalopram and probably escitalopram would not be expected to interact and an *in vitro* study supports this suggestion.

Propafenone + Terbinafine ⚠

In vitro studies suggest that terbinafine is an inhibitor of CYP2D6. It may therefore be expected to increase the plasma levels of other drugs that are substrates of this enzyme, such as propafenone.

Until more is known it would seem wise to be aware of the possibility of an increase in adverse effects if propafenone is given with terbinafine and consider a dose reduction if necessary.

Propafenone + Warfarin and other oral anticoagulants ⚠

The anticoagulant effects of warfarin are increased by propafenone (mean 7 second rise in prothrombin time, which was considered to be clinically significant). Case reports suggest that phenprocoumon and fluindione interact similarly.

Monitor the anticoagulant effect if propafenone is added or withdrawn. This interaction appears to start in the first week of concurrent use.

Protease inhibitors

The protease inhibitors are extensively metabolised by cytochrome P450, particularly CYP3A4. All of the protease inhibitors inhibit CYP3A4, with ritonavir being the most potent inhibitor, followed by indinavir, nelfinavir, amprenavir, and saquinavir. The protease inhibitors therefore have the potential to interact with other drugs metabolised by CYP3A4, and are also affected by CYP3A4 inhibitors and inducers. Ritonavir and nelfinavir also affect some other cytochrome P450 isoenzymes. In addition, protease inhibitors are substrates as well as inhibitors of P-glycoprotein. The plasma level of protease inhibitors is thought to be critical in maintaining efficacy and minimising the potential for development of viral resistance. Therefore even modest reductions in levels are potentially clinically important.

Protease inhibitors + **Proton pump inhibitors** ❌

The levels of atazanavir/ritonavir and nelfinavir are reduced by omeprazole: all proton pump inhibitors are expected to interact similarly. However, in some patients taking omeprazole the levels of nelfinavir were *raised*. Indinavir levels are also reduced however the addition of ritonavir may negate this effect. Tipranavir reduces esomeprazole and omeprazole levels.

> It has been said that omeprazole should probably not be used with indinavir unless ritonavir is used to boost the indinavir levels. This would be likely to apply to other proton pump inhibitors used with indinavir as well. Atazanavir or atazanavir/ritonavir, and nelfinavir should not be given with proton pump inhibitors. Similar caution would seem prudent with amprenavir. The use of tipranavir with omeprazole or esomeprazole is not recommended, but if both drugs are given, consider increasing the dose of the proton pump inhibitor, according to response.

Protease inhibitors + **Quinidine** ❌

The protease inhibitors are generally expected to increase quinidine levels.

> The following protease inhibitors are contraindicated with quinidine: amprenavir (UK), atazanavir/ritonavir (UK), darunavir/ritonavir (UK), fosamprenavir (UK), nelfinavir, ritonavir, saquinavir/ritonavir (US) tipranavir/ritonavir. Caution, with monitoring of quinidine levels, is recommended for indinavir, lopinavir/ritonavir and saquinavir/ritonavir (UK).

Protease inhibitors + **Rifabutin** ⚠

The bioavailability of rifabutin is increased by amprenavir, atazanavir, indinavir, nelfinavir, and especially ritonavir, with an increased risk of toxicity. Rifabutin decreases the bioavailability of indinavir, nelfinavir, and particularly saquinavir (with an increased risk of therapeutic failure) but has no effect on amprenavir, atazanavir and ritonavir-boosted fosamprenavir.

> The combination of rifabutin with protease inhibitors may be used, but large dosage reductions of rifabutin and/or increases in the doses of the protease inhibitors are often necessary. The treatment of tuberculosis in patients taking antiretrovirals is complex and up-to-date guidelines should be consulted.

Protease inhibitors + **Rifampicin (Rifampin)** ❌

Rifampicin bioavailability is increased by indinavir, but amprenavir has no effect. Rifampicin markedly reduces the bioavailability of amprenavir, atazanavir, indinavir, lopinavir, nelfinavir and saquinavir.

> The use of many of the protease inhibitors with rifampicin is contraindicated. The treatment of tuberculosis in patients taking antiretrovirals is complex and up-to-date guidelines should be consulted.

Protease inhibitors + **Rimonabant** ⚠

Ketoconazole doubles the AUC of rimonabant. Other drugs that are potent inhibitors of CYP3A4, such as ritonavir, are predicted to interact similarly.

The manufacturers of rimonabant recommend caution. Monitor for signs of increased rimonabant adverse effects.

Protease inhibitors + **Sirolimus** ⚠

Nelfinavir increased the levels of sirolimus in one patient. Other protease inhibitors are predicted to raise sirolimus levels.

Sirolimus levels and effects (e.g. on renal function) should be monitored as a matter of routine, but it would be prudent to increase monitoring if protease inhibitors are given.

Protease inhibitors + **Solifenacin** ⚠

Ketoconazole increases solifenacin levels 2- to 3-fold by inhibiting CYP3A4. The manufacturers say other potent CYP3A4 inhibitors (such as the protease inhibitors) will have the same effect.

The manufacturers limit the daily dose of solifenacin to 5 mg if it is given with potent inhibitors of CYP3A4. In addition, in patients with severe renal impairment or moderate hepatic impairment, concurrent use is contraindicated.

Protease inhibitors + **SSRIs** ⚠

Fluoxetine modestly raises the levels of ritonavir. A few cases of serotonin syndrome have been attributed to the use of fluoxetine and ritonavir. Darunavir/ritonavir and fosamprenavir/ritonavir reduced paroxetine levels and darunavir/ritonavir reduced sertraline levels. Fluoxetine would be expected to be similarly affected. These *reductions* in SSRI levels are opposite to the effect originally predicted.

It would be prudent to anticipate some reduction in efficacy when starting these protease inhibitors (and probably any ritonavir-boosted protease inhibitors) in patients taking fluoxetine, sertraline or paroxetine. Monitor the clinical effect and increase the SSRI dose as necessary. The general relevance of the few cases of serotonin syndrome, page 392, is also uncertain.

Protease inhibitors + **Statins**

Atorvastatin ⚠

The levels of atorvastatin appear to be markedly increased by darunavir/ritonavir, lopinavir/ritonavir, nelfinavir, and saquinavir/ritonavir. The manufacturers of atazanavir/ritonavir and amprenavir state that they may also increase atorvastatin levels.

It is generally recommended that atorvastatin is used at low doses (i.e. 10 mg) and with care in patients taking protease inhibitors. Patients should be counselled regarding myopathy (e.g. report any unexplained muscle pain, tenderness or weakness). The manufacturers of atazanavir and tipranavir advise avoiding concurrent use.

Simvastatin or Lovastatin ✖

The levels of simvastatin appear to be markedly increased by nelfinavir, ritonavir and saquinavir/ritonavir. Two cases of rhabdomyolysis have been attributed to the use of ritonavir with simvastatin. The manufacturers of atazanavir, amprenavir and fosamprenavir state that they may increase simvastatin and lovastatin levels.

It is generally recommended that simvastatin and lovastatin be avoided in patients taking any protease inhibitor. The manufacturers of amprenavir and fosamprenavir recommend fluvastatin or pravastatin as alternatives.

Other statins ⚠

Fluvastatin, pravastatin and rosuvastatin are not predominantly metabolised by CYP3A4, so it seems unlikely that dosage adjustments will be needed if they are given with protease inhibitors. However, there is some limited evidence to suggest that moderate increases in the levels of some statins may occur and an increase in some muscle disorders has been reported. The manufacturers of rosuvastatin note that during clinical studies there was an increase in myositis and myopathy in patients also taking protease inhibitors.

Patients should be counselled regarding myopathy (e.g. report any unexplained muscle pain, tenderness or weakness). Note that some manufacturers recommend starting with the lowest doses of pravastatin or rosuvastatin.

Protease inhibitors + Tacrolimus ⚠

Protease inhibitors are predicted to inhibit the metabolism of tacrolimus and increase its blood levels. Case reports have described this interaction with lopinavir, nelfinavir and saquinavir/ritonavir.

When protease inhibitors are given to patients taking tacrolimus, careful monitoring and probably a reduction in the dose of tacrolimus is required. Note that in one case tacrolimus was dosed just once weekly to achieve appropriate levels.

Protease inhibitors + Theophylline ⚠

Ritonavir can reduce the serum levels of theophylline by up to 57%.

Monitor the effect of concurrent use on theophylline levels. It may be necessary to increase the theophylline dose. Note that the interaction may take a week to fully develop.

Protease inhibitors + Tolterodine ⚠

Ketoconazole raises the AUC of tolterodine by more than 2-fold in some patients. Other potent inhibitors of CYP3A4, such as the protease inhibitors, are predicted to interact similarly.

The UK manufacturers advise avoiding concurrent use. The US manufacturers suggest reducing the tolterodine dose to 1 mg twice daily, which seems practical. It may be prudent to assess experience of adverse effects in these patients, and to reduce the dose further or withdraw the drug if it is not tolerated.

Protease inhibitors + Trazodone ▲

Ritonavir increases the AUC of trazodone by more than 2-fold and sedation and fatigue were increased. Two cases of serotonin syndrome, page 392, have been reported in patients taking trazodone and ritonavir or indinavir. Other protease inhibitors may interact similarly.

A lower dose of trazodone should be considered if it is given with potent CYP3A4 inhibitors such as ritonavir and indinavir, although note that in the UK it has been suggested that the combination should be avoided where possible.

Protease inhibitors + Tricyclics ▲

Ritonavir raises desipramine levels and is predicted to also raise the levels of other tricyclic antidepressants. *In vitro* evidence suggests that other protease inhibitors may interact similarly, but to a lesser extent.

A lower starting dose of desipramine has been suggested, and monitoring is advisable if tricyclic antidepressants are given to patients taking protease inhibitors.

Protease inhibitors + Triptans ✗

The manufacturer of eletriptan predicts that indinavir, nelfinavir and ritonavir will increase eletriptan levels. This seems reasonable, based on the way other CYP3A4 inhibitors interact. It seems possible that all protease inhibitors may interact, although probably to a lesser degree.

The manufacturers of eletriptan say that the concurrent use of indinavir, nelfinavir and ritonavir should be avoided.

Protease inhibitors + Venlafaxine ▲

In a single-dose study venlafaxine lowered indinavir levels by over 35%.

Monitor concurrent use to confirm that the effects of indinavir remain adequate.

Protease inhibitors + Warfarin and other oral anticoagulants ❓

Ritonavir has been predicted to raise warfarin levels and INRs. This was confirmed by one case report, whereas two others found entirely the opposite. A case report suggests that indinavir might cause a moderate reduction in anticoagulation. There is also a report of a marked reduction in anticoagulation in a patient taking acenocoumarol with ritonavir or nelfinavir. An isolated report describes a gradual INR rise in an elderly patient taking warfarin with saquinavir.

It would seem prudent to monitor any anticoagulant/protease inhibitor combination for an alteration in anticoagulant effect, although current evidence tends to suggest that a clinically significant interaction is rare.

P

Proton pump inhibitors

Proton pump inhibitors + SSRIs ⚠

Fluvoxamine inhibits the metabolism of lansoprazole, omeprazole and rabeprazole in some patients. Theoretically other proton pump inhibitors will be similarly affected. Omeprazole (and therefore probably esomeprazole) increases escitalopram (and therefore probably citalopram) levels by 50%.

Monitor concurrent use for adverse effects (such as nausea, diarrhoea, dry mouth, palpitations). The manufacturers of escitalopram say that dose adjustments may be necessary, but this would seem unlikely in most patients.

Proton pump inhibitors + Tacrolimus ⚠

Lansoprazole may increase tacrolimus levels in patients with low CYP2C19 levels. Omeprazole (and therefore probably esomeprazole) and pantoprazole are predicted to interact similarly.

It would seem prudent to consider monitoring tacrolimus levels as it is unlikely that CYP2C19 metaboliser status is known. Rabeprazole may be a suitable alternative proton pump inhibitor, as limited evidence suggests that it does not interact, and nor would it be expected to do so.

Proton pump inhibitors + Warfarin and other oral anticoagulants ❓

Raised INRs and/or bleeding have been seen in patients taking warfarin with esomeprazole, lansoprazole or omeprazole, and acenocoumarol with omeprazole, but on the whole the proton pump inhibitors do not appear to have any clinically significant interactions with these anticoagulants.

Any interaction seems rare, but bear the possibility in mind in case of an excessive response to anticoagulation.

Pyrimethamine

Pyrimethamine + Sulfonamides ⚠

Serious pancytopenia and megaloblastic anaemia have been described in patients given pyrimethamine and either co-trimoxazole (which contains sulfamethoxazole) or other sulfonamides.

Pyrimethamine is usually given with a sulfonamide for toxoplasmosis and malaria. Nevertheless, caution should be used in prescribing the combination, especially in the presence of other drugs (e.g. methotrexate) or disease states that may predispose to folate deficiency. When high-dose pyrimethamine is used for the treatment of toxoplasmosis, the manufacturer recommends that all patients should receive a folate supplement. Note that the manufacturer of sulfadoxine/pyrimethamine recommends that the concurrent use of sulfonamides (including co-trimoxazole) should be avoided.

Pyrimethamine + Trimethoprim ⚠

Serious pancytopenia and megaloblastic anaemia have been described in patients given pyrimethamine and co-trimoxazole (which contains trimethoprim).

Caution should be used in prescribing the combination, especially in the presence of other drugs (e.g. methotrexate) or disease states that may also affect folate metabolism. When high-dose pyrimethamine is used for the treatment of toxoplasmosis, the manufacturer recommends that all patients should receive a folate supplement.

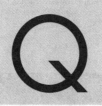

Quinidine

Quinidine + Rifabutin ⚠

The serum levels of quinidine and its therapeutic effects can be markedly reduced by *rifampicin*. In one case quinidine levels were reduced from 4 to 0.5 micrograms/mL. Rifabutin is predicted to interact similarly, but probably to a lesser extent.

> A quinidine dosage increase may be necessary if rifabutin is given. Monitor concurrent use and adjust the dose as necessary.

Quinidine + Rifampicin (Rifampin) ⚠

The serum levels of quinidine and its therapeutic effects can be markedly reduced by rifampicin. In one case quinidine levels were reduced from 4 to 0.5 micrograms/mL.

> The dosage of quinidine will need to be increased (possibly more than doubled in some patients) if rifampicin is given concurrently. The quinidine dose will need to be reduced when the rifampicin is stopped. Monitor the serum levels where possible.

Quinidine + Tricyclics ⚠

Quinidine can significantly reduce the clearance of some tricyclics (desipramine, imipramine, nortriptyline and trimipramine), thereby increasing their serum levels.

> Monitor for signs of tricyclic adverse effects. Additive QT-prolonging effects are also possible, see drugs that prolong the QT interval, page 237.

Quinidine + Warfarin and other oral anticoagulants ❓

In one study and one retrospective analysis, quinidine had no effect on the anticoagulant control with warfarin. However, a few isolated cases of increased anticoagulant effect with bleeding have been reported. Limited evidence suggests that quinidine does not alter phenprocoumon pharmacokinetics.

No interaction would normally be anticipated.

Quinine

Quinine + **Rifampicin (Rifampin)** ⚠

Rifampicin increases the clearance of quinine 6-fold.

It has been suggested that rifampicin should not be given with quinine for the treatment of malaria. Patients receiving rifampicin who also require quinine for malaria may need increased doses of quinine.

Quinine + **Warfarin and other oral anticoagulants** ❓

Normally no significant interaction occurs between warfarin and quinine but 2 women required warfarin dosage reductions and one man developed extensive haematuria after drinking large amounts of quinine-containing tonic water.

Any interaction seems rare, but bear it in mind in case of unexpected bleeding.

Quinolones

The quinolones are generally considered to be inhibitors of CYP1A2; however, it should be noted that they varying in the strength of their effect. Quinolones that are more potent inhibitors of CYP1A2 are likely to have greater effects on substrates of this isoenzyme, and therefore their use seems more likely to be associated with greater clinical consequences. Caffeine is used as a probe substrate for CYP1A2. Therefore the magnitude of the effect the quinolones have on caffeine can be used as a guide to the strength of their effect on CYP1A2. The interactions of the quinolones with caffeine suggests that enoxacin has the greatest effects, ciprofloxacin and pipemidic acid have moderate effects, while gatifloxacin, levofloxacin, lomefloxacin, moxifloxacin, nalidixic acid, norfloxacin, ofloxacin, pefloxacin, rufloxacin and sparfloxacin only inhibit CYP1A2 to a small or clinically irrelevant extent.

Quinolones + **Sevelamer** ⚠

Sevelamer reduced the bioavailability of ciprofloxacin by 48% in one study.

The manufacturers advise that ciprofloxacin should be taken at least 1 hour before or 3 hours after sevelamer. It seems possible that other quinolones could be similarly affected.

Quinolones + **Strontium** ✗

The manufacturer of strontium predicts that it will form a complex with quinolones, and therefore prevent their absorption.

It is recommended that when treatment with a quinolone is required, strontium ranelate therapy should be temporarily suspended.

Quinolones + **Sucralfate** ⚠

Sucralfate causes a marked reduction in the absorption of ciprofloxacin, moxifloxacin, lomefloxacin, ofloxacin, norfloxacin, and sparfloxacin, which may lead to therapeutic failure. It seems possible that other quinolones could be similarly affected.

The interaction is reduced if sucralfate is given 2 to 6 hours after the quinolone. Proton pump inhibitors and H_2-receptor antagonists do not normally interact and may therefore be possible alternatives in some patients.

Q

Quinolones + **Theophylline** ⚠

Theophylline levels can be markedly increased in some patients by ciprofloxacin, and possibly pefloxacin. Norfloxacin and ofloxacin normally cause a much smaller rise in theophylline levels, although serious toxicity has been seen in a few patients taking norfloxacin. Convulsions have been reported with theophylline and ciprofloxacin or norfloxacin. With some of these cases it is difficult to know whether what happened was due to increased theophylline levels, to patient pre-disposition, to potential additive effects on the seizure threshold, or to all three factors combined.

The dose should be modified based on the theophylline level on day 2 of ciprofloxacin treatment. It may be prudent to follow similar precautions with ofloxacin and norfloxacin. Seizures resulting from concurrent use are relatively rare. Gatifloxacin, levofloxacin, lomefloxacin, moxifloxacin, nalidixic acid and sparfloxacin appear not to significantly affect theophylline levels.

Quinolones + **Tizanidine** ✗

Ciprofloxacin increases the AUC of tizanidine tenfold, which increases the hypotensive and sedative effects of tizanidine. Other quinolones may also interact, see quinolones, page 382.

Anticipate the need to reduce the tizanidine dose before starting ciprofloxacin, and closely monitor adverse effects such as marked hypotension, bradycardia, and sedation. Note that in the manufacturers contraindicate the combination.

Quinolones + **Triptans** ⚠

Quinolones are predicted to raise zolmitriptan levels.

The manufacturer recommends a dose reduction of zolmitriptan to a maximum of 5 mg in 24 hours in patients taking quinolones such as ciprofloxacin. Other quinolones may interact to varying extents, see quinolones, page 382.

Quinolones + **Warfarin and other oral anticoagulants** ⚠

The quinolones do not normally alter the effects of coumarin anticoagulants in most patients, but increased effects and even bleeding have been seen in some patients.

It would be prudent to monitor the effects of concurrent use. In one large review serious problems were identified at about 5 days so it may be prudent to measure the INR just before this point.

Quinolones + **Zinc** ⚠

Limited evidence suggests zinc interacts like iron, page 292, to reduce serum quinolone levels.

Since the quinolones are rapidly absorbed, taking them 2 hours before the zinc should minimise the risk of admixture in the gut and largely avoid this interaction.

Q

Raloxifene

Raloxifene + Warfarin and other oral anticoagulants ⚠

A single-dose study found that when raloxifene was given with warfarin the pharmacokinetics of both drugs were not altered.

Despite the lack of pharmacokinetic interaction, modest decreases in prothrombin times have been seen, which may develop over several weeks. The manufacturers therefore recommend that prothrombin times should be checked. They extend this recommendation to cover the use of all coumarins.

Reboxetine

Reboxetine + SSRIs ❌

The manufacturers of reboxetine predict that potent inhibitors of CYP3A4 will reduce its metabolism. They name fluvoxamine, but note that fluvoxamine is more usually considered a potent inhibitor of CYP1A2 and is generally considered a weak inhibitor of CYP3A4.

The manufacturers say that concurrent use of fluvoxamine should be avoided.

Rifabutin

Rifabutin + Sirolimus ❌

Rifampicin (*rifampin*) greatly decreases sirolimus levels. Rifabutin is predicted to interact similarly.

The manufacturers say that concurrent use is not recommended.

Rifabutin + **Tacrolimus** ⚠

Rifampicin (rifampin) increases the clearance and decreases the bioavailability of tacrolimus. Rifabutin is expected to interact similarly, although to a lesser extent.

Tacrolimus levels and effects (e.g. on renal function) should be monitored as a matter of routine, but it is advisable to increase monitoring if rifabutin is started or stopped.

Rifabutin + **Warfarin and other oral anticoagulants** ⚠

The manufacturers and the CSM in the UK warns that rifabutin may reduce the effects of anticoagulants.

Expect any interaction to occur within 7 days of starting rifabutin. It may persist for several weeks after the rifabutin is stopped. Monitor the INR closely.

Rifampicin (Rifampin)

Rifampicin (Rifampin) + **Rimonabant** ❓

The manufacturers predict that potent inducers of CYP3A4 such as rifampicin may lower the serum levels of rimonabant. This is based on the fact that potent *inhibitors* of CYP3A4 *increase* rimonabant levels (see under azoles, page 122).

Caution is recommended with concurrent use of rifampicin and rimonabant and patients should be monitored to ensure rimonabant remains effective.

Rifampicin (Rifampin) + **Sirolimus** ✖

A clinical study found that multiple doses of rifampicin increased the clearance of sirolimus 5.5-fold, and reduced the maximum serum levels by 71%.

The manufacturers say that concurrent use is not recommended.

Rifampicin (Rifampin) + **Solifenacin** ⚠

Ketoconazole increases solifenacin levels 2- to 3-fold by *inhibiting* CYP3A4. The manufacturers predict that potent CYP3A4 *inducers* (e.g. rifampicin) will decrease solifenacin levels.

Be alert for a reduction in the efficacy of solifenacin in patients taking rifampicin.

Rifampicin (Rifampin) + SSRIs ❓

In two cases rifampicin decreased the efficacy of citalopram and sertraline. In theory rifampicin could affect other SSRIs but there appear to be no reports of this.

Information is limited. The dosage adjustment of any SSRI on starting or stopping rifampicin should be guided by clinical effect. Be alert for evidence of SSRI withdrawal symptoms of loss of effect.

Rifampicin (Rifampin) + Statins ⚠

Limited evidence suggests that rifampicin may reduce atorvastatin, fluvastatin, pravastatin, and simvastatin levels.

The general significance of this interaction is unclear but it would be prudent to monitor the outcome of concurrent use to ensure that the statin remains effective.

Rifampicin (Rifampin) + Sulfonamides ⚠

Rifampicin modestly reduces the AUC of sulfamethoxazole (given as co-trimoxazole) by 28% in HIV-positive subjects.

The effect of rifampicin on other sulfonamides does not appear to have been studied. Consider also co-trimoxazole, page 214.

Rifampicin (Rifampin) + Tacrolimus ⚠

Rifampicin increases the clearance and decreases the bioavailability of tacrolimus. In some cases a 10-fold increase in the tacrolimus dose has been needed to manage this interaction.

Tacrolimus levels and effects (e.g. on renal function) should be monitored as a matter of routine, but it is advisable to increase monitoring if rifampicin is started or stopped.

Rifampicin (Rifampin) + Terbinafine ⚠

Rifampicin doubles the clearance of terbinafine and halves its AUC.

Terbinafine seems likely to be less effective in the presence of rifampicin. Monitor carefully and consider increasing the terbinafine dose.

R

Rifampicin (Rifampin) + Tetracyclines ⚠

Rifampicin may cause a marked reduction in doxycycline levels (AUC reported to be reduced by 60% in one study), which has led to treatment failures in some cases.

Monitor the effects of concurrent use and increase the doxycycline dosage as necessary.

Rifampicin (Rifampin) + Theophylline ⚠

Rifampicin increases the clearance of theophylline by 45%. In one study rifampicin (with isoniazid) increased theophylline clearance during the initial few days of tuberculosis treatment, but another study suggested that these antituberculars decreased theophylline clearance within 4 weeks.

Monitor theophylline levels. An effect has been seen within 36 hours of starting rifampicin. Expect to need to increase the theophylline dose. The picture is less clear when isoniazid is also taken. In this situation it would seem prudent to monitor theophylline levels closely for the first month of treatment.

Rifampicin (Rifampin) + Tibolone ❓

The manufacturers of tibolone warn that rifampicin may increase its metabolism and thereby reduce its effects.

The clinical significance of this warning is unclear. There appear to be no reports of an interaction in practice.

Rifampicin (Rifampin) + Toremifene ⚠

Rifampicin increases the metabolism of toremifene (peak plasma levels more than halved), and might be expected to reduce its efficacy.

Monitor the outcome of concurrent use to ensure the effects of toremifene are adequate.

Rifampicin (Rifampin) + Trimethoprim ⚠

Rifampicin reduces the AUC of trimethoprim (given as co-trimoxazole) by 56% in HIV-positive subjects, but apparently has no effect on trimethoprim in healthy subjects.

The interaction between rifampicin and trimethoprim seems unlikely to be relevant in subjects who are not infected with HIV. Consider also co-trimoxazole, page 214.

Rifampicin (Rifampin) + Warfarin and other oral anticoagulants ⚠

The anticoagulant effects of acenocoumarol, phenprocoumon and warfarin are markedly reduced by rifampicin.

A marked reduction occurs within 5 to 7 days of starting rifampicin, persisting for up to 5 weeks after the rifampicin is stopped. Monitor the INR closely. The warfarin dosage may need to be at least doubled.

R

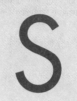

Salbutamol (Albuterol) and related bronchodilators

Salbutamol (Albuterol) and related bronchodilators + Theophylline ❓

The concurrent use of theophylline and beta$_2$ agonist bronchodilators such as salbutamol is a useful option in the management of asthma and chronic obstructive pulmonary disease, but potentiation of some adverse reactions can occur. The most serious of these are hypokalaemia and tachycardia, particularly with high-dose theophylline. Some patients may show a significant fall in serum theophylline levels if given oral or intravenous salbutamol or intravenous isoprenaline (isoproterenol).

Potassium should be monitored, particularly in acutely unwell patients receiving high-dose intravenous treatment. The CSM in the UK particularly recommends monitoring potassium levels in those with severe asthma as the hypokalaemic effects of beta$_2$ agonists can be potentiated by theophylline, corticosteroids, diuretics and hypoxia.

Sevelamer

Sevelamer + Tacrolimus ⚠

Sevelamer reduced the absorption of tacrolimus in one patient (AUC *increased* 2.4-fold when sevelamer *stopped*).

The manufacturers advise that tacrolimus should be taken at least 1 hour before or 3 hours after sevelamer.

Sibutramine

Sibutramine + SSRIs ⊗

Serotonin syndrome has been seen in 2 cases when sibutramine was taken with SSRIs.

The manufacturers advise that concurrent use should be avoided, or only undertaken with appropriate monitoring, see serotonin syndrome, page 392.

Sibutramine + Triptans ⊗

Sibutramine inhibits serotonin uptake. The serious serotonin syndrome, page 392, has, rarely, been seen when sibutramine has been taken with serotonergic drugs. The manufacturers therefore say that sibutramine should not be taken with any serotonergic drugs and specifically name sumatriptan.

The combination need not be avoided, but monitor carefully if any triptan is also given.

Sibutramine + Tryptophan ⊗

Central and peripheral toxicity developed in a number of patients taking *fluoxetine* with tryptophan. On theoretical grounds an adverse reaction (such as serotonin syndrome, page 392) seems possible between any serotonergic drug (such as sibutramine) and tryptophan.

The combination need not be avoided, but monitor carefully if tryptophan is also given.

Sirolimus

Sirolimus + Vaccines ⊗

The body's immune response is suppressed by sirolimus. The antibody response to vaccines may be reduced and the use of live attenuated vaccines may result in generalised infection.

For many inactivated vaccines even the reduced response seen is considered clinically useful and, in the case of renal transplant patients, influenza vaccination is actively recommended. If a vaccine is given, it may be prudent to monitor the response, so that alternative prophylactic measures can be considered where the response is inadequate. Note that even where effective antibody titres are produced, these may not persist as long as in healthy subjects, and more frequent booster doses may be required. The use of live vaccines is generally considered to be contraindicated.

SSRIs

Although the SSRIs are likely to share pharmacodynamic interactions (for example development of the serotonin syndrome with other serotonergic drugs) they do have differing effects on cytochrome P450, which leads to different metabolic actions. Fluvoxamine is a potent inhibitor of CYP1A2, whereas fluoxetine, paroxetine, and possibly sertraline, have moderate inhibitory effects on CYP2D6.

Serotonin syndrome

Serotonin syndrome is thought to result from the over-stimulation of the 5-HT$_{1A}$ and 5-HT$_{2A}$ receptors and possibly other serotonin receptors in the central nervous system. It can, exceptionally, occur with the use of one drug, but much more usually it develops when two or more drugs with serotonergic actions are given together. The characteristic symptoms fall into three main areas, namely altered mental status (agitation, confusion, mania), autonomic dysfunction (diaphoresis, diarrhoea, fever, shivering) and neuromuscular abnormalities (hyperreflexia, incoordination, myoclonus, tremor). Serotonin syndrome usually resolves within about 24 hours if the offending drugs are withdrawn and supportive measures given. Most patients recover uneventfully, but there have been a few fatalities. Many drugs have serotonergic actions, but the advice on concurrent use of these drugs varies greatly between manufacturers. The SSRIs are amongst the most commonly implicated drugs, and the concurrent use of serotonergic drugs with SSRIs is generally cautioned. The most practical approach therefore seems to be to monitor for potential symptoms, and to seek medical advice should they occur.

SSRIs + Tacrine ⚠

Fluvoxamine can increase the AUC of tacrine by up to 8-fold. Tacrine adverse effects (nausea, vomiting, diarrhoea, sweating) are increased.

> A decrease in the tacrine dose is likely to be needed. Other SSRIs such as fluoxetine, paroxetine, or sertraline may be suitable alternatives, as these are unlikely to inhibit tacrine metabolism.

SSRIs + Terbinafine ❓

Although terbinafine modestly increases paroxetine levels one study found no increase in paroxetine adverse effects. Other SSRIs may interact similarly.

> The clinical relevance of this interaction is unclear. Be alert for an increase in SSRI adverse effects, and consider reducing the dose if these become troublesome.

SSRIs + Theophylline ⚠

Theophylline serum levels can be markedly and rapidly increased by the concurrent use of fluvoxamine. Toxicity has occurred.

> Ideally concurrent use should be avoided. If this is not possible, reduce the theophylline dose and monitor theophylline levels. Some preliminary clinical evidence suggests that fluoxetine and citalopram (and therefore probably escitalopram) may not interact with theophylline, and *in vitro* evidence suggests

that paroxetine and sertraline are also unlikely to interact. They may therefore be suitable alternatives.

SSRIs + Tizanidine ✗

Fluvoxamine causes a very marked 33-fold increase in tizanidine levels with a consequent increase in its hypotensive and sedative effects.

The combination is potentially hazardous and should be avoided.

SSRIs + Trazodone ❓

Trazodone and fluoxetine have been used concurrently with advantage, although fluoxetine may modestly increase the levels of trazodone and some patients may develop increased adverse effects. Additive adverse effects such as sedation are predicted to possibly occur with other SSRIs.

It may be prudent to monitor for excessive sedation when trazodone is used with an SSRI.

SSRIs + Tricyclics ⚠

The levels of the tricyclic antidepressants can be raised by the SSRIs, but the extent varies greatly, from 20% to 10-fold. Tricyclic toxicity has been seen in a number of cases. Tricyclics may increase the levels of citalopram and possibly fluvoxamine, but the significance of this is unclear. There are several case reports of the serotonin syndrome, page 392, following concurrent and even sequential use of the SSRIs and tricyclics.

The increased tricyclic antidepressant levels can be beneficial. However, it has been suggested that patients given fluoxetine should have their tricyclic dose reduced to a quarter. Similar recommendations have been made with fluvoxamine (reduction in tricyclic dose to one-third) and sertraline. It would also seem prudent to consider a dosage reduction of the tricyclic if paroxetine is added. Some suggest that a small initial dose of the SSRI should also be used. Patients taking any combination of tricyclic and SSRI should be monitored for adverse effects (e.g. dry mouth, sedation, confusion) with tricyclic levels monitored where possible. Note that the active metabolite of fluoxetine has a half-life of 7 to 15 days, and so any interaction may persist for some time after the fluoxetine is withdrawn, and may therefore occur on sequential use.

SSRIs + Triptans ⚠

The concurrent use of a triptan and an SSRI is normally uneventful, but adverse reactions (such as serotonin syndrome, page 392, reported with sumatriptan and some SSRIs) do occasionally occur. Fluvoxamine has been shown to increase the blood levels of frovatriptan by 27 to 49%, and is predicted to increase the levels of zolmitriptan.

The combination need not be avoided, but monitor carefully, especially if other serotonergic drugs are also used. The manufacturers of zolmitriptan recommend a dosage reduction to a maximum of 5 mg in 24 hours in the presence of fluvoxamine.

S

SSRIs + Tryptophan ⚠

Central and peripheral toxicity developed in a number of patients taking fluoxetine with tryptophan. On theoretical grounds an adverse reaction (such as serotonin syndrome, page 392) seems possible between any SSRI and tryptophan.

> The combination is probably best avoided, as advised by the manufacturers of tryptophan. If tryptophan is given with an SSRI, the SSRI should be started at a low dose and tryptophan gradually introduced starting with a low dose. Patients should be closely monitored for adverse effects.

SSRIs + Venlafaxine ⚠

The manufacturer of venlafaxine cautions its use with SSRIs because of the potential risks of serotonin syndrome, page 392. Cases of this reaction have been reported. Additive antimuscarinic effects have also been seen.

> Monitor concurrent use carefully for symptoms including agitation, confusion and tremor.

SSRIs + Warfarin and other oral anticoagulants ❓

Warfarin plasma levels can be increased by fluvoxamine and raised INRs have been seen in several cases. Isolated reports describe raised INRs and/or haemorrhage in patients taking acenocoumarol with citalopram or paroxetine, and warfarin with fluoxetine or paroxetine. SSRIs alone have, rarely, been associated with bleeding.

> Studies have not demonstrated a consistent interaction, perhaps with the exception of fluvoxamine and warfarin. It may be prudent to monitor the INR when fluvoxamine is first added, being alert for the need to decrease the anticoagulant dosage. Consider monitoring with other SSRIs, but note only a few patients appear to have demonstrated this interaction. Any interaction appears to occur in about the first 2 weeks of treatment.

Statins

Lovastatin and simvastatin are extensively metabolised by CYP3A4 so that drugs that inhibit this enzyme can cause marked rises in statin levels. Atorvastatin is also metabolised by CYP3A4, but to a lesser extent than lovastatin or simvastatin. Fluvastatin is metabolised primarily by CYP2C9, rosuvastatin by CYP2C9 and CYP2C19, while the cytochrome P450 system does not appear to be involved in the metabolism of pravastatin. Therefore the statins tend to interact differently. In order to reduce the risk of myopathy the CSM in the UK advises that statins should be used with care in patients who are at increased risk of this adverse effect, such as those taking interacting drugs. They also recommend that patients should be made aware of the risks of myopathy and rhabdomyolysis, and asked to promptly report muscle pain, tenderness or weakness, especially if accompanied by malaise, fever or dark urine.

Statins + Warfarin and other oral anticoagulants

Fluvastatin and Rosuvastatin ⚠

Studies have suggested that fluvastatin and rosuvastatin can increase warfarin levels and/or effects. Not all patients are affected.

> Increased monitoring is required when starting or stopping fluvastatin or rosuvastatin, or changing the dose.

Other statins ✓

Studies with atorvastatin, lovastatin, pravastatin, and simvastatin suggest that they do not usually significantly alter the effects of warfarin, although cases of bleeding have been seen when these statins were given with coumarins and fluindione.

> It has been suggested that it would be prudent to monitor the early stages of concurrent use of statins and anticoagulants in all patients, or if the dosage of statin is changed, being alert for the need to adjust the anticoagulant dosage. However, this interaction has only been clinically significant in a handful of patients, so monitoring every patient may be over-cautious.

S

Strontium

Strontium + Tetracyclines ✗

The manufacturer of strontium ranelate predicts that it will complex with tetracyclines, and therefore prevent their absorption.

> It is recommended that when treatment with a tetracycline is required, strontium ranelate therapy should be temporarily suspended.

Sucralfate

Sucralfate + Tetracyclines ⚠

On theoretical grounds the absorption of tetracycline may possibly be reduced by sucralfate, but clinical confirmation of this appears to be lacking.

> The manufacturers suggest that they should be given 2 hours apart to minimise their admixture in the gut.

Sucralfate + Warfarin and other oral anticoagulants ❓

Case reports describe a marked reduction in the effects of warfarin in patients given sucralfate. Other evidence suggests that this interaction is uncommon.

Concurrent use need not be avoided but bear this interaction in mind if a patient has a reduced anticoagulant response to warfarin. Information about other anticoagulants is lacking, but be aware that a similar interaction is possible.

Sulfinpyrazone

Sulfinpyrazone + Theophylline ✓

Sulfinpyrazone causes a small 22% increase in the clearance of theophylline.

This seems unlikely to be clinically relevant in most patients but bear this interaction in mind in case of an unexpected response to treatment.

Sulfinpyrazone + Warfarin and other oral anticoagulants ⚠

The anticoagulant effects of warfarin and acenocoumarol are markedly increased by sulfinpyrazone and serious bleeding has occurred.

The INR should be well monitored and suitable anticoagulant dosage reductions made. Halving the dosage of warfarin and reducing the acenocoumarol dosage by one-fifth has proven to be adequate in some patients.

Sulfonamides

Sulfonamides + Warfarin and other oral anticoagulants ⚠

The anticoagulant effects of warfarin, acenocoumarol, and phenprocoumon are increased by co-trimoxazole (sulfamethoxazole with trimethoprim). Bleeding may occur if the anticoagulant dosage is not reduced appropriately. There is also evidence that sulfaphenazole, sulfafurazole (sulfisoxazole) and sulfamethizole may interact like co-trimoxazole.

The incidence of the interaction with co-trimoxazole appears to be high. If bleeding is to be avoided the INR should be well monitored and the warfarin, acenocoumarol, or phenprocoumon dosage should be reduced. Phenindione is said not to interact. The other interactions are poorly documented. However, it would seem prudent to follow the precautions suggested for co-trimoxazole if any sulfonamide is given with an oral anticoagulant.

S

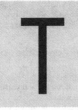

Tacrine

Tacrine + Theophylline ⚠

Limited evidence suggests that tacrine reduces the clearance of theophylline by 50%.

Until more is known it may be prudent to monitor theophylline levels if tacrine is started or stopped.

Tacrolimus

Tacrolimus + Vaccines ❌

The body's immune response is suppressed by tacrolimus. The antibody response to vaccines may be reduced and the use of live attenuated vaccines may result in generalised infection.

For many inactivated vaccines even the reduced response seen is considered clinically useful and, in the case of renal transplant patients, influenza vaccination is actively recommended. If a vaccine is given, it may be prudent to monitor the response, so that alternative prophylactic measures can be considered where the response is inadequate. Note that even where effective antibody titres are produced, these may not persist as long as in healthy subjects, and more frequent booster doses may be required. The use of live vaccines is generally considered to be contraindicated.

Tamoxifen

Tamoxifen + **Warfarin and other oral anticoagulants** ✕

The anticoagulant effects of acenocoumarol and warfarin are markedly increased by tamoxifen and bleeding has been seen.

> Monitor the effects closely if tamoxifen is added to treatment with warfarin or acenocoumarol and reduce the dosage as necessary. Reports indicate that a reduction of between one-half to two-thirds may be needed for warfarin but some patients may need much larger reductions. The dosage reduction needed for acenocoumarol is not known. In the US, when tamoxifen is being used for the primary prevention of breast cancer, the manufacturer specifically contraindicates concurrent use with warfarin.

T

Terbinafine

Terbinafine + **Tricyclics** ?

Terbinafine markedly increased the AUC of desipramine in one study. Case reports describe increases in the serum levels of amitriptyline, desipramine, imipramine, and nortriptyline, with associated toxicity, in patients given oral terbinafine.

> Monitor for any increase in the adverse effects of the tricyclic, and be aware that the dosage may need to be decreased, sometimes substantially. Note that an interaction may occur for a number of weeks after stopping terbinafine, because it has a long half-life.

Terbinafine + **Venlafaxine** ?

The metabolism of venlafaxine to its active metabolite *O*-desmethylvenlafaxine is reduced in the presence of terbinafine. However, the combined AUC of venlafaxine and its metabolite is only raised by a modest 22%.

> Until more is known, it may be prudent to be alert for any indication of increased venlafaxine adverse effects (e.g. nausea, insomnia, dry mouth) in patients also taking terbinafine.

Tetracyclines

Tetracyclines + Warfarin and other oral anticoagulants ❓

The effects of the anticoagulants are not usually altered to a clinically relevant extent by the concurrent use of tetracyclines, but a few patients have shown increases in anticoagulant effect, and a handful have bled.

The clinical importance of this interaction is unknown, but bear it in mind in case of an excessive response to anticoagulant treatment.

Tetracyclines + Zinc ⚠️

The absorption of tetracyclines is inhibited by up to 50% by zinc. All tetracyclines (with perhaps the exception of doxycycline) are expected to interact similarly.

Separate administration. In the case of *iron*, which interacts by the same mechanism, 2 to 3 hours is sufficient. Doxycycline may be a useful non-interacting alternative.

Theophylline

Theophylline is metabolised by cytochrome P450 in the liver, principally by CYP1A2. Many drugs interact with theophylline by inhibition or potentiation of its metabolism. Theophylline has a narrow therapeutic range, and small increases in serum levels can result in toxicity. Moreover, symptoms of serious toxicity such as convulsions and arrhythmias can occur before minor symptoms suggestive of toxicity. Furthermore, age, cigarette smoking, chronic obstructive airways disease, congestive heart failure, and liver disease (cirrhosis, acute hepatitis) can also affect theophylline clearance. Within the context of interactions, aminophylline is expected to behave like theophylline, because it is a complex of theophylline with ethylenediamine.

Theophylline + Ticlopidine ⚠️

Ticlopidine reduces the clearance of theophylline by about 40%, and is expected to raise its serum levels.

Monitor concurrent use for theophylline toxicity (headache, nausea, palpitations), particularly when levels are already at the top end of the range.

Theophylline + Vaccines ❓

BCG vaccine appears to slightly increase the half-life of theophylline. Normally influenza vaccines (whole-virion, split-virion and surface antigen) do not interact with theophylline, but raised theophylline levels and toxicity have been seen in occasional cases.

It seems possible that the occasional patient may develop some signs of theophylline toxicity, especially if their serum levels are already towards the top end of the therapeutic range, but most patients are unlikely to be affected.

Theophylline + Zafirlukast ❓

A single case report describes a rapid rise in theophylline levels after the addition of zafirlukast. Zafirlukast levels are modestly reduced by theophylline, but this does not appear to be clinically important.

The clinical significance of the case is unclear. Bear this interaction in mind in case of an unexpected response to treatment.

Ticlopidine

Ticlopidine + Warfarin and other oral anticoagulants ❌

In one study ticlopidine increased warfarin levels, although the INR appeared to be unchanged. There is some evidence that liver damage may occur in a small number of patients given warfarin with ticlopidine. The anticoagulant effects of acenocoumarol are modestly reduced by ticlopidine.

The manufacturers of ticlopidine strongly advise avoiding the concurrent use of anticoagulants because of the possible increased bleeding risks. If both drugs are essential they recommend monitoring the anticoagulant effect.

Toremifene

Toremifene + Warfarin and other oral anticoagulants ❌

The anticoagulant effects of acenocoumarol and warfarin are markedly increased by *tamoxifen* and bleeding has been seen. Toremifene is expected to interact similarly.

Monitor the effects closely if toremifene is added to treatment with warfarin or acenocoumarol and reduce the dosage as necessary. Note that the manufacturers contraindicate concurrent use (UK), or advise increased monitoring (US).

Tricyclics

Tricyclics + **Valproate** ❓

Amitriptyline and nortriptyline plasma levels can be increased by sodium valproate. Status epilepticus has been attributed to elevated clomipramine levels in a patient taking valproic acid.

> It would seem prudent to monitor for tricyclic adverse effects (such as dry mouth, blurred vision and urinary retention) and reduce the dosage of the tricyclic if necessary. Tricyclics can lower the convulsive threshold and should therefore be used with caution in patients with epilepsy.

Tricyclics + **Venlafaxine** ⚠

Venlafaxine can cause a marked increase in the antimuscarinic adverse effects of clomipramine, desipramine and nortriptyline. An isolated report describes seizures in a patient taking venlafaxine with trimipramine, and serotonin syndrome, page 392, developed in patients taking venlafaxine and amitriptyline, with or without pethidine (meperidine).

> Be alert for any evidence of increased antimuscarinic adverse effects. Although there appears to be only one report, the possibility of an increased risk of seizures with concurrent use should be borne in mind, especially in those already at risk of seizures. It may be necessary to withdraw one or other of the two drugs. The reports of the serotonin syndrome highlight the need for caution when one or more serotonergic drugs are given.

Tricyclics + **Warfarin and other oral anticoagulants** ❓

Amitriptyline and possibly other tricyclics can cause unpredictable increases or decreases in prothrombin times, which can make stable anticoagulation difficult.

> There is insufficient evidence to recommend an increased frequency of INR monitoring, but it would at least seem prudent to bear this interaction in mind when prescribing anticoagulants and tricyclics.

Triptans

Triptans + **Venlafaxine** ⚠

The manufacturers caution the use of drugs that affect serotonergic transmission, such as the triptans. This is because of the possible risks of serotonin syndrome, page 392.

> Monitor concurrent use carefully for symptoms including agitation, confusion and tremor.

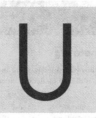

No interactions have been included for drugs beginning with the letter U.

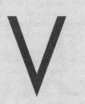

Vaccines

Vaccines + **Warfarin and other oral anticoagulants** ❓

The concurrent use of warfarin and influenza vaccine is usually safe and uneventful, but there are reports of bleeding in a handful of patients (life-threatening in one case) attributed to an interaction. Acenocoumarol also does not normally interact.

This interaction seems rare, but bear it in mind in case of unexpected bleeding.

Venlafaxine

Venlafaxine + **Warfarin and other oral anticoagulants** ❓

There are a handful of isolated case reports indicating that the effects of warfarin are occasionally increased by venlafaxine. These reports describe increased prothrombin times, raised INRs and bleeding (haematuria, gastrointestinal bleeding, melaena, haemarthrosis).

It would seem prudent to increase INR monitoring if venlafaxine is added or withdrawn from treatment with warfarin.

Vitamins

Vitamins + **Warfarin and other oral anticoagulants** ⚠️

The effects of these anticoagulants can be reduced or abolished by vitamin K. This effect can be used to manage overdosage, but unintentional and unwanted antagonism has occurred in patients after taking some proprietary chilblain preparations, health foods, food supplements, enteral feeds or exceptionally large amounts of some green vegetables, seaweed, or green tea, which can contain significant amounts of vitamin K.

The drug intake and diet of any patient who shows warfarin resistance' should be investigated for the possibility of this interaction. It can be accommodated either by increasing the anticoagulant dosage, or by reducing the intake of vitamin K. However, patients taking vitamin K-rich diets should not change their eating habits without at the same time reducing the anticoagulant dosage, because excessive anticoagulation and bleeding may occur.

V

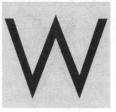

Warfarin and other oral anticoagulants

Warfarin, phenprocoumon and acenocoumarol are racemic mixtures of *S*- and *R*-enantiomers. The *S*-enantiomers of these coumarins have several times more anticoagulant activity than the *R*-enantiomers. The *S*-enantiomer of warfarin is metabolised primarily by CYP2C9. The metabolism of *R*-warfarin is more complex but this enantiomer is primarily metabolised by CYP1A2, CYP3A4, and CYP2C19. There is much more known about the metabolism of warfarin compared to other anticoagulants but it is established that *S*-phenprocoumon and *S*-acenocoumarol are also substrates for CYP2C9. Whilst the metabolism of the coumarins, especially warfarin, is well known, the numerous interaction pathways and the variability in patient responses makes the clinical consequences of alterations in metabolism difficult to predict.

Warfarin and other oral anticoagulants +
Zafirlukast ⚠

Zafirlukast increases the anticoagulant effects of warfarin and bleeding has been seen.

If zafirlukast is given to patients stabilised on warfarin, monitor prothrombin times closely and be alert for the need to reduce the warfarin dosage to avoid over-anticoagulation.

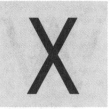

No interactions have been included for drugs beginning with the letter X.

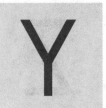

No interactions have been included for drugs beginning with the letter Y.

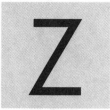

No interactions have been included for drugs beginning with the letter Z.

Index